846

D1434586

DATE DUE

16 12 14	
20 8 15	
1/11/17	
1/12/17	

Essentials of Gastroenterology

Edited by

Shanthi V. Sitaraman, MD, PhD[†]

Professor of Medicine and Pathology
Division of Digestive Diseases
Department of Medicine
Emory University School of Medicine
Atlanta, GA, USA

Lawrence S. Friedman, MD

Professor of Medicine, Harvard Medical School, Boston
Professor of Medicine, Tufts University School of Medicine, Boston
Chair, Department of Medicine, Newton-Wellesley Hospital, Newton
Assistant Chief of Medicine, Massachusetts General Hospital, Boston
MA, USA

Foreword by

Daniel K. Podolsky, MD

President, University of Texas Southwestern Medical Center
Professor of Medicine
Philip O'Bryan Montgomery, Jr, MD Distinguished Presidential Chair in Academic
Administration
Doris and Bryan Wildenthal Distinguished Chair in Medical Science
University of Texas Southwestern Medical Center
Dallas, TX, USA

[†]Deceased

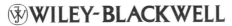

WILEY-BLACKWELL

A John Wiley & Sons, Ltd., Publication

1   2012

To the memory of Shanthi V. Sitaraman, MD, PhD

Contents

Contributor list

Frank A. Anania, MD, FACP, AGAF
Professor of Medicine
Acting Director
Division of Digestive Diseases, Department of Medicine
Emory University School of Medicine
Atlanta, GA, USA

Muhammad Fuad Azrak, MD, MPH
Assistant Professor of Medicine
Wayne University
Oakwood Hospital and Medical Center
Dearborn, MI, USA

Qiang Cai, MD, PhD, FASGE, FACG
Professor of Medicine
Director, Advanced Endoscopy Fellowship
Division of Digestive Diseases
Emory University School of Medicine
Atlanta, GA, USA

Jennifer Christie, MD
Assistant Professor of Medicine
Director of Gastrointestinal Motility
Division of Digestive Diseases
Emory University School of Medicine
Atlanta, GA, USA

Abhijit Datir, MD, FRCR, DMRE
Fellow
Department of Radiology
Emory University Hospital
Atlanta, GA, USA

Nader Dbouk, MD
Fellow
Division of Digestive Diseases
Emory University School of Medicine
Atlanta, GA, USA

Tanvi Dhere, MD
Assistant Professor of Medicine
Division of Digestive Diseases
Emory University School of Medicine
Atlanta, GA, USA

Wayne M. Fleishmann, MD
Fellow
Division of Digestive Diseases
Emory University School of Medicine
Atlanta, GA, USA

Ryan M. Ford, MD
Assistant Professor of Medicine
Division of Digestive Diseases
Emory University School of Medicine
Atlanta, GA, USA

Lawrence S. Friedman, MD
Professor of Medicine, Harvard Medical School and Tufts University
School of Medicine
Chair, Department of Medicine
Newton-Wellesley Hospital
Newton, MA;
Assistant Chief of Medicine
Massachusetts General Hospital
Boston, MA, USA

Anthony Gamboa, MD
Resident
Department of Medicine
Emory University School of Medicine
Atlanta, GA, USA

Sagar Garud, MD, MS
Fellow
Division of Digestive Diseases
Emory University School of Medicine
Atlanta, GA, USA

Nicole M. Griglione, MD
Fellow
Division of Digestive Diseases
Emory University School of Medicine
Atlanta, GA, USA

Melanie S. Harrison, MD
Assistant Professor of Medicine
Division of Digestive Diseases
Emory University School of Medicine;
Atlanta Veterans Administration Medical Center
Atlanta, GA, USA

Steven Keilin, MD
Assistant Professor of Medicine
Division of Digestive Diseases
Emory University School of Medicine
Atlanta, GA, USA

Jan-Michael A. Klapproth, MD
Associate Professor of Medicine
Emory University School of Medicine;
Atlanta Veterans Administration Medical Center
Atlanta, GA, USA

Edward Lin, DO, MBA, FACS
Associate Professor of Surgery
Department of Surgery
Emory University School of Medicine
Atlanta, GA, USA

Julia Massaad, MD
Assistant Professor of Medicine
Division of Digestive Diseases
Emory University School of Medicine
Atlanta, GA, USA

Pardeep Mittal, MD
Assistant Professor of Radiology
Department of Radiology
Emory University School of Medicine
Atlanta, GA, USA

Kamil Obideen, MD
Atlanta Gastroenterology Associates
Northside Forsyth Hospital
Cumming, GA, USA

Henry C. Olejeme, MD
Assistant Professor of Medicine
Emory University School of Medicine;
Chief of Gastroenterology Service
Grady Memorial Hospital
Atlanta, GA, USA

Samir Parekh, MD
Assistant Professor of Medicine
Division of Digestive Diseases
Emory University School of Medicine
Atlanta, GA, USA

Douglas C. Parker, MD, DDS
Assistant Professor of Pathology and Dermatology
Departments of Pathology and Dermatology
Emory University School of Medicine;
Grady Memorial Hospital
Atlanta, GA, USA

Neal R. Patel, MD
Resident
Department of Medicine
Emory University School of Medicine
Atlanta, GA, USA

Meena Prasad, MD
Resident
Department of Medicine
Emory University School of Medicine
Atlanta, GA, USA

Emad Qayed, MD
Fellow
Division of Digestive Diseases
Emory University School of Medicine
Atlanta, GA, USA

Preeti A. Reshamwala, MD
Southern California Liver Centers
Coronado, CA, USA

Zakiya P. Rice, MD
Clinical Associate
Department of Dermatology
Department of Pediatrics
Emory University School of Medicine
Atlanta, GA, USA

Robin E. Rutherford, MD
Associate Professor of Medicine
Clinical Director, Division of Digestive Diseases
Emory University School of Medicine
Atlanta, GA, USA

Sonali S. Sakaria, MD
Assistant Professor of Medicine
Division of Gastroenterology
Thomas Jefferson University
Philadelphia, PA, USA

Charles W. Sewell, MD
Professor of Pathology
Department of Pathology
Emory University School of Medicine
Atlanta, GA, USA

Andrew J. Simpson, MD
Assistant Professor of Medicine
Division of Digestive Diseases
Department of Medicine and Emory Transplant Center
Emory University School of Medicine
Atlanta, GA, USA

Shanthi V. Sitaraman, MD, PhD[†]
Professor of Medicine and Pathology
Division of Digestive Diseases
Department of Medicine
Emory University School of Medicine
Atlanta, GA, USA

William Small, MD, PhD
Professor of Radiology
Director of Abdominal Imaging
Department of Radiology and Imaging Sciences
Emory University School of Medicine
Atlanta, GA, USA

Marc B. Sonenshine, MD
Fellow
Division of Digestive Diseases
Emory University School of Medicine
Atlanta, GA, USA

Shanthi Srinivasan, MD
Associate Professor of Medicine
Emory University School of Medicine;
Atlanta Veterans Administration Medical Center
Atlanta, GA, USA

Ram Subramanian, MD
Assistant Professor of Medicine and Surgery
Departments of Medicine and Surgery
Emory University School of Medicine
Atlanta, GA, USA

Robert A. Swerlick, MD
Alecia Leizman Stonecipher Professor and Chairman
Department of Dermatology
Emory University School of Medicine;
Staff Physician
Atlanta Veterans Administration Medical Center
Atlanta, GA, USA

[†]Deceased

Mohammad Wehbi, MD
Assistant Professor of Medicine
Emory University School of Medicine;
Associate Program Director, Fellowship Program
Section Chief, Gastroenterology
Atlanta Veterans Administration Medical Center
Atlanta, GA, USA

Field F. Willingham, MD, MPH
Assistant Professor of Medicine
Director of Endoscopy
Division of Digestive Diseases
Emory University School of Medicine
Atlanta, GA, USA

Vincent W. Yang, MD, PhD
Professor and Chair
Department of Medicine
Stony Brook University School of Medicine
Stony Brook, NY, USA

Xuan Zhu, MD
Director and Professor of Gastroenterology
The First Affiliated Hospital of Nanchang University
Nanchang
People's Republic of China

Foreword

In an age when information on any subject is but a few clicks away – the Internet offering seemingly unlimited information to be found in response to any inquiry as well as democratization of information through social media – it is reasonable to question the need for any textbook, much less a new one. Textbooks as resources for definitive information are inherently archival in nature. The deliberate process necessary to produce a textbook, which helps ensure the accuracy that readers expect, makes them less agile as an information resource than the many electronic vehicles that are now nearly ubiquitous.

Ironically, the importance of textbooks may actually be more sharply defined by the immediate access to massive amounts of information through the Internet and other electronic vehicles. That role is to provide trusted core knowledge for a learner new to the field in need of focused, credible information. In the unregulated environment of the Internet, *caveat emptor* is implicit. Without foundational knowledge the learner approaches a search for insight or answers without the ability to distinguish the reliable from the unreliable.

The general importance of textbooks as a source of validated information in this era is especially relevant to medicine, in which the tension between the immediacy of the Internet to disseminate new information and the textbook to provide a source of vetted knowledge is particularly acute. The expansion of medical knowledge has reached a seemingly exponential rate, and the textbook is hardly the medium to reflect that almost daily evolution. However, as breakthroughs are reported and then often quickly superseded by contradictory reports or are otherwise intermixed with misinformation in the virtual world, a reference for core knowledge that has been truly validated as a foundation for the student or practitioner of medicine remains the province of the textbook.

What, then, is the need for a *new* textbook when libraries are already replete with reference works in every field? An answer to this second important question has an implicit criterion: that the new book differs from existing textbooks in fulfilling an inadequately met need for a particular formulation of a body of knowledge.

The present new volume clearly fulfills that requirement. The field of gastroenterology has the benefit of a number of excellent, comprehensive textbooks. They provide the reader in-depth information about the field and can serve as a resource for the practitioner to find detailed knowledge around a specific question that may have arisen in the course of practice or research. These textbooks, however, do not as effectively serve the needs of the medical student, trainee, or other early career health care professional. In the early stages of education or training, the essential need is for a coherent and concise, yet substantive, formulation of the foundational knowledge of gastrointestinal medicine and the most important and common clinical problems encountered in the field.

Essentials of Gastroenterology has taken a creative approach to orient the reader to the key problems of clinical gastroenterology and provides an approach that will resonate with the student or trainee who is first encountering the challenges of this field. Edited by two outstanding experts with broad experience, this volume has been developed using the frame of reference of the students, to whom they have dedicated their careers in parallel with their commitment to patients. The result is a wonderful resource in which the reader moves quickly from an initial basic understanding of the clinical topic to an understanding of the science underpinning the clinical approach and ultimately clinical management itself.

Each chapter pivots on an initial clinical vignette, which immediately captures the interest of the reader and provides an almost palpable sense of the clinical specialty as a springboard to the rest of the chapter. This is especially effective in giving life to the chapters that focus on the more fundamental aspects of anatomy and physiology of the digestive system. The book also includes chapters covering key ancillary aspects of digestive disease and the modalities used in the practice of gastroenterology. Vivid images provide an especially vibrant view of the field to the reader.

This textbook gives a resounding answer to both questions posed in this foreword with respect to the role of textbooks. In an era in which use of "just-in-time" learning tools increasingly dominate teaching rounds and the clinical environment, this textbook provides the essential context by which more focused information of momentary relevance can be properly assimilated. Further, this textbook does indeed fulfill a distinct and important need that is not met by larger comprehensive textbooks of gastroenterology. The result is fresh: with crisp presentation, the information is accessible in a way that is well matched to the needs of its intended readers.

I note finally that this has been a labor of love for all those involved but especially the two editors, with whom I have had the pleasure of working as colleagues in years past. Dr. Friedman has brought his encyclopedic knowledge and broad experience as clinician and teacher to ensure the sharpened focus that is evident throughout this book. For Dr. Shanthi Sitaraman this book was the culminating reflection of her passion for teaching that was matched by the deep humanity that was evident in all of her efforts, including the care of patients and leadership of a research laboratory. Sadly, Shanthi did not live to see the publication of this textbook; she passed away after a long illness shortly after all of the chapters had been finalized. Her steadfast determination to see this textbook through to what is now a wonderful result is testament to her spirit. Although the field of gastroenterology has been deprived of Shanthi's continuing contributions, this textbook serves as an important and, I am sure, enduring legacy.

Daniel K. Podolsky, MD
UT Southwestern Medical Center

Preface

Essentials of Gastroenterology was conceived, developed, and co-edited by Shanthi V. Sitaraman, MD, PhD, who tragically passed away after a long illness as the book was nearing completion. The book reflects Shanthi's dream and vision to create a textbook of gastroenterology targeted specifically to medical students but useful as well to residents rotating on a gastroenterology service and fellows and practitioners preparing for certification examinations and desiring a focused overview of the state-of-the-art of the field. To achieve these goals, Shanthi enlisted contributions from her colleagues in the Division of Digestive Diseases and the Departments of Pathology and Surgery at the Emory University School of Medicine, where Shanthi was Professor of Medicine (with Tenure) and Professor of Pathology. The book is, in fact, based on the highly acclaimed lectures given by Shanthi and her colleagues to the medical students during their pathophysiology course and clinical rotations in gastroenterology. Shanthi herself was an award-winning teacher who was beloved by the students, residents, fellows, and faculty at Emory. She was a recipient of the Silver Pear Mentoring Award from the Department of Medicine, the Student Association Teaching Award and Dean's Teaching Award from the School of Medicine, and the Attending of the Year designation and the Mentor Award from the Division of Digestive Diseases at Emory, among numerous other honors. Many of her colleagues who contributed to this volume have also been recipients of awards for outstanding contributions to medical education.

The book reflects Shanthi's high standards and commitment to clear exposition, proper organization, and clarifying figures and tables. The 28 chapters are organized into five sections, each edited or co-edited by one of her colleagues. These sections are entitled Luminal Gastrointestinal Tract, Liver, Pancreas and Biliary System, Common Problems in Gastroenterology, and Picture Gallery. Each chapter covers a key clinical issue in the practice of gastroenterology, and the Picture Gallery provides the proverbial "textbook" examples of classic pathology, radiology, and dermatology findings in gastroenterology. The chapters are written in an easy-to-read outline format that covers the basics of pathophysiology, clinical features, diagnosis, natural history, prognosis, and treatment of the common disorders seen in the practice of gastroenterology. Figures and tables illustrate and highlight key information. Shaded boxes draw attention to important practice points, and a concluding segment in each chapter in the first four sections provides a list of "pearls" useful in clinical practice. Illustrative cases begin each chapter in the first four sections, and multiple-choice questions pertaining to these clinical vignettes and to the content of the chapter provide an opportunity for the reader to test his or her knowledge of the subject matter at the end of each chapter. A few key references and web links are provided. The aim is to make the information as clear, concise, and "digestible" as possible. Medical students will find the information relevant and readily understandable, while more senior trainees will be able to obtain a quick and practical overview of the field in a short amount of time. Readers should find the book useful and focused without being overwhelming.

For me, it was a particular, though poignant, privilege to work with Shanthi, a former fellow of mine, on this book. Her love of gastroenterology and passion for teaching were evident throughout the entire project and shine in this book. She was a brilliant and dedicated physician–scientist who, as a faculty member at Emory, made numerous contributions to education, research, and clinical practice. Her work in inflammatory bowel diseases resulted in over 200 publications that advanced our understanding of basic mechanisms of inflammation and led to novel approaches to therapy. Her devotion to patients was legendary, and as recently as 2011, she received the Crohn's and Colitis Foundation of America Premier Physician Award in Georgia. She mentored and taught countless medical students, residents, fellows, and junior faculty, and her humanitarian service to the greater Atlanta community was inspiring. *Essentials of Gastroenterology* is both a fitting tribute to and a wonderful legacy of an exceptional educator, colleague, and friend.

Lawrence S. Friedman, MD

Acknowledgments

Every chapter in this book was personally edited by Dr. Shanthi V. Sitaraman, whose labor of love is reflected in every page. She received invaluable assistance and support from her colleagues at the Emory University School of Medicine and particularly from members of the Division of Digestive Diseases. Their adherence to deadlines, attention to detail, and commitment to excellence were essential to the successful completion of this book. I am particularly grateful to Dr. Frank A. Anania, Director of Hepatology and now Acting Chief of the Division of Digestive Diseases at Emory, and Dr. Vincent W. Yang, Chief of the Division of Digestive Diseases at Emory and now Chair of the Department of Medicine, Stony Brook University School of Medicine, for their extraordinary support of this project. Each and every contributor to this book deserves acknowledgment for his or her effort. Shanthi would particularly want to acknowledge the devotion and love of her husband, Professor Suresh Sitaraman, and her son Karthik. I am grateful for the support of my own family, including my wife, Mary Jo Cappuccilli, son Matthew Friedman, and grandson Christopher Friedman. The support of our publisher Wiley-Blackwell, including Oliver Walter, Senior Editor for Health Sciences, Kate Newell, Senior Development Editor, Cathryn Gates, Senior Production Editor, and Ruth Swan, Project Manager at Toppan Best-set, was phenomenal, and I personally cannot thank them enough. We are especially grateful to Dr. Daniel Podolsky, a mentor to both Shanthi and me, who graciously prepared the Foreword for this book. We also acknowledge the remarkable efforts of our Assistants, Carla Fairclough for Shanthi and Alison Sholock for me, who served as surrogate editors for the book. For me, the opportunity to work with Shanthi Sitaraman on this book was a once-in-a-lifetime experience that I will always treasure.

Lawrence S. Friedman, MD

Luminal Gastrointestinal Tract

Jan-Michael A. Klapproth and Shanthi Srinivasan

Gastroesophageal Reflux Disease

Jennifer Christie

CHAPTER 1

Clinical Vignette

A 40-year-old man with a history of hypertension presents with a 2-month history of chest discomfort. He describes the discomfort as a burning and occasionally a pressure sensation in the mid-sternal area. The discomfort often occurs 30 minutes after eating a meal and lasts for about 2 hours, gradually improving thereafter. He occasionally awakens in the morning with a sore throat and bitter taste is his mouth. He has tried over-the-counter ranitidine with only minimal relief. He was recently seen in the emergency department for an episode of severe chest pain. A cardiac work-up, including an electrocardiogram, cardiac enzymes, and a stress echocardiogram, was negative. Physical examination reveals a well built, well nourished man in no apparent distress. The blood pressure is 137/84 mmHg, pulse rate 72/min, respiratory rate 14/min, and body mass index 30. The physical examination is otherwise unremarkable.

General

- Gastroesophageal reflux disease (GERD) is defined as symptoms or tissue damage due to the reflux of gastric contents into the esophagus.
- GERD is a common disorder, affecting almost half of the US population, with varying severity. Forty percent of the US population experiences reflux symptoms about once per month, 20% complain of symptoms once per week, and 7–10% report daily symptoms.

Essentials of Gastroenterology, First Edition. Edited by Shanthi V. Sitaraman, Lawrence S. Friedman.
© 2012 John Wiley & Sons, Ltd. Published 2012 by John Wiley & Sons, Ltd.

• GERD affects 10–20% of western populations. It is less common in Asian and African countries.

> The most common symptoms of GERD are heartburn and regurgitation. GERD is the most common cause of noncardiac chest pain.

Risk Factors

• Advancing age (>65 years)
• Obesity
• Genetic factors.

Spectrum of GERD

• The clinical spectrum of GERD ranges from nonerosive reflux disease (NERD) to esophagitis (Figure 1.1). NERD is defined as symptoms of acid reflux without evidence of esophageal damage on esophagogastroduodenoscopy (upper endoscopy).
• A small proportion of patients will develop metaplasia of the squamous esophageal epithelium into columnar epithelium (called Barrett's esophagus). Barrett's esophagus is a risk factor for adenocarcinoma (see later).

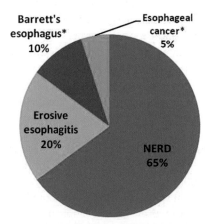

Figure 1.1 Clinical spectrum of GERD. (*May be associated with erosive esophagitis; NERD, nonerosive esophageal reflux disease.)

- Some patients presenting with heartburn have "functional" heartburn. Functional heartburn is defined as a burning retrosternal discomfort in the absence of gastroesophageal reflux or esophageal motor disorder.

Pathophysiology

- Transient lower esophageal sphincter relaxations (TLESRs):
  - The etiology of GERD is multifactorial; however, "aberrant" TLESRs are the major pathophysiologic factor in many patients with GERD.
  - A TLESR is defined as the relaxation of the lower esophageal sphincter in response to gastric distension. In healthy persons, TLESRs occur in the absence of a swallow, last 10–30 seconds, and result in physiologic gastroesophageal reflux.
  - TLESRs are regulated by the neurotransmitter γ-aminobutyric acid (GABA) acting on GABA type B receptors located in the peripheral nervous system as well as in the brainstem.
  - In many cases, GERD is thought to be caused by an increased number of or prolonged TLESRs.
- Gastric factors:
  - Increased gastric acid production as well as delayed gastric emptying with distention may trigger TLESRs.
- Diminished esophageal clearance:
  - Poor esophageal clearance due to defects in primary or secondary esophageal peristalsis allows prolonged exposure of the esophageal mucosa to acid.
- Diet and medications:
  - Dietary factors such as acidic foods, caffeine, alcohol, peppermint, and chocolate may reduce lower esophageal sphincter (LES) tone or increase gastric acid production.
  - Medications such as calcium channel blockers, hormones (e.g., progesterone, cholecystokinin, secretin), and barbiturates can decrease LES tone, thereby predisposing to gastroesophageal reflux.
  - Smoking has also been associated with a predisposition to gastroesophageal reflux.
- Hiatal hernia:
  - A hiatal hernia usually occurs when there is a defect in the diaphragmatic hiatus that allows the proximal stomach to herniate above the diaphragm and into the thorax. It is unclear how this predisposes to gastroesophageal reflux; however, it is thought that the barrier function of the LES to prevent the reflux of gastric contents into the esophagus is disrupted. Large hiatal hernias also lead to increased acid dwell times in the distal esophagus.

Clinical Features

- Thorough history taking detailing the onset and duration of symptoms and the association of symptoms with meals and diet should be performed. "Alarm symptoms" such as vomiting, gastrointestinal bleeding, weight loss, dysphagia, and symptoms of cardiac disease should be elicited.
- Patients may present with typical (classic) or atypical symptoms.
- Typical symptoms:
  - **Heartburn** is described as a burning sensation in the substernal area that may radiate to the neck and/or back.
  - **Regurgitation** is the feeling of stomach contents traveling retrograde from the stomach up to the chest and often into the mouth.
  - **Dysphagia** (difficulty swallowing) is reported in about 30% of patients with GERD, even in the absence of a stricture.
  - Less common symptoms associated with GERD include water brash, burping, hiccups, nausea, and vomiting. Water brash is the sudden appearance of a sour or salty fluid in the mouth and represents secretions from the salivary glands in response to acid reflux. Odynophagia occurs when there is severe esophagitis.
  - The sensitivity of typical symptoms for detecting GERD is poor.
- Atypical symptoms:
  - Patients may present with chest pain, chronic cough, difficult-to-treat asthma, and laryngeal symptoms such as hoarseness, throat clearing, or throat pain.
  - Patients with atypical symptoms are less likely than patients with typical symptoms to have endoscopic evidence of esophagitis or Barrett's esophagus. They also have a less predictable response to therapy. Ambulatory esophageal pH testing (see later) is not as sensitive for diagnosing GERD in patients with atypical symptoms as it is in patients with typical symptoms.
- In uncomplicated GERD, physical findings are minimal or absent.

> GERD as the etiology of chest pain should be pursued only after potentially life-threatening cardiac etiologies have been excluded.

Diagnosis

Trial of Proton Pump Inhibitor (PPI) Therapy
- A PPI trial is the simplest approach to diagnosing GERD and evaluating symptom response to treatment.

- A 30-day trial of a PPI (omeprazole, lansoprazole, rabeprazole, pantoprazole, esomeprazole) twice daily (taken 1 hour before breakfast and before dinner) is recommended. If the patient has GERD, symptoms will usually improve within 1–2 weeks.
- The pooled sensitivity of a PPI trial for diagnosing GERD is 78% with a specificity of 54% when compared with 24-hour pH testing.

A PPI trial is recommended as the initial diagnostic and therapeutic intervention in patients with uncomplicated GERD. In patients who fail a PPI trial, additional testing is recommended.

Barium Esophagogram
- This is a radiographic test that can detect reflux of barium contrast into the esophagus after the patient drinks the contrast solution (see Chapter 27).
- A barium esophagogram (swallow) can evaluate other potential mechanical causes for the symptoms (e.g., stricture, neoplasm); however, the test lacks sensitivity (20–30%) to assess mucosal damage and to diagnose GERD.

Upper Endoscopy
- Upper endoscopy allows direct visualization of the esophageal mucosa.
- The test has a high sensitivity (90–95%) for diagnosing GERD, but the specificity is only 50%.
- The spectrum of findings on upper endoscopy in persons with GERD includes normal mucosa, esophageal inflammation characterized by erythema, erosions, mucosal breaks, bleeding, and ulceration of the esophageal mucosa (see Chapter 2).
- Upper endoscopy is recommended for patients with alarm symptoms such as weight loss, dysphagia, hematemesis, and bleeding.
- Upper endoscopy is useful for detecting complications of GERD such as stricture or Barrett's esophagus and other upper gastrointestinal disorders (e.g., peptic ulcer).
- Los Angeles classification of erosive esophagitis:
  - grade A: greater than 1 mucosal break, <5mm long;
  - grade B: greater than 1 mucosal break, >5mm long;
  - grade C: greater than 1 mucosal break, bridging tops of folds but <75% of the circumference of the esophagus;

○ grade D: greater than 1 mucosal break, bridging tops of folds and >75% of the circumference of the esophagus;
○ Most patients have mild (LA grade A–B) esophagitis.

> Endoscopic mucosal biopsies should be obtained in all patients with dysphagia to exclude eosinophilic esophagitis (see Chapter 2).

Ambulatory Esophageal pH Testing

- pH monitoring is the gold standard for detecting acid reflux and correlating reflux with the patient's symptoms.
- A pressure catheter is inserted transnasally and advanced to 5 cm above the manometrically determined LES. The catheter is attached to a data logger that records pH values of the distal esophagus for 24 hours. The patient records his/her meals, positioning (upright/supine), and symptoms. The patient returns the data logger, and the pH data are downloaded onto a computer that transforms the data into a 24-hour tracing.
- The sensitivity of pH monitoring ranges from 79–96%, with a specificity of 85–100% in patients with typical symptoms of gastroesophageal reflux.
- A wireless ambulatory pH capsule placed endoscopically allows for 48 hours of pH data recording. The sensitivity of this technique is greater than that of conventional pH monitoring.
- Many patients (25–60%) with noncardiac chest pain will have an abnormal ambulatory pH study result.
- Clinical indications for pH monitoring include:
  ○ refractory gastroesophageal reflux symptoms;
  ○ atypical symptoms;
  ○ typical symptoms and a normal upper endoscopy;
  ○ preoperatively before a fundoplication;
  ○ follow-up of antireflux therapy (see later).
- The most sensitive parameter used to determine pathologic acid reflux includes the percentage of time the pH remains <4 and the correlation with symptoms. A pH <4 suggests that active pepsin may be a part of the refluxate, leading to erosion of the esophageal mucosa and symptoms.
- Some patients continue to have reflux symptoms despite documentation of a negative 24-hour pH test. Weakly acidic (pH = 4–7) as well as nonacidic (pH >7) reflux can produce reflux symptoms. **Multichannel impedance testing** combined with pH testing can be used to assess acidic, weakly acidic, and nonacidic reflux and the relationship of reflux events to symptom events.

Complications

Esophageal Stricture
- The frequency of esophageal strictures (also called peptic strictures) in patients with GERD is 0.1%.
- Esophageal strictures are generally smooth, scarred, circumferential narrowings usually in the distal esophagus (see Chapter 2).
- Patients usually present with progressive dysphagia for solids that generally is not associated with weight loss, as occurs with malignant strictures (see Chapter 2).
- Esophageal peptic strictures are treated with per-endoscopic dilation. Dysphagia improves once the esophageal luminal diameter reaches 15 mm or above.

Barrett's Esophagus
- Prolonged esophageal acid exposure can result in damage to the esophageal mucosa leading to metaplasia of the squamous epithelium of the distal mucosa into specialized columnar mucosa with goblet cells; this is referred to as intestinal metaplasia.
- In some persons **intestinal metaplasia** may progress to dysplasia and esophageal adenocarcinoma. The risk of progression to adenocarcinoma has been estimated to be 0.5–1.0% per year but may be as low as 0.12% per year.
- The prevalence of Barrett's esophagus is highest in Caucasian men over 50 years of age.
- The diagnosis of Barrett's esophagus is suspected on upper endoscopy by the detection of salmon-colored mucosa extending above the gastroesophageal junction (Z-line) (Figure 1.2). The diagnosis is confirmed by histologic examination (see Chapter 26).

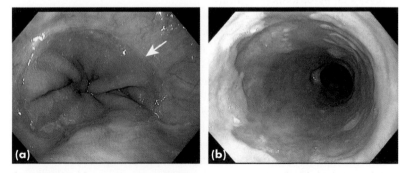

Figure 1.2 Endoscopic images of the normal esophagus and Barrett's esophagus. (a) Normal esophagus showing the squamocolumnar junction (arrow); (b) Barrett's esophagus: intestinal metaplasia is seen as salmon-colored mucosa that extends above the gastroesophageal junction.

- High-dose acid suppression therapy with a PPI is prescribed for symptoms but has not been proven to prevent progression to dysplasia in patients with Barrett's esophagus. In selected patients, endoscopic therapy (especially radiofrequency ablation) or surgical therapy may be used to treat Barrett's esophagus complicated by dysplasia.
- Periodic endoscopic surveillance with mucosal biopsies of Barrett's esophagus to detect dysplasia is widely practiced, although the benefit of this approach is controversial at this time. Adjunct techniques such as chromoendoscopy (application of vital dye to the mucosa to enhance visualization of dysplastic mucosa) appears to increase the yield of surveillance endoscopy.

Treatment

Treatment of GERD depends on the severity of symptoms. Therapy includes lifestyle modifications, medication, surgery, or a combination of these.

Lifestyle Modifications
- In patients with mild and infrequent symptoms, lifestyle modifications can decrease the frequency and severity of symptoms and are considered first-line therapy. Recommended changes include weight loss, avoidance of late-night meals, raising the head of the bed to at least a 30-degree angle in an attempt to minimize acid reflux, avoidance of spicy and greasy foods, acidic foods such as tomato-based products, and citrus juices, cessation of smoking, and a reduction in alcohol consumption and caffeinated products such as chocolate.
- Weight loss and elevation of the head of the bed seem to be the most beneficial lifestyle interventions.

Antacids
- Antacids neutralize gastric acid, thereby raising the pH above 4 and decreasing reflux symptoms.
- The onset of action is approximately 5 minutes after ingestion, and the effect lasts for 90 minutes.
- Over-the counter antacids and alginates have been found to be helpful in patients with mild, infrequent GERD.
- Side effects include diarrhea with magnesium-containing products and constipation with aluminum-containing formulations.

Histamine H2 Receptor Antagonists (H2RAs)
- H2RAs block histamine H2 receptors on parietal cells of the stomach, thereby inhibiting histamine binding to the cell and decreasing gastric acid production.

- They have a rapid onset of action with a duration of effect between 6 and 10 hours.
- The healing rate for esophagitis is 50% compared with 24% in a placebo group.
- These drugs are effective in patients with mild, infrequent GERD.

PPIs

- PPIs bind covalently and irreversibly with the hydrogen/potassium adenosine triphosphatase (H^+/K^+-ATPase) pump on the apical surface of parietal cells in the stomach.
- PPI therapy is the mainstay of treatment for moderate to severe GERD and is used as maintenance therapy.
- Usually, once-a-day dosing is effective. PPIs have been shown to maintain intragastric pH above 4 for 15–21 hours. Occasionally twice daily dosing is necessary for patients with severe symptoms or those with erosive esophagitis.
- PPIs have been shown to be superior to H2RAs in healing esophagitis at 8 weeks (83–96% for PPIs vs. 50% for H2RAs).
- Reasons for a failure to respond to a PPI include poor adherence, inadequate acid suppression with breakthrough acid secretion, weakly acidic reflux as the cause of symptoms, duodenogastroesophageal reflux, delayed gastric emptying, or functional heartburn.
- The most common side effects of PPIs include diarrhea, headache, and abdominal pain. Chronic PPI use has been associated with a slightly increased susceptibility to enteric infections, including *Clostridium difficile* colitis, as well as hip fractures.
- Although there may be slight differences among the various PPIs with respect to potency, the choice of PPI is best made on the basis of prescription plan coverage and a history of adverse side effects.

Additional Medications

- Prokinetic agents such as metoclopramide, a dopamine antagonist, may be effective as an adjunct to PPIs in persons with delayed gastric emptying. Prokinetic agents have no effect in improving esophageal clearance. Side effects include tremors, Parkinson-like symptoms, and tardive dyskinesia. The US Food and Drug Administration (FDA) has not approved metoclopramide for GERD.
- GABA agonists such as baclofen inhibit TLESRs and reflux episodes. The side effects include drowsiness, nausea, and an increased risk of seizures. Baclofen has not been approved by the FDA for the treatment of GERD.

Endoscopic Therapy

- The goals of therapy are to reduce reflux, alter neural response to acid, and improve symptoms.

- Endoscopic approaches include delivery of radiofrequency energy to the gastroesophageal junction, injection of bulking agents in the LES, suturing near the gastroesophageal junction, and implantion of a prosthetic device into the LES.
- Following such therapy, patients often must continue acid suppression therapy because of persistent, although often less severe, symptoms.
- Endoscopic approaches to the treatment of GERD are still considered experimental and currently are not recommended for routine treatment of GERD.

Surgical Therapy

- Antireflux surgery corrects the mechanical factors that contribute to GERD. The most common surgical procedure performed is the Nissen fundoplication. The technique involves wrapping the upper portion of the stomach (fundus) around the distal esophagus 360° to enhance the integrity of the LES (see also Chapter 4). This prevents gastric contents from flowing retrograde into the esophagus, therby reducing GERD symptoms and allowing the esophageal mucosa to heal. In a patient with a hiatal hernia, the hernia is reduced back into the abdomen during surgery.
- A partial wrap (Toupet fundoplication) is performed in patients who have poor esophageal motility.
- These procedures are most often done laparoscopically to reduce the length of the hospital stay and operative morbidity.
- Surgery does not appear to reduce the rate of progression of Barrett's esophagus to adenocarcinoma.
- Surgery is as effective as PPIs in controlling symptoms in the short term (5 years).
- Common adverse effects of a fundoplication include dysphagia (19.4% in one study) due to a too tight a wrap at the LES and gas and bloating (gas–bloat syndrome) due to difficulty in expelling air from the stomach. Half of patients who undergo fundoplication will still require acid suppression medication.
- Surgical fundoplication is a good alternative to PPI treatment in patients who:
  ○ respond to PPI therapy but want a permanent treatment or do not tolerate PPIs;
  ○ respond to PPIs in terms of a decrease in heartburn but continue to have regurgitation;
  ○ develop recurrent complications of GERD such as a stricture or respiratory complications.

An algorithm for the management of GERD is shown in Figure 1.3.

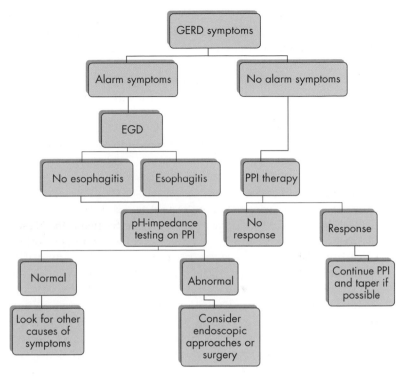

Figure 1.3 Algorithm for the management of GERD. (EGD, esophagogastroduodenoscopy; PPI, proton pump inhibitor.)

Pearls

GERD is a common chronic gastrointestinal disorder.

Most patients have mild or moderate symptoms that respond to lifestyle modifications and antacid therapy. However, some patients have severe, daily as well as night-time symptoms that can reduce the patient's quality of life significantly.

In patients with typical symptoms (heartburn, regurgitation), a PPI is the mainstay of therapy.

In patients with atypical or refractory symptoms, ambulatory pH testing and, in some cases, impedance testing are helpful in determining if the symptoms are truly related to gastroesophageal reflux.

Surgical treatment is appropriate in patients who do not wish to be on long-term medications or who continue to have complications of GERD. Early recognition of GERD can result in a reduction in both symptoms and complications of GERD and an improved quality of life.

Questions

Questions 1 and 2 relate to the clinical vignette at the beginning of this chapter.

1. Which of the following management strategies would you recommend for this patient?
   A. Schedule an upper endoscopy
   B. Continue ranitidine as needed
   C. Start a proton pump inhibitor
   D. Order a barium esophagogram
   E. Order a 24-hour pH study

2. Six months later, the patient reports intermittent difficulty swallowing solid food such as bread or rice. He denies odynophagia, weight loss, vomiting, or other symptoms. Which of the following is the most likely cause of his dysphagia?
   A. Achalasia
   B. Esophageal stricture
   C. Esophageal cancer
   D. Barrett's esophagus
   E. Hiatal hernia

3. Which of the following is considered to be the major pathophysiologic factor in GERD?
   A. Hiatal hernia
   B. Smoking
   C. Poor esophageal motility
   D. Transient lower esophageal sphincter relaxations
   E. Obesity

4. Long-standing GERD is a risk factor for which of the following?
   A. Squamous cell cancer of the esophagus
   B. Adenocarcinoma of the esophagus
   C. Peptic ulcer disease
   D. Gastric adenocarcinoma
   E. Achalasia

5. Surgical fundoplication for GERD has been shown to result in which of the following?
   A. Greater improvement in symptoms of GERD than therapy with a PPI
   B. Greater improvement in symptoms of GERD in patients with persistent regurgitation despite therapy with a PPI
   C. Improvement in esophageal clearance
   D. Reduction in the frequency of adenocarcinoma in patients with Barrett's esophagus
   E. Reduction in gastric acid production

Answers

1. C

The patient presents with symptoms of GERD, including heartburn, chest discomfort, a sore throat, and a bitter taste in the mouth. GERD may cause chest pain that can be indistinguishable from ischemic cardiac pain, and the first priority often is to rule out heart disease as the etiology. In this patient, a cardiac work-up was negative. An upper endoscopy may be a reasonable choice if the patient is >50 years of age (risk of Barrett's esophagus and adenocarcinoma increases with age), has alarm symptoms such as unintentional weight loss, gastrointestinal bleeding, vomiting, or dysphagia, or does not respond to a trial of a PPI. The most cost-effective diagnostic test for GERD in a younger person is a trial of a PPI. A barium esophagogram is not sensitive to diagnose GERD. A 24-hour pH study may be obtained if the patient does not respond to a trial of a PPI.

2. B

The most common complication of GERD is an esophageal stricture, which occurs in 0.1% of patients with GERD. Esophageal cancer (adenocarcinoma) is a possibility in a patient with long-standing GERD but is less likely in the absence of alarm symptoms. Patients with Barrett's esophagus are often asymptomatic or have symptoms of GERD. A hiatal hernia contributes to GERD but does not cause dysphagia. Achalasia is a motility disorder of the esophagus that generally presents with progressive dysphagia for both solids and liquids.

3. D

The etiology of GERD is multifactorial; smoking, poor esophageal motility, obesity, and hiatal hernia may contribute to GERD. Transient lower esophageal sphincter relaxations are the major etiologic factor in most patients with GERD.

4. B

5. B

Surgical fundoplication (wrapping or plicating of the stomach around the esophagus) is as effective as PPI therapy in controlling symptoms in the short term (5 years). It is a good alternative to PPI treatment in patients who have persistent regurgitation or develop complications of GERD such as a stricture or respiratory complications. Surgical fundoplication does not decrease the rate of progression of Barrett's esophagus to adenocarcinoma and does not affect gastric acid secretion.

Further Reading

Boeckxstaens, G.E. (2005). The lower esophageal sphincter. *Neurogastroenterology and Motility*, 17 (Suppl.1), 13–21.

Hvid-Jensen, F., Pedersen, L., Drewes, A.M., *et al.* (2011). Incidence of adenocarcinoma among patients with Barrett's esophagus. *New England Journal of Medicine,* 365, 1375–1383.

Pandolfino, J. (2008) The pathophysiologic basis for epidemiologic trends in gastroesophageal reflux disease. *Gastroenterology Clinics of North America,* 37, 827–843.

Richter, J. (2007) The many manifestations of gastroesophageal reflux disease: presentation, evaluation and treatment. *Gastroenterology Clinics of North America,* 37, 577–599.

Richter, J.E. and Friedenberg, F.K. (2010) Gastroesophageal reflux disease, in *Sleisenger and Fordtran's Gastrointestinal and Liver Disease: Pathophysiology/ Diagnosis/Management,* 9th edn (eds M. Feldman, L.S. Friedman, L.J. Brandt). Saunders Elsevier, Philadelphia, pp. 705–730.

Wang, C. and Hunt, R. (2008) Medical management of gastroesophageal reflux disease. *Gastroenterology Clinics of North America,* 37, 879–899.

Weblinks

http://www.nlm.nih.gov/medlineplus/gerd.html
http://www.acg.gi.org/physicians/guidelines/GERDTreatment.pdf
http://www.gastrojournal.org/article/S0016-5085(08)01605-3/fulltext

Dysphagia

Emad Qayed and Shanthi Srinivasan

CHAPTER 2

Clinical Vignette

A 55-year-old man is seen in the office for difficulty swallowing for the past 6 months. Food "sticks" in the middle of his chest in the mid-sternal area. This sensation has been worsening over the past several months. For the past 5 years he has had occasional heartburn. He has no difficulty swallowing liquids and denies odynophagia, choking, cough, or shortness of breath during swallowing. He denies nausea, vomiting, or abdominal pain. His weight has been stable. His past medical and surgical history is unremarkable. He takes ranitidine as needed for his heartburn but no other medications. His family history is unremarkable. He works as a consultant in a computer software company. He is married and has three children, all of whom are healthy. He drinks a few beers on the weekends and does not smoke cigarettes. He has no history of illicit drug use. A colonoscopy done 4 years ago was unremarkable. Physical examination reveals a well nourished middle-aged man with a blood pressure of 128/88 mmHg, pulse rate 72/min, temperature 98.5 °F (37 °C), and body mass index 29. Examination of the oral cavity reveals no lesions, and there are no palpable lymph nodes or swelling in his neck. The chest, cardiac, and abdominal examinations are unremarkable. The neurologic examination is normal. When asked to swallow a sip of water, he swallows normally without choking or coughing. Routine laboratory tests show a normal complete blood count and comprehensive metabolic panel.

Essentials of Gastroenterology, First Edition. Edited by Shanthi V. Sitaraman, Lawrence S. Friedman.
© 2012 John Wiley & Sons, Ltd. Published 2012 by John Wiley & Sons, Ltd.

General

- **Dysphagia** refers to difficulty swallowing. The condition results from impeded transport of liquids, solids, or both, from the pharynx to the stomach.
- **Odynophagia** refers to pain during swallowing and is frequently associated with dysphagia.
- Swallowing disorders can occur in all age groups, but the frequency of dysphagia is higher in the elderly. Approximately 7–10% of adults older than 50 years of age, up to 25% of hospitalized patients, and 30–40% of nursing home residents experience problems with swallowing.
- Dysphagia is classified as oropharyngeal and esophageal dysphagia. *Oropharyngeal* dysphagia, or transfer dysphagia, refers to difficulty transferring food (solids, liquids, or both) from the oropharynx to the esophagus. *Esophageal* dysphagia refers to difficulty passing food through the esophagus into the stomach.

Physiology of Swallowing

- Normal swallowing is a smooth, coordinated process that involves a complex series of voluntary and involuntary neuromuscular contractions (Figure 2.1). The process of swallowing typically is divided into three distinct phases: oral, pharyngeal, and esophageal. Impairment of any of these phases results in dysphagia.
- The *oral* phase involves preparing and propelling the food from the anterior oral cavity into the oropharynx where an involuntary swallowing reflex is initiated. The oral phase is the only voluntary phase

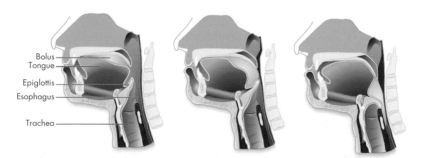

Bolus
Tongue
Epiglottis
Esophagus
Trachea

Figure 2.1 Oral and pharyngeal phases of swallowing. The diagram shows the transfer of a bolus of food from the mouth to the oropharynx to the upper esophagus.

of swallowing and requires coordinated contractions of the tongue and striated muscles of mastication.

- The *pharyngeal* phase involves overlapping events that are critical to protect the airway while allowing the bolus to transfer to the esophagus. The food bolus is propelled into the pharyngeal cavity, while the soft palate elevates and closes the nasal aperture and the larynx begins to elevate. The food bolus is then propelled into the hypopharynx by pharyngeal contractions. The larynx closes and the soft palate and the posterior pharyngeal wall oppose the posterior aspect of the tongue to prevent reflux of food into the oral cavity. The last step involves opening of the upper esophageal sphincter to allow the passage of food to the esophageal lumen.
  - ○ Alteration of any of the steps of the oral or pharyngeal phases of swallowing, due to mechanical obstruction or a neuromuscular condition, results in oropharyngeal dysphagia.
- In the *esophageal* phase, the food bolus is propelled down the esophagus by peristaltic contractions.
  - ○ Once the food reaches the esophageal lumen, primary peristaltic contractions propel the food bolus down the length of the esophagus to the distal esophagus. This is accompanied by relaxation of the lower esophageal sphincter and emptying of the esophageal contents into the gastric lumen.
  - ○ Residual food in the esophagus causes local distension and triggers secondary peristaltic contractions that clear the esophagus of remaining food in the lumen.
  - ○ Altered esophageal peristaltic contractions or failure of the lower esophageal sphincter to relax can result in esophageal dysphagia.
  - ○ Another important mechanism of esophageal dysphagia is mechanical obstruction of the esophagus. This can be secondary to intraluminal obstruction or extrinsic compression.

Etiology

Oropharyngeal Dysphagia
Oropharyngeal dysphagia can be caused by mechanical obstruction or neuromuscular disease (Table 2.1).

Esophageal Dysphagia
Esophageal dysphagia can be caused by mechanical obstruction of the esophageal lumen or can be secondary to dysmotility of the esophagus or lower esophageal sphincter (Figure 2.2).

- **Mechanical obstruction**. The most common cause of esophageal dysphagia is mechanical obstruction of the esophageal lumen (Table

Table 2.1 Causes of oropharyngeal dysphagia.

Category	Etiologies
Structural lesions	Benign or malignant tumors Candidal infection (thrush) Caustic ingestion Cervical spondylosis Peritonsillar abscess Radiation Retropharyngeal abscess or mass Thyromegaly Zenker's diverticulum

Neuromuscular causes	Diseases of the cerebral cortex and cranial nerves:
	  Alzheimer's disease
	  Bulbar and pseudobulbar palsy
	  Cerebral palsy
	  CNS tumors (benign or malignant)
	  Multiple sclerosis
	  Metabolic encephalopathy
	  Parkinson's disease
	  Stroke
	  Vascular dementias
	
	Neuromuscular disorders:
	  Botulism
	  Myositis (polymyositis, dermatomyositis)
	  Myasthenia gravis
	  Primary myopathies (myotonic dystrophy, oculopharyngeal myopathy)

CNS, central nervous system.

2.2) due to intraluminal (intrinsic) lesions or extrinsic compression. Dysphagia usually occurs when the diameter of the esophageal lumen is 13 mm or less. The symptoms depend on the degree of obstruction. For example, mild narrowing of the esophageal lumen causes symptoms only with large boluses of food, whereas more complete obstruction results in dysphagia for both solids and liquids. Intraluminal causes of dysphagia include the following:

○ Esophageal cancer: patients with esophageal cancer present with dysphagia that is progressive, from solids to liquids, and associated with constitutional symptoms such as weight loss and anorexia. Patients may have risk factors such as smoking and alcohol use in

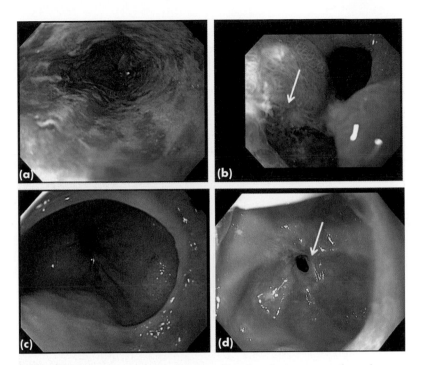

Figure 2.2 Endoscopic images of various disorders that cause esophageal dysphagia. (a) Reflux esophagitis: superficial ulcerations, edema, and erythema are seen in a continuous fashion from the gastroesophageal junction to proximal esophagus in a patient with chronic gastroesophageal reflux. (b) Pill-induced esophagitis: a discrete deep ulcer with sharply demarcated edges and necrotic center (arrow) is seen in a patient with a history of tetracycline use. (c) An esophageal ring is seen as a fibrotic circumferential ring in the lower esophagus. (d) An esophageal stricture leads to severe narrowing of the esophageal lumen (arrow) with dilatation of the proximal esophagus in a patient with history of lye ingestion.

the case of squamous cell carcinoma or longstanding gastroesophageal reflux disease in the case of adenocarcimona.

○ Esophageal stricture: esophageal strictures can be caused by caustic ingestion, certain medications, gastroesophageal reflux disease, and radiation therapy.
○ Esophageal rings and webs: rings or webs typically cause intermittent nonprogressive dysphagia.
○ Esophagitis: dysphagia caused by esophagitis is usually accompanied by odynophagia. Medications known to cause esophagitis include aspirin and other nonsteroidal anti-inflammatory drugs,

Table 2.2 Causes of esophageal dysphagia.

Category	Etiology

Mechanical obstruction	Intrinsic narrowing:
	    Benign strictures: gastroesophageal reflux, caustic substances, medications, postsurgical, radiation therapy
	    Cricopharyngeal hyperplasia/bar
	    Esophagitis: infectious, eosinophilic, pill-induced, gastroesophageal reflux disease
	    Esophageal rings and webs
	    Esophageal diverticula
	    Tumors: benign or malignant
	
	Extrinsic compression:
	    Anterior mediastinal mass
	    Vascular lesions:
	        Congenital (dysphagia lusoria): aberrant right subclavian artery, right-sided aorta
	        Acquired: aortic aneurysm, left atrial enlargement, right-sided aorta

Esophageal motility disorders	Achalasia Diffuse (distal) esophageal spasm: high amplitude, nonpropagating, presents with chest pain and dysphagia Hypertensive peristalsis (nutcracker esophagus) presents with chest pain Hypotensive peristalsis: scleroderma

doxycycline or tetracycline, bisphosphonates, and potassium preparations.
○ Eosinophilic esophagitis is an increasingly recognized cause of dysphagia.

Eosinophilic esophagitis typically causes intermittent dysphagia with food or pill impactions. This condition can present without endoscopic changes. The diagnosis is confirmed by esophageal mucosal biopsies and is most common in persons younger than 45 years of age.

• **Motility disorders**. Esophageal motility disorders are a less common cause of dysphagia than mechanical causes. Dysphagia due to esophageal dysmotility typically results in difficulty swallowing both solids and liquids.

○ Achalasia: characteristic manometric features of achalasia include absence of esophageal peristalsis and failure of the lower esophageal sphincter to relax with swallowing. The etiology of achalasia is unknown. A selective loss of postganglionic inhibitory neurons innervating smooth muscle of the esophagus is typically seen and is thought to result in a hypertensive lower esophageal sphincter that fails to relax with swallowing and leads to a functional obstruction.

○ Certain diseases mimic clinical, radiologic, and manometric features of achalasia. Such conditions are termed pseudoachalasia. An example of psuedoachalasia is gastric adenocarcinoma of the cardia.

○ Spastic motility disorders have been termed diffuse (or distal) esophageal spasm and so-called nutcracker esophagus. Patients with these disorders usually present with chest pain in addition to dysphagia.

○ Systemic diseases such as scleroderma can present with dysphagia. Scleroderma causes hypomotility of the esophagus along with a hypotensive lower esophageal sphincter and aperistalsis. Patients often present with gastroesophageal reflux in addition to dysphagia.

Clinical Features

• The clinical history is extremely important in evaluating the cause of dysphagia. In addition to dysphagia, a history of odynophagia should be elicited. Dysphagia should be distinguished from *globus sensation*, which refers to a constant feeling of a lump or tightness in the throat without any demonstrable abnormality in swallowing. Important questions to ask the patient with dysphagia include the time of onset of symptoms, progression, severity, and pattern (intermittent or constant) of symptoms, presence of heartburn, type of food that induces symptoms (liquids or solids, or both), history of head and neck malignancy or surgery, and associated neurologic disorders. A careful medication history should be obtained.

• Typical symptoms of oropharyngeal dysphagia include choking, cough, or shortness of breath with swallowing. Patients often have difficulty initiating a swallow and point to the throat as the location where the food is stuck. In some patients, liquids are regurgitated through the nose. Other associated symptoms include dysarthria, nasal speech, hoarseness, weight loss, and recurrent pulmonary infections.

- Symptoms of esophageal dysphagia include a sensation that food is stuck in the chest or throat. Most patients will point to the lower or mid sternum as the location of their symptoms. However, this localization often does not correlate with the anatomic level of the abnormality. Other associated symptoms include heartburn, odynophagia, hematemesis, chest pain, sensitivity to hot or cold liquids, and weight loss.
- Esophageal dysphagia to both solids and liquids suggests a motility disorder of the esophagus, whereas dysphagia to solids that progresses over time to involve liquids suggests a mechanical obstruction. Odynophagia suggests esophagitis.
- Physical examination:
  - Important elements of the physical examination include the patient's general appearance and nutritional status and an assessment of respiratory distress as well as a mental status examination.
  - Examination of the cranial nerves (especially V and VII–XII) should be performed.
  - Systemic examination should focus on skin and nail, respiratory, and abdominal findings. *Tylosis* is a genetic syndrome characterized by hyperkeratosis of the palm and soles associated with a high frequency of squamous cell carcinoma of the esophagus.
  - It is usually helpful to ask the patient to take a sip of water while being observed for symptoms of oropharyngeal dysphagia.

Diagnosis

- In most patients the distinction between oropharyngeal and esophageal dysphagia as well as among mechanical, motility, and neuromuscular causes can be made by careful history taking and physical examination. An approach to the diagnosis of esophageal dysphagia is shown in Figure 2.3.
- **Video-radiographic studies (video fluoroscopy).** If the clinical history and physical examination suggest oropharyngeal dysphagia, especially with a risk of aspiration (e.g., neurologic impairment), video-radiographic studies are performed to identify the presence, nature, and severity of oropharyngeal swallowing dysfunction. This test is performed by a team composed of a radiologist, otolaryngologist, and speech pathologist.
- **Barium studies.** A barium esophagogram (barium swallow) is recommended as the initial test for esophageal dysphagia. It can help identify a structural or obstructive lesion of the esophagus such as Zenker's diverticulum, caustic injury, benign or malignant stricture, or tumor. A barium esophagogram can show the location of a lesion and the

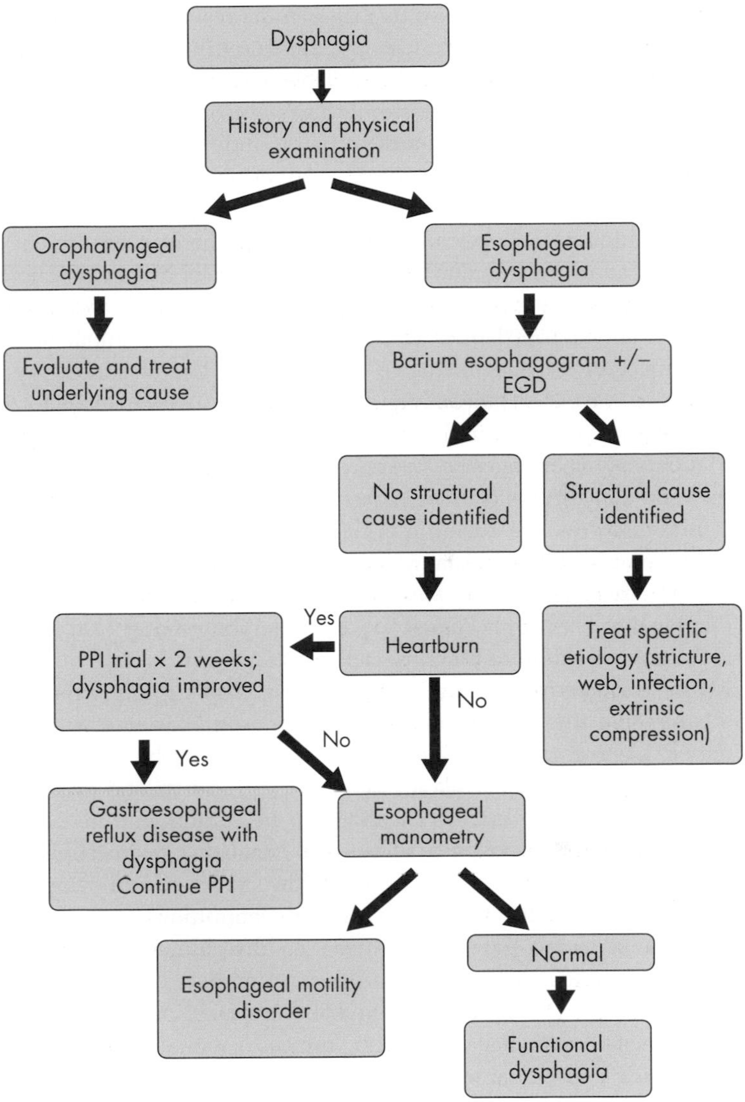

Figure 2.3 Algorithm for the diagnostic evaluation of esophageal dysphagia. (EGD, esophagogastroduodenoscopy; PPI, proton pump inhibitor)

complexity of a stricture and is a safer initial test than esophagogas-troduodenoscopy (upper endoscopy) in this setting. A barium esoph-agogram with a solid bolus (barium tablet or marshmallow) is useful in detecting extrinsic compression or a subtle esophageal ring that can be missed by endoscopy. A double-contrast study provides better visu-alization of the esophageal mucosa than a single-contrast study (see Chapter 27).

- **Upper endoscopy**. Upper endoscopy provides the best assessment of the esophageal mucosa and allows diagnostic (e.g., biopsy of lesions) and therapeutic (e.g., dilation of a stricture, removal of impacted food bolus) intervention. Upper endoscopy should be the initial test in patients with dysphagia due to a food impaction. If endoscopy is normal, some experts recommend esophageal biopsies to evaluate for the presence of eosinophilic esophagitis.

- **Manometry**. Esophageal manometry assesses the motor function of the esophagus. A nasogastric catheter with electronic probes is used to measure pressure during esophageal contractions and upper and lower esophageal body and sphincter responses to swallowing. Manometry is indicated in patients with dysphagia in whom a barium esophagogram or upper endoscopy reveals no abnormality. Manometry is the gold standard to diagnose achalasia.

- **pH measurements**. Although cumbersome, esophageal pH monitor-ing remains the gold standard for diagnosing patients with sus-pected gastroesophageal reflux disease. A pH probe is placed in the patient's esophagus via a nasogastric catheter or endoscopically and detects acid reflux. (pH testing can be combined with imped-ance testing to assess both acidic and nonacidic gastroesophageal reflux.) The patient is asked to record the occurrence of symptoms over a 24-hour period, and the patient's symptoms are compared with the recorded pH measurements to determine if gastric acid reflux correlates with the symptoms. Combined recordings of esophageal pH levels and intraluminal esophageal pressure may aid in diagnosing patients with reflux-induced esophageal spasm. pH monitoring and manometry are usually available through referral to gastroenterologists.

A barium esophagogram is the first step in evaluating patients with symptoms of esophageal dysphagia, especially if an obstructive lesion is suspected. Upper endoscopy is the recommended initial study in patients with acute obstruction such as an impacted food bolus.

Treatment

See also Chapters 1 and 4.

Oropharyngeal Dysphagia

The goals of management in oropharyngeal dysphagia are to provide adequate nutrition, improve the patient's ability to eat and swallow, and prevent tracheobronchial aspiration. Therapy is individualized based on the functional and structural abnormalities and the initial response to treatment observed at the patient's bedside or during a video-radiographic study.

Esophageal Dysphagia

- Mechanical obstruction can be relieved by surgery (e.g., tumors or diverticula) or by endoscopic dilation (e.g., strictures, rings, webs).
- If the results of a barium esophagogram and upper endoscopy are normal and the patient has symptoms of heartburn or regurgitation associated with dysphagia, a therapeutic trial of a proton pump inhibitor (PPI) taken twice daily for 2 weeks is recommended. Improvement in symptoms suggests that the dysphagia is related to the presence of gastroesophageal reflux (see Table 2.1).

Achalasia and Other Esophageal Motility Disorders

Definitive treatment of achalasia is surgical esophagomyotomy (Heller myotomy, see Chapter 4). A trial of nitrates or calcium channel blockers may be useful in patients with diffuse esophageal spasm.

Pearls

A detailed history can help identify the cause of dysphagia in approximately 80% of patients.

Intermittent symptoms and dysphagia to both liquids and solid food are features that most strongly suggest a motility disorder.

A trial of therapy for reflux symptoms should be undertaken before further diagnostic evaluation of dysphagia in patients who are thought to have gastroesophageal reflux disease.

Questions

Questions 1–3 relate to the clinical vignette at the beginning of this chapter.

1. The differential diagnosis of the patient's dysphagia includes all of the following EXCEPT:
   A. Esophageal stricture
   B. Esophageal adenocarcinoma
   C. Achalasia
   D. Eosinophilic esophagitis
   E. Gastroesophageal reflux disease

2. Which of the following is the next step in the management of this patient?
   A. Upper endoscopy
   B. Computed tomography of the chest
   C. Barium esophagogram
   D. A trial of a proton pump inhibitor for 8 weeks
   E. Reassurance and follow-up

3. A barium esophagogram does not reveal any abnormalities. The patient undergoes upper endoscopy, which is completely normal. The next step in the management of this patient is which of the following?
   A. Test and treat for *Helicobacter pylori* infection
   B. A trial of a proton pump inhibitor for 2 weeks
   C. Video-radiographic study
   D. Upper endoscopy
   E. Esophageal manometry

4. Which of the following neurons is selectively lost in achalasia?
   A. Preganglionic neurons containing nitric oxide
   B. Postganglionic neurons containing nitric oxide
   C. Preganglionic neurons containing acetylcholine
   D. Postganglionic neurons containing acetylcholine

5. An 80-year-old man presents with progressive dysphagia for solid food over the past 3 months. He reports a weight loss of 20 lb (9 kg). He has had gastroesophageal reflux symptoms for the past 15 years. The differential diagnosis of his dysphagia includes all of the following EXCEPT:
   A. Benign esophageal ("peptic") stricture
   B. Adenocarcinoma of the esophagus
   C. Squamous cell carcinoma of the esophagus
   D. Parkinson's disease

6. A 65-year-old man presents with progressive dysphagia for liquids and solids over the past few weeks. He has episodes of choking when he swallows liquids. His symptoms are intermittent and have not resulted in weight loss. He does not take any medications. In addition to dysphagia, he notes mild weakness of his left arm and leg. The most likely cause of dysphagia in this patient is which of the following?

A. Reflux esophagitis
B. Neurologic dysfunction
C. Squamous cell carcinoma of the esophagus
D. Adenocarcinoma of the esophagus

7. The best test to establish the diagnosis in the patient presented in Question 6 is which of the following?
   A. Upper endoscopy
   B. Barium esophagogram
   C. Esophageal pH testing
   D. Video-radiographic study

8. The best diagnostic test to establish the diagnosis of achalasia is which of the following?
   A. Upper endoscopy
   B. Esophageal manometry
   C. Esophageal pH testing
   D. Video-radiographic study

9. A 65-year-old man with intermittent dysphagia is noted to have an esophageal ring on upper endoscopy. The patient denies any symptoms of gastroesophageal reflux. Which of the following is the best treatment option for his dysphagia?
   A. Endoscopic dilation
   B. Proton pump inhibitor
   C. Surgical resection
   D. Dietary modification

Answers

1. C
2. C
3. B

   The patient has classic symptoms of esophageal dysphagia, likely due to mechanical obstruction. In the setting of a prior long-term history of heartburn, the differential diagnosis includes reflux esophagitis, peptic stricture, or adenocarcinoma of the esophagus. Barium esophagogram with a tablet is the first test of choice. If the test is normal, the next step is to perform upper endoscopy. If upper endoscopy, with mucosal biopsies to evaluate for eosinophilic esophagitis, is normal, the patient should be treated empirically for gastroesophageal reflux disease with a proton pump inhibitor twice daily for 2 weeks. If the patient does not respond to a trial of a proton pump inhibitor, esophageal manometry should be performed to rule out an esophageal motor disorder.

(Continued)

4. B

   In achalasia the postganglionic nitric oxide-containing neurons are lost, thereby resulting in failure of relaxation of the lower esophageal sphincter.

5. D

   The patient has symptoms of esophageal dysphagia. His recent weight loss raises concern about esophageal cancer. His symptoms are also consistent with a benign stricture, given his longstanding reflux symptoms. Parkinson's disease is usually associated with oropharyngeal dysphagia, and patients complain of cough, choking, or neurologic symptoms.

6. B

   The patient has symptoms of oropharyngeal dysphagia including coughing and a choking sensation after eating. This presentation could be secondary to stroke, particularly in light of the weakness on his left side. Esophageal cancer is usually associated with weight loss and progressive dysphagia for solid food. Reflux esophagitis is typically associated with heartburn and odynophagia. Dysphagia for solids and liquids is uncommon in patients with reflux esophagitis.

7. D

   A video-radiographic study is used to observe the process of deglutition. Abnormalities in oropharyngeal dysphagia can be detected using this test. When esophageal dysphagia is suspected, one should perform a barium esophagogram with or without an upper endoscopy. In a patient in whom gastroesophageal reflux is a suspected cause of dysphagia, pH testing may be performed.

8. B

   Achalasia is a motility disorder characterized by loss of myenteric ganglion inhibitory neurons leading to loss of relaxation of the lower esophageal sphincter. Manometry is the best test to establish this diagnosis. Upper endoscopy may reveal a tight lower esophageal sphincter but is not diagnostic for achalasia. A video-radiographic study is useful for the evaluation of oropharyngeal dysphagia. Upper endoscopy is useful for detection of a structural lesion causing dysphagia. Esophageal pH testing can help in establishing the role of gastroesophageal reflux as a cause of dysphagia.

9. A

   The best treatment option for an esophageal ring is to perform an endoscopic dilation. In the absence of reflux symptoms, a trial of a proton pump inhibitor is not recommended. Surgical resection is not a treatment option for an esophageal ring. Dietary modification is generally not beneficial for an esophageal ring.

Further Reading

DeVault, K.D. (2010) Symptoms of esophageal disease, in *Sleisenger and Fordtran's Gastrointestinal and Liver Disease: Pathophysiology/Diagnosis/Management*, 9th edn (eds M. Feldman, L.S. Friedman and L.J. Brandt), Saunders Elsevier, Philadelphia, pp. 173–179.

Galmiche, J.P., Clouse, R.E., Balint A., *et al.* (2006) Functional esophageal disorders. *Gastroenterology*, 130, 1459–1465.

Kahrilas, P.J. and Smout, A.J.P.M. (2010) Esophageal disorders. *American Journal of Gastroenterology*, 105, 747–756.

Weblinks

http://www.merckmanuals.com/professional/sec02/ch012/ch012b.html?qt=dysphagia&alt=sh
http://emedicine.medscape.com/article/324096-overview

Peptic Ulcer Disease

Shanthi V. Sitaraman and Lawrence S. Friedman

CHAPTER 3

Clinical Vignette

A 43-year-old African-American woman is seen in the office for epigastric discomfort of 8 months' duration. She describes the discomfort as a constant dull ache that usually occurs postprandially and is associated with nausea but not vomiting. The pain abates spontaneously after a few hours. She has no nocturnal pain, diarrhea, rectal bleeding, or weight loss. At age 40, she had a colonoscopy for rectal bleeding, which was unremarkable except for hemorrhoids. Her past medical and surgical history is unremarkable except for seasonal allergies. She takes antihistamines and ibuprofen 1–2 tablets several times a month for headaches. She does not take any prescription medications. Her parents are alive and well, and her two siblings are healthy. Her paternal grandfather died of colon cancer at age 80. She works as an administrative assistant, is married, and has two children. She drinks a glass of wine with dinner and does not smoke. She has no history of illicit drug use. Physical examination reveals a blood pressure of 114/80 mmHg, pulse rate 67/min, and body mass index 22. She is afebrile. The remainder of the examination including an abdominal examination is unremarkable. Rectal examination reveals brown stool that is negative for occult blood. A complete blood count is normal.

General

- The lifetime prevalence of peptic ulcer disease (PUD) is approximately 10%.
- PUD affects approximately 4.5 million people in the US annually.

Essentials of Gastroenterology, First Edition. Edited by Shanthi V. Sitaraman, Lawrence S. Friedman.
© 2012 John Wiley & Sons, Ltd. Published 2012 by John Wiley & Sons, Ltd.

Etiology and Pathogenesis

> The majority (95%) of gastric and duodenal ulcers are caused by *Helicobacter pylori* or nonsteroidal anti-inflammatory drugs (NSAIDs).

- *Helicobacter pylori*:
  - ○ Seventy percent of gastric ulcers and 80–95% of duodenal ulcers are attributed to *H. pylori* infection.
  - ○ Approximately 15% of *H. pylori*-infected persons will develop PUD.
  - ○ In the US the estimated prevalence of *H. pylori* infection is 20% in persons younger than 30 years and 50% of those older than 60 years of age. The prevalence is higher in African-American and Hispanic people.
  - ○ *H. pylori* is a Gram-negative microaerophilic bacterium that colonizes the surface of epithelial cells of the gastric antrum. If found in the duodenum, *H. pylori* is associated with metaplastic gastric epithelium. The bacterium produces urease, which breaks down urea to ammonia and carbon dioxide and is required for the survival of *H. pylori* in an acidic environment (and is the basis of diagnostic tests, see below).
  - ○ Duodenal and gastric ulcers result as a consequence of both destruction of antral epithelial cells by *H. pylori* and production of gastric acid, induced by the bacteria, that overwhelms the intrinsic defense mechanisms in the stomach and duodenum. The inflammatory response to *H. pylori* colonization induces hyperplasia of antral G cells, which in turn secrete gastrin, thereby causing a further increase in gastric acid production.
- NSAIDs:
  - ○ Account for 10% of duodenal ulcers and 15–30% of gastric ulcers.
  - ○ NSAIDs (including aspirin) inhibit cyclooxygenase-1, the enzyme that catalyzes the synthesis of prostaglandins (which act as mucosal protectants). NSAIDs are also weak acids that, when protonated by gastric acid, penetrate the epithelial cell membrane and cause rapid epithelial cell death and mucosal erosion.

> Risk factors for developing NSAID-induced ulcers include age >60 years, concomitant use of glucocorticoids, use of multiple or high doses (≥2× normal) of NSAIDs, prior history of PUD, and anticoagulant use.

- Malignancy (can cause gastric or duodenal ulceration): adenocarcinoma, lymphoma, gastrointestinal stromal tumor (GIST).
- Less common causes: gastrin hypersecretory states such as gastrinoma (Zollinger-Ellison syndrome), mastocytosis, antral G cell hyperplasia.
- Rare causes: Crohn's disease, eosinophilic gastroenteritis, viruses (cytomegalovirus, herpes virus).

In many patients with ulcer-like symptoms (dyspepsia), no ulcer (or other "organic" disorder) is identified. Such patients are considered to have functional (or non-ulcer) dyspepsia.

Clinical Features

- Typical symptoms (occur in <20% of patients) include dyspepsia (epigastric pain, fullness, or bloating, often with nausea and eructation). The discomfort is often described as gnawing or burning in nature. With duodenal ulcer, the discomfort often occurs 1–3 hours after a meal and is relieved by food or antacids. With gastric ulcer, the discomfort is often exacerbated by food. Nocturnal symptoms may occur. In many patients, symptoms are nonspecific and vague.
- Physical examination: in uncomplicated PUD, physical findings are minimal or absent. When present, findings include epigastric tenderness and occult blood in the stool or melena (black or maroon stools resulting from gastrointestinal bleeding). Peritoneal signs (rebound abdominal tenderness, guarding, and rigidity) signify a perforated ulcer, and a succussion splash is seen with partial or complete gastric outlet obstruction.

Diagnosis

- In most patients with uncomplicated PUD, routine laboratory tests are not usually helpful.
- Confirmation of PUD is best made by an upper endoscopy (esophagogastroduodenoscopy [EGD]) (Figure 3.1). Guidelines for the approach to patients presenting with dyspepsia are shown in Figure 3.2.

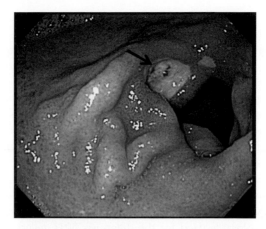

Figure 3.1 Endoscopic image of a pyloric channel ulcer (arrow).

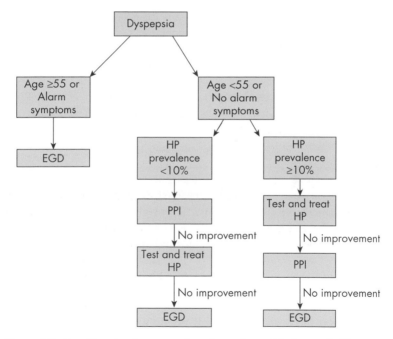

Figure 3.2 Algorithm for the approach to the patient with dyspepsia (American College of Gastroenterology, 2005). Alarm symptoms include unintentional weight loss, iron deficiency anemia, persistent vomiting, NSAID use, and gastrointestinal bleeding. (EGD, esophagogastroduodenoscopy; HP, *Helicobacter pylori*; NSAID, nonsteroidal anti-inflammatory drug; PPI, trial of proton pump inhibitor; Test and treat indicates testing for *H. pylori* and treating the infection, if present.)

Tests for *H. pylori*

- Invasive (require endoscopy):
  - **Rapid urease test**: done on a mucosal biopsy specimen from the antrum, body, or fundus of the stomach (95% sensitive and specific).
  - **Histology**: organisms can be visualized on histologic examination of the surface of epithelial cells in gastric mucosal biopsy specimens. The absence of chronic gastritis (inflammation) on histologic examination of a gastric mucosal biopsy specimen is good evidence of the absence of *H. pylori*.
  - **Culture and sensitivity**: seldom performed.
- Noninvasive (do not require endoscopy):
  - **Serology**: antibodies to *H. pylori* (sensitivity 90%, specificity 70–80%). Serology is used for the diagnosis of *H. pylori* in previously untreated persons. It is not as useful in confirming eradication of *H. pylori* following treatment.
  - **Urea breath test**: radiolabeled urea is ingested by the patient, and isotope-labeled carbon dioxide generated by the bacterial urease is measured in exhaled breath (sensitivity and specificity >95%). This test may be used as an initial diagnostic test or to confirm eradication.
  - **Stool antigen**: the test is based on the amplification of *H. pylori* RNA shed in stool (sensitivity >90%, specificity 80–90%). The test may be used as an initial diagnostic test or to confirm eradication.

> Tests based on urease activity of the bacteria may yield false-negative results in the setting of recent antibiotic use or treatment with a proton pump inhibitor (PPI), histamine H2 receptor antagonist (H2RA), or a bismuth-containing compound. Testing should be repeated if necessary 4 weeks after discontinuation of antibiotics and 2 weeks after discontinuation of a PPI or H2RA.

Serum Gastrin Level

- Usually measured if gastrinoma (Zollinger–Ellison syndrome) is suspected (on the basis of recurrent peptic ulcer, severe and multiple ulcers, and concomitant diarrhea).
- Other conditions associated with an elevated serum gastrin level include use of a PPI and atrophic gastritis. *H. pylori* infection may raise the serum gastrin level slightly.
- A serum gastrin level >1000 pg/mL is highly suggestive of gastrinoma. If the level is elevated but <1000 pg/mL, gastric pH measurement may be performed (pH measurement is done on gastric fluid obtained via endoscopy or insertion of a nasogastric tube). A gastric pH <3.0 is

consistent with a gastrinoma or antral *H. pylori* infection. A secretin stimulation test will confirm gastrinoma if the rise in serum gastrin after intravenous administration of secretin is >200 pg/mL. A gastric pH ≥3.0 is seen with the use of a PPI or in atrophic gastritis.

Treatment

- Antisecretory agents: administered orally (8 weeks for duodenal ulcer and 8–12 weeks for gastric ulcer), these are the primary drugs used to treat PUD:
  - **H2RAs**: block H2 receptors on parietal cells of the stomach; can heal 90% of ulcers in 8 weeks; can be given as a single nighttime dose.
  - **PPIs**: bind covalently and irreversibly with the hydrogen/potassium-adenosine triphosphatase enzyme (H^+/K^+ -ATPase pump) on parietal cells in the stomach; more potent acid-suppressing agents than H2RAs; heal >95% of ulcers. Side effects include headache, diarrhea, constipation, nausea, and acid "rebound" on withdrawal.
- Mucosal protectants (not used as first-line therapy for PUD):
  - **Sucralfate**: after oral ingestion, forms a cross-linking, viscous, paste-like material that coats the ulcer bed; in an acidic environment, binds to proteins such as albumin, pepsin, and fibrinogen to form stable insoluble complexes on the surface of an ulcer.
  - **Misoprostol**: stimulates gastric mucus and bicarbonate secretion after oral ingestion; its primary use is in ulcer prevention, for example, in a patient taking an NSAID who has a high risk of developing PUD; side effects include diarrhea; the drug is contraindicated in pregnancy.
  - **Antacids**: neutralize gastric acid after oral ingestion; multiple daily doses are required to heal ulcer. Side effects depend on the formulation: magnesium-containing, diarrhea; aluminum-containing, constipation; calcium-containing, gastric acid "rebound" when antacid is discontinued.
- Discontinue NSAIDs:
  - If an NSAID is required despite PUD, consider prophylactic PPI treatment concomitantly. Alternatively, consider administration of a more selective cyclooxygenase-2 (COX-2) inhibitor instead of a non-selective NSAID.
- *H. pylori* eradication (Table 3.1):
  - Treatment is given orally for 10–14 days. A four-drug combination, either sequential or concomitant, or a bismuth-containing regimen is recommended. Concomitant treatment consists of a PPI, amoxicillin, clarithromycin, and a nitroimidazole (metronidazole or tinidazole); sequential treatment consists of a 10-day regimen in which a PPI plus amoxicillin is given for 5 days followed by a PPI plus

Table 3.1 Treatment regimens for *H. pylori* eradication.

Concomitant treatment 14 days

PPI	BID
Amoxicillin	1000 mg BID
Clarithromycin	500 mg BID
Metronidazole or tinidazole	500 mg BID

Sequential treatment 10 days

PPI	BID for all 10 days
Amoxicillin	1000 mg BID for the first 5 days
Clarithromycin	500 mg BID on days 5–10
Metronidazole or tinidazole	500 mg TID or 400 mg QID on days 5–10

Bismuth-containing regimen 14 days

PPI	BID
Bismuth subsalicylate	2 tablets QID
Metronidazole or tinidazole	500 mg TID or 400 mg QID
Tetracycline HCl	500 mg QID

PPI, proton pump inhibitor, e.g., esomaprazole 40 mg, lansoprazole 30 mg, omeprazole 20 mg, pantoprazole 40 mg, rabeprazole 20 mg; BID, twice daily; TID, three times a day; QID, four times a day.

clarithromycin and a nitroimidazole (metronidazole or tinidazole) for 5 days. These regimens are associated with an *H. pylori* eradication rates of >90%.

Confirmation of *H. pylori* eradication is indicated in patients with PUD associated with complications such as bleeding and in those in whom symptoms recur after treatment.

- *H. pylori* eradication and NSAID use:
  - *H. pylori* eradication in chronic NSAID users is insufficient to prevent NSAID-related ulcer disease. Prophylaxis with a PPI is recommended in high-risk patients.
  - Patients taking an NSAID in whom bleeding from PUD develops should be tested for *H. pylori* and treated for the infection, if present. If such patients require long-term NSAID use, a PPI should also be administered long term.
- Discontinue smoking.

Complications

- The most common (15–20%) complication is bleeding (see Chapter 22). Others include perforation or penetration into the pancreas (5–7%) and gastric outlet obstruction (<5%).
- Persons with *H. pylori* infection have a 3- to 6-fold higher incidence of gastric adenocarcinoma.
- Mucosa-associated lymphoid tissue (MALT) lymphoma is associated with *H. pylori* infection. Treatment of *H. pylori* infection results in regression or cure in >90% of patients if the lymphoma is diagnosed at an early stage.
- Gastroesophageal reflux disease (see Chapter 1) appears to increase in frequency and/or severity after eradication of *H. pylori*.

Prognosis

The majority of peptic ulcers heal with antisecretory therapy in combination with treatment of *H. pylori* infection and/or discontinuation of NSAIDs. The frequency of recurrence of an *H. pylori*-related ulcer is 4–10%.

Pearls

Because a small percentage of gastric ulcers are actually ulcerated gastric carcinomas, all gastric ulcers must be assessed carefully to distinguish a benign from a malignant ulcer.

Endoscopy should be repeated to ensure that a gastric ulcer (not related to NSAID use), particularly if it is >2 cm, has healed.

Questions

Questions 1 and 2 relate to the clinical vignette at the beginning of this chapter.
1. The next step in the management of the patient is which of the following?
   A. Upper endoscopy
   B. *H. pylori* test and eradication
   C. Antacids for 8 weeks
   D. Reassurance and follow-up
   E. Proton pump inhibitor (PPI) for 8 weeks

(Continued)

2. The patient returns to your office in 12 weeks stating that she felt better initially after taking a PPI but that her symptoms recurred after discontinuing the PPI and despite avoiding NSAIDs. The next step in the management of this patient is which of the following?
   A. Upper endoscopy
   B. Measure serum gastrin
   C. Increase the dose of the PPI to twice daily
   D. Switch to another PPI
   E. Test the urine for surreptitious NSAID use

3. A 57-year-old man presents with epigastric pain of 2 months' duration. An upper endoscopy reveals a duodenal ulcer. In advising the patient of complications of the duodenal ulcer, you explain that the most common complication is which of the following?
   A. Perforation
   B. Bleeding
   C. Obstruction
   D. Pancreatitis
   E. Cholecystitis

4. A 40-year-old man who has osteoarthritis of his knee requires long-term use of a nonsteroidal anti-inflammatory drug (NSAID). The patient is concerned about PUD as a result of NSAID use. What would you advise this patient?
   A. Stop smoking
   B. Use cholestyramine
   C. Test for *Helicobacter pylori* and eradicate if present
   D. Use amoxicillin
   E. Upper endoscopy

5. Which of the following statements regarding *Helicobacter pylori* is true?
   A. It is the cause of only a small proportion of duodenal ulcers
   B. It invades the gastric mucosa and rarely can cause systemic infection
   C. It colonizes surface epithelial cells in the antrum of the stomach
   D. It causes a decrease in the number of antral G cells
   E. It increases the risk of gastroesophageal reflux disease

6. A 30-year-old man presents to the emergency department with the sudden onset of severe abdominal pain. He states that he has been training for a marathon and has been taking ibuprofen for myalgias. Physical examination reveals a distended, rigid abdomen, and rebound tenderness. Bowel sounds are absent. You suspect perforation of a gastric or duodenal ulcer. Which of the following tests can confirm a perforation?
   A. Upright abdominal film
   B. Chest x-ray
   C. Computed tomography (CT) of the abdomen
   D. All of the above

Answers

1. B

2. A

This patient presents with dyspepsia. She has no alarm symptoms and is less than 55 years of age. The prevalence of *H. pylori* is increased in African-Americans, and the next step in the management of this patient is to test for and, if present, treat *H. pylori* infection. If *H. pylori* is not found, a trial of a PPI for 8 weeks is appropriate. If the symptoms do not improve with a trial of a PPI, upper endoscopy should be performed. The patient uses NSAIDs infrequently, and discontinuation of the NSAID alone is insufficient in the management of this patient's symptoms.

3. B

Gastrointestinal bleeding is seen in 15–20% of patients with PUD. The next most common complication (5–7%) is perforation. The remainder of the choices are uncommon complications of PUD.

4. A

This patient has no risk factors (age > 60 years, concomitant use of glucocorticoids, use of multiple or high doses (≥2X normal) of NSAIDs, prior history of PUD, or anticoagulant use) for developing PUD from the use of NSAIDs. *H. pylori* eradication in NSAID users is insufficient to prevent NSAID-related ulcer disease. On the other hand, smoking cessation has been shown to reduce the incidence of NSAID-induced PUD. Cholestyramine is a bile-acid binding agent and has no role in the management of PUD. Amoxicillin has not been shown to prevent NSAID-induced PUD. Upper endoscopy is not indicated in this patient.

5. C

6. D

Any of the tests listed can detect signs of a perforated ulcer (free air in the abdomen). The most sensitive test is CT of the abdomen (see Chapter 27).

Further Reading

Graham, D.Y. and Fischbach, L. (2010) *Helicobacter pylori* treatment in the era of increasing antibiotic resistance. *Gut*, 59, 1143–1153.

Talley, N.J. and Vakil, N. (2005) Guidelines for the management of dyspepsia. Practice Parameters Committee of the American College of Gastroenterology. *American Journal of Gastroenterology*, 100, 2324–2337.

Vakil, N. (2010) Peptic ulcer disease, in *Sleisenger and Fordtran's Gastrointestinal and Liver Disease: Pathophysiology/Diagnosis/Management*, 9th edn (eds M. Feldman, L.S. Friedman and L.J. Brandt), Saunders Elsevier, Philadelphia, pp. 861–886.

Weblinks

http://www.merckmanuals.com/professional/sec02/ch013/ch013e.html
http://hopkins-abxguide.org/diagnosis/gi/h._pylori-related_peptic_ulcer_disease.html?contentInstanceId=255373

Common Upper Gastrointestinal Surgeries

Marc B. Sonenshine and Edward Lin

CHAPTER 4

Billroth I and Billroth II Gastroenterostomy

Clinical Vignette

A 53-year-old man undergoes an esophagogastroduodenoscopy (EGD) for nausea and abdominal discomfort associated with melena and an 8-lb (3.6-kg) weight loss. On endoscopy, a 1.5-cm mass lesion in the stomach is found to be an adenocarcinoma on histologic examination. Endoscopic ultrasonography (EUS) reveals neither submucosal invasion nor lymphadenopathy, and computed tomography (CT) confirms antral thickening without surrounding lymphadenopathy.

Procedure

- Surgical resection of gastric neoplasms or for complicated peptic ulcer disease involves partial resection of the stomach and re-establishment of gastrointestinal continuity by reconnecting the gastric remnant directly to the duodenum (Billroth I gastroenterostomy) or closing the duodenal stump and creating a gastrojejunostomy (Billroth II gastroenterostomy) (Figure 4.1).
- The Billroth I procedure is an end-to-end gastroduodenostomy. The duodenal bulb, gastric pylorus, antrum, and a small portion of the body of the stomach are resected and an anastomosis between the gastric remnant and proximal portion of the remaining duodenum is made, thereby preserving physiologic flow of chyme.
- The Billroth II gastroenterostomy is a side-to-side gastrojejunostomy with partial gastric and proximal duodenal resection. The remaining

Essentials of Gastroenterology, First Edition. Edited by Shanthi V. Sitaraman, Lawrence S. Friedman.
© 2012 John Wiley & Sons, Ltd. Published 2012 by John Wiley & Sons, Ltd.

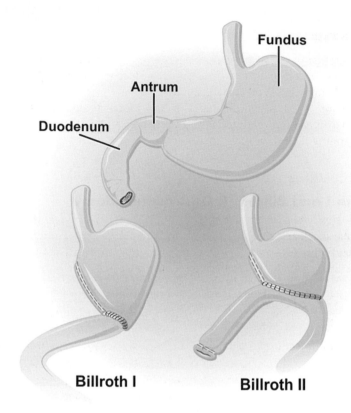

Figure 4.1 Billroth I and II gastroenterostomies.

duodenum containing the ampulla of Vater is created into an afferent limb that drains into the stomach; a loop of jejunum connected by a side-to-side anastomosis to the stomach forms the efferent limb.
- A modification of the Billroth II to reduce alkaline reflux is a Roux-en-Y gastrojejunostomy in which the afferent limb is anastomosed approximately 40–60 cm distal to the gastrojejunostomy, leaving a gastrojejunostomy that empties distally.
- In the case of a gastrectomy for malignancy, lymphadenectomy is often added, which involves removal of the pyloric, portal, celiac, splenic, and cardiac lymph nodes.
- In the case of a gastrectomy for ulcer disease, truncal vagotomy may be performed. Vagotomy is not required when gastrectomy is performed for gastric adenocarcinoma because the patients are often achlorhydric.

Indications

* Complicated peptic ulcer disease: defined as an ulcer associated with bleeding, perforation, or gastric outlet obstruction or refractory to medical and endoscopic management.
* Malignant antral adenocarcinoma (stages I–III – limited local and regional spread on computed tomography [CT] and endoscopic ultrasonography [EUS]); or other tumors.

Complications

Anastomotic Dehiscence

This is a dreaded postoperative complication that can result in peritonitis and septic shock and that can be fatal. Early management is imperative, and occurrence in a patient with a Billroth I gastroenterostomy often requires conversion to a Billroth II gastroenterostomy.

Postgastrectomy Syndrome

This includes multiple entities that frequently occur after Billroth I or Billroth II gastroenterostomies:
* **Postvagotomy diarrhea** likely results from colonic hypersecretion due to excess bile acids and salts that are unabsorbed in the small intestine (see Chapter 20). Treatment with an oral bile acid binding agent such as cholestyramine is usually effective in reducing diarrhea.
* **Alkaline reflux gastritis** results from the reflux of bile into the gastric remnant. Sucralfate, a bile-salt binding agent such as cholestyramine, or a proton pump inhibitor (PPI) may be used for symptomatic relief. In patients who do not respond to medical therapy for alkaline reflux gastritis, the gastrojejunostomy can be converted to a Roux-en-Y configuration.
* **Dumping syndrome** is defined as a constellation of symptoms that include lightheadedness, palpitations, hypoglycemia, and diarrhea that occurs after a meal. Dumping syndrome results from the reduced capacity of the stomach and a dysregulated hormonal response to calorie-dense nutrients.
  ◦ "Early" dumping syndrome typically occurs 15–30 minutes after a meal due to rapid emptying of hyperosmolar chyme into the small intestine, thereby leading to intravascular shifts of fluid into the small intestinal lumen.
  ◦ "Late" dumping occurs 2–3 hours after a meal due to a hyperinsulinemic response to the large carbohydrate load.
  ◦ Dietary modifications that include avoidance of simple carbohydrates and frequent small meals consisting of complex carbohydrates

and high-fiber foods and avoidance of drinking beverages with meals are the mainstays of treatment.
• **Afferent loop syndrome** results from obstruction of the afferent limb that prevents emptying of biliary and pancreatic fluid into the stomach. The obstruction, caused by a stricture, kinking of the bowel, adhesions, or narrowing of the anastomosis (due to recurrent ulcer or malignancy), may lead to bowel ischemia, pancreatitis, or cholangitis.

Whipple Resection

Clinical Vignette

A 62-year-old woman is evaluated for jaundice, dark urine, and weight loss of 10 lb (4.5 kg) over the previous 2 months. Her past medical history is unremarkable. She takes no prescription or over-the-counter medications. Physical examination shows conjunctival icterus and a painless palpable gallbladder (Courvoisier's sign). Laboratory tests reveal a serum total bilirubin level of 6 mg/dL (direct 5.8 mg/dL) and alkaline phosphatase 280 U/L. The remainder of the routine laboratory tests are normal. Abdominal CT reveals a 3-cm mass in the head of the pancreas and dilated intra- and extrahepatic bile ducts. An EUS-guided biopsy of the mass confirms adenocarcinoma. The tumor does not involve lymph nodes or invade vascular structures or distant organs.

Procedure

• A Whipple resection is a pancreaticoduodenoctomy (Figure 4.2).
• A conventional Whipple resection involves resection of the head and uncinate process of the pancreas, distal third (antrum and pylorus) of the stomach, duodenum, gallbladder, and distal bile duct.
• Three anastomoses are created to restore intestinal continuity:
  ○ end-to-side gastrojejunostomy;
  ○ end-to-side hepaticojejunostomy;
  ○ end-to-end or end-to-side pancreaticojejunostomy.

Indications

• A malignant tumor of the head of the pancreas is the most common indication for performing a Whipple resection:
  ○ Resectability of malignant lesions is determined by the absence of invasion of surrounding arteries and lack of distant metastatic spread.
  ○ Unlike arterial invasion, invasion of the portal venous structures is no longer considered an absolute contraindication to resection

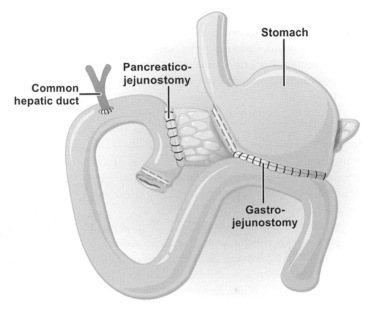

Figure 4.2 Whipple resection.

because harvested vein grafts or prosthetic vascular conduits may be used to re-establish portal blood flow.
• Other reasons for performing a Whipple resection include duodenal tumors, symptomatic benign tumors of the head of the pancreas, chronic pancreatitis, and premalignant or malignant lesions of the ampulla of Vater or distal bile duct.

Complications

• The two most frequent immediate complications seen after a Whipple resection are delayed gastric emptying and pancreatic fistula formation.
  ○ Approximately 25% of patients experience delayed gastric emptying after a Whipple resection. Delayed gastric emptying is diagnosed by the requirement for a nasogastric tube for more than 10 postoperative days as well as continued inability to tolerate oral feeding on postoperative day 14. Delayed gastric emptying is managed with a nasojejunal tube, gastrojejunal tube, or total parental nutrition. Gastric emptying is restored in 4–6 weeks in most patients. Persistent delayed gastric emptying beyond this timeframe requires surgical intervention.
  ○ Pancreatic fistula is defined by leakage of pancreatic secretions into the surgical bed, as confirmed by a fluid collection and an elevated serum amylase level. A fistula is often suspected because of a large

output from surgical drains. A fistula is more common in patients having a Whipple resection for causes other than a malignant pancreatic head mass. Patients with a pancreatic fistula are at higher risk of developing a biliary fistula, bile leak, intra-abdominal abscess, and prolonged hospitalization, and they therefore have an increased mortality rate.

- Longterm complications of a Whipple resection are generally related to reduced exocrine and endocrine function of the remaining pancreas.
  - Patients with diabetes mellitus prior to the procedure often require escalating therapy for glucose control. Those without diabetes mellitus preoperatively typically develop glucose intolerance or diabetes mellitus postoperatively.
  - Intestinal malabsorption of fat (including fat-soluble vitamins A, D, E, and K) can occur due to the lack of exocrine pancreatic enzymes, with resulting steatorrhea and malnutrition. Pancreatic enzyme and vitamin supplements should be provided routinely to patients who have undergone a Whipple resection.
- All patients who have undergone a Whipple procedure should be prescribed supplementation of iron, calcium, and copper, which are normally absorbed in the duodenum.

Nissen Fundoplication

Clinical Vignette

A 42-year-old man complains of a persistent burning sensation in the epigastrium, acid taste in his mouth, and intermittent regurgitation. Physical examination is unremarkable except for a body mass index of 26. Initially, diet, lifestyle modifications, and daily PPI therapy provided symptomatic relief, but the symptoms have slowly recurred. Despite a maximum dose of antisecretory medication, upper endoscopy shows Los Angeles Class B esophagitis and a small hiatal hernia (see Chapter 1). A 24-hour ambulatory esophageal pH study correlates the symptoms with reflux episodes. Esophageal manometry indicates a decreased lower esophageal sphincter pressure. The patient is concerned about the long-term use of medications and wants a surgical procedure for his gastroesophageal reflux disease (GERD).

Procedure

The classic Nissen fundoplication entails ligating the short gastric vessels and mobilizing the entire gastric fundus so that it can be delivered

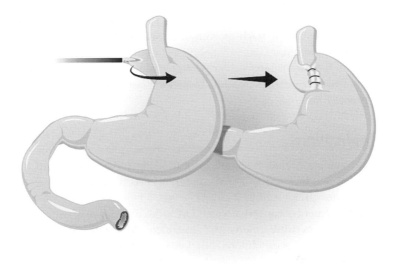

Figure 4.3 Nissen fundoplication.

behind the gastroesophageal junction to create a 360-degree wrap of the distal 3–4 cm of the esophagus (Figure 4.3). The fundoplication essentially increases the pressure of the lower esophageal sphincter.

Indications

- Persistent gastroesophageal reflux despite maximal medical therapy to suppress gastric acid secretion is the most common indication for a fundoplication:
  - Young patients with GERD who respond symptomatically to PPI treatment may consider surgery to defer long-term costs and associated concerns about chronic PPI use (such as a possible increased risk of osteoporosis and an increased risk of *Clostridium difficile* colitis [see Chapter 1]).
  - Patients in whom symptoms correlate with reflux episodes during an ambulatory esophageal pH evaluation have the best outcome following a fundoplication.
- Large hiatal or paraesophageal hernias often require surgery to reposition the stomach back within the abdominal cavity. To prevent future herniation of the stomach into the thoracic cavity, some surgeons believe that a fundoplication that serves as a buttress must be performed after repair of the diaphragmatic crura; however, postsurgical dysphagia may occur following fundoplicaton.

- A fundoplication may also be considered for nongastrointestinal manifestations of GERD, such as cough, asthma, laryngeal stenosis, and aspiration pneumonia.
  - Many lung transplant center protocols offer a fundoplication at the time of lung transplantation to prevent aspiration into the transplanted lung(s).

Complications

- Gas-bloat syndrome, a sensation of needing to belch but with difficulty, occurs in less than 5% of patients and seems to dissipate as time progresses after surgery.
  - Management is conservative and includes avoidance of caffeine, use of a straw to drink liquids, and simethicone. In some patients, motility agents or even balloon dilation may be necessary to improve symptoms.
- Dysphagia occurs in approximately 20% of patients in the early postoperative period (first 12 weeks). Dysphagia is managed by modifying the diet to consist mostly of liquids until the symptoms resolve.
  - Persistent dysphagia requiring frequent dilations and even reoperation to convert a 360-degree complete wrap into a 270-degree or 180-degree partial wrap occurs in 5–15% of patients.
  - In some patients, antisecretory medications may be necessary.

Heller Cardiomyotomy

Clinical Vignette

A 28-year-old woman presents with acid reflux and a 15-lb (6.8-kg) weight loss over 4 months. EGD demonstrates a dilated esophagus with retained food debris. A barium swallow demonstrates esophageal dysmotility and a bird's beak appearance of the lower esophageal sphincter. A 12.5-mm barium tablet becomes lodged at the gastroesophageal junction. Esophageal manometry shows aperistalsis, an elevated resting lower esophageal sphincter (LES) pressure, and inability of the LES to relax with a swallow, consistent with achalasia (see Chapter 2).

Procedure

- The initial esophageal mobilization is similar to a fundoplication, as described above. Prior to closing the diaphragmatic crura, the muscular layer of the lower esophagus and the seromuscular layer of the

gastric cardia are completely divided, leaving the mucosal layer intact. To avoid an incomplete myotomy, it is recommended that the myotomy extend at least 6 cm above the squamocolumnar junction and 2 cm below the squamocolumnar junction. The crura are then closed after the myotomy is performed.
- Whenever possible, a partial fundoplication is performed to reduce the amount of acid reflux into the esophagus.

Indication

- Myotomy of the LES is curative for achalasia.
  - ○ Young patients and persons with early achalasia tend to have better outcomes with a Heller myotomy than older patients or those in whom the disease has progressed to a megaesophagus.

Complications

- Immediate postmyotomy complications include gastric or esophageal perforations.
- Persistent dysphagia, even several months after surgery, may be the result of an incomplete myotomy or adhesion formation. Treatment options include endoscopic dilation and repeat myotomy.
- GERD occurs in up to 40% of patients undergoing myotomy without an associated antireflux procedure.
- Barrett's esophagus may occur with longstanding gastroesophageal reflux disease. Postsurgical endoscopic surveillance for Barrett's esophagus should be performed.

Weight-Loss Surgery

Clinical Vignette

A 30-year-old man with morbid obesity, diabetes mellitus, hypertension, and dyslipidemia presents for a routine annual health check-up. He complains of arthralgias of his knees that limit his physical activities. He routinely visits a nutritionist but is unable to lose weight despite aggressive dietary modifications.

Procedure

Roux-en-Y Gastric Bypass (RYGB)
- A small, 15–30-mL gastric pouch is separated from the larger, remnant stomach. The pouch is then connected to a jejunal limb to create a

gastrojejunal anastomosis. The gastrojejunostomy (Roux) limb is connected downstream (75–100 cm) to the biliopancreatic limb via a Roux-en-Y reconstruction (Figure 4.4).

- Weight loss occurs due to the restrictive nature of the gastric pouch as well as malabsorption. There is no absorption within the Roux limb, and caloric and nutrient absorption can be further reduced by creating a longer Roux limb.
- A longer Roux limb portends greater malabsorption; thus, patients need life-long micronutrient and vitamin supplementation. The procedure provides sustained, continued weight loss over many years.

Laparoscopic Adjustable Gastric Band (LAGB)

- A restrictive band is placed circumferentially around the cardia of the stomach to create a small reservoir. The band is connected to a reservoir port placed under the abdominal skin pad. The port can be

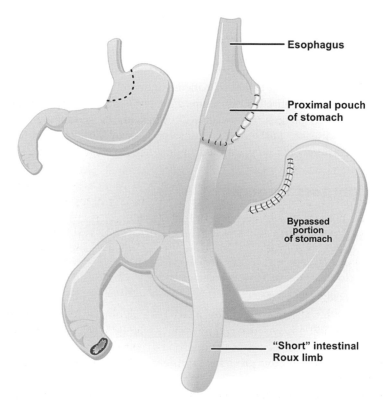

Figure 4.4 Roux-en-Y gastric bypass.

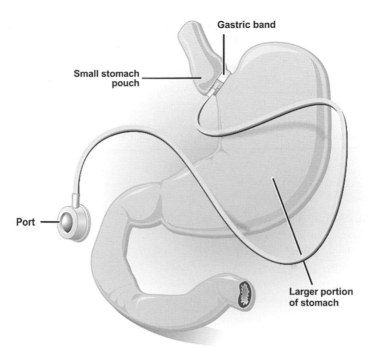

Figure 4.5 Laparoscopic adjustable gastric band.

accessed by a needle containing saline, and the band can be tightened or loosened to constrict or enlarge, respectively, the size of the stoma (Figure 4.5).

- No anastomoses are created, and therefore, it is a less morbid procedure than the others.
- Because the procedure has no malabsorptive properties and is solely restrictive, patients who continue on a soft, liquid, high-caloric diet may not lose weight despite a restricted gastric capacity.
- Weight loss is also not as profound as for a RYGB and is frequently temporary due to the ability of the stomach to distend despite repeated tightening of the band.

Sleeve Gastrectomy
- This is a restrictive procedure in which a significant portion of the fundus and greater curve (approximately 65–80% of the stomach) is removed to create a tubular stomach reservoir (Figure 4.6).
- As solely a restrictive procedure, nutrient malabsorption is less severe than after a RYGB.
- The sleeve gastrectomy tends to result in more persistent weight loss than the LAGB because the entire stomach is reduced in size;

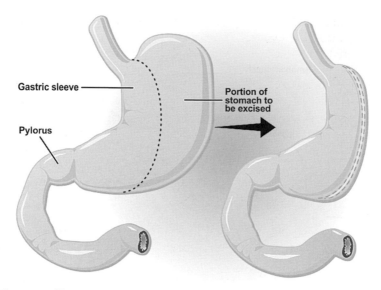

Figure 4.6 Sleeve gastrectomy.

in the LAGB, restriction is limited to the upper aspect of the stomach.

Indications

- Morbidly obese persons (BMI >40) and moderately obese persons (BMI >35) with significant comorbidities (e.g., diabetes mellitus, hypertension, coronary artery disease) are candidates for a weight-loss procedure.
- Prior to bariatric surgery, patients must have attempted and failed prior weight-loss programs, including strict compliance with a low-calorie diet as well as an aggressive exercise program.
- Mental illness is the most common contraindication to a weight-loss procedure.

Complications

- Vitamin and mineral deficiencies are the most significant complications associated with malabsorptive weight-loss procedures, particularly the RYGB:

- ○ Vitamin B12 deficiency occurs when the fundus and body of the stomach are removed. Intrinsic factor, the peptide necessary for intestinal absorption of vitamin B12, is synthesized by the parietal cells of the stomach.
- ○ Iron deficiency arises from bypass of the proximal duodenum (RYGB) or decreased acid production as a result of parietal cell loss due to resection of the fundus (sleeve gastrectomy).
- ○ Like iron absorption, calcium absorption occurs in the proximal duodenum, and procedures that bypass the duodenum require that the patient takes supplements to try to prevent osteoporosis.
- ○ Malabsorption of vitamins A and D may occur due to disruption of the enterohepatic circulation (see Chapter 20).
- Others:
  - ○ Because of multiple anastomoses, a RYGB is associated with an increased risk of anastomotic leak, ulceration, and stomal stenosis.
  - ○ The LAGB procedure is associated with the highest rate of failure to lose weight due to distention of the stomach pouch proximal to the band, band slippage, and high-calorie nutrient intake. Band erosions through the stomach wall can also occur with the LABG and can be detected by endoscopy or a skin port-site infection.

Table 4.1 presents a comparison of weight-loss procedures.

Pearls

When evaluating a patient after any gastrointestinal surgical procedure, it is important to understand the anatomy and the physiologic consequences. For example, a Whipple resection or RYGB leads to absent duodenal nutrient absorption and therefore to micronutrient (e.g., iron, calcium) deficiency.

Most patients with peptic ulcer disease are now effectively treated with a combination of endoscopic procedures, aggressive acid suppression, avoidance of nonsteroidal anti-inflammatory drugs, and eradication of *Helicobacter pylori*. Persistent ulcer disease not responsive to conservative management or complications of peptic ulcer disease can be treated with either a Billroth I or II procedure.

A Whipple resection, most commonly performed for pancreatic adenocarcinoma, entails an extensive resection that leaves patients with consequences from altered gastrointestinal luminal anatomy as well as pancreatic exocrine and endocrine deficiencies.

(Continued)

Patient selection is critical for a good outcome from a surgical procedure; understanding the indications while explaining possible complications and side effects of a procedure to the patient will help create reasonable expectations.

The RYGB remains the gold standard for weight-loss surgery because it leads to persistent and predictable weight loss, but the LAGB and sleeve gastrectomy continue to grow in popularity because of their lower morbidity despite less predictable weight loss.

Table 4.1 Comparison of weight-loss procedures.

	Roux-en-Y gastric bypass	Laparoscopic adjustable gastric band	Sleeve gastrectomy
Weight-loss mechanism	Restrictive + malabsorption	Restrictive	Restrictive
Weight loss and other outcomes	50–70% in 3–8 years; gold standard; weight loss is permanent, sustained, and predictable	25–80% in 3–8 years; high failure rate; weight loss is reversible because band may be removed	Data beyond 5 years are not available; weight loss is permanent but may not be sustained
Nutrient deficiencies	Minerals absorbed in duodenum or requiring acid; fat-soluble vitamins	None	Vitamin B12, iron, calcium
Complications	Anastomotic leak, ulceration, or stenosis	Weight loss failure; band erosion or infection	Gastroesophageal reflux

Questions

1. A 42-year-old man is diagnosed with gastric adenocarcinoma. Four weeks after curative surgery, he presents with palpitations, headache, and lightheadedness that occur approximately 30 minutes after each meal. Which of the following is the most appropriate recommendation for this patient?
   A. Referral to a cardiologist
   B. High-caloric, large meals
   C. Frequent, small meals with reduced simple carbohydrates
   D. Referral for exploratory laparotomy
   E. Referral to a neurologist

2. A 19-year-old male college football player presents to the emergency department with melena and fatigue. He had been taking ibuprofen 1–2 g every 6 hours following a knee injury. Upper endoscopy reveals a large ulcer in the duodenal bulb without bleeding stigmata but with surrounding edema creating gastric outlet obstruction. Despite intensive gastric acid suppression with a proton pump inhibitor for 8 weeks as well as empiric antibiotic therapy to eradicate *Helicobacter pylori*, he develops refractory nausea and vomiting, followed by recurrent melena and fatigue. Imaging studies are consistent with gastric outlet obstruction. Which of the following surgical procedures should be considered?
   A. Billroth I gastroenterostomy
   B. Billroth II gastroenterostomy
   C. Whipple resection
   D. Roux-en-Y bypass
   E. Heller cardiomyotomy

3. Which of the following interventions in a morbidly obese person results in the most predictable and sustained weight loss?
   A. Laparoscopic gastric banding
   B. Roux-en-Y bypass surgery
   C. Sleeve gastrectomy
   D. 800-kcal diet and intensive exercise program

4. A 53-year-old woman is lost to follow-up after gastric bypass surgery until she presents years later with numbness in her fingertips, fatigue, and confusion. Which of the following tests will likely reveal the cause of her symptoms?
   A. Serum vitamin B12 level
   B. Serum thyroid stimulating hormone level
   C. Serum protein electrophoresis
   D. Hemoglobin A1c level
   E. Serum folic acid level

(Continued)

5. A surgeon is consulted on a patient with dysphagia and weight loss despite maximum gastric acid suppressive therapy. Upper endoscopy is unremarkable. The surgeon agrees with the gastroenterologist's concern for achalasia. Which combination of diagnostic tests and therapeutic procedures is indicated?
   A. Esophageal manometry and Nissen fundoplication
   B. Esophageal manometry and Heller cardiomyotomy
   C. Bravo pH probe and Heller cardiomyotomy
   D. Barium esophagogram and Heller cardiomyotomy
   E. Barium esophagogram and Nissen fundoplication

Answers

1. C
   The patient likely has early dumping syndrome following a Billroth gastrectomy to resect the tumor. Dumping syndrome results from rapid gastric emptying that leads to fluid shifts into the small intestine as a result of high-caloric luminal contents. Smaller meals with reduced simple carbohydrates that result in lower osmolality are recommended to alleviate symptoms. The patient does not need referral to a cardiologist, neurologist, or surgeon at this time. Large meals will worsen his symptoms.

2. B
   A Billroth II gastroenterostomy includes resection of the duodenal bulb and gastric pylorus and antrum and is appropriate treatment for refractory gastric outlet obstruction. A Billroth I gastroenterostomy involves resection the gastric antrum and pylorus, which may not be sufficient in this patient. The other procedures are not indicated for complicated ulcer disease.

3. B
   The Roux-en-Y bypass surgery remains the gold-standard weight-loss procedure due to its restrictive and malabsorptive effects. The LAGB and sleeve gastrectomy are both restrictive procedures and do not result in malabsorption.

4. A
   This patient likely has vitamin B12 deficiency as a result of the gastric bypass surgery. Parietal cells synthesize intrinsic factor, which is required for intestinal absorption of vitamin B12. Although other diseases such as hyper- or hypothyroidism, multiple myeloma, and diabetes mellitus may cause the symptoms experienced by this patient, the most likely cause after weight-loss surgery is vitamin B12 deficiency.

5. B

Esophageal manometry is the gold standard test for diagnosing achalasia. Characteristic manometric findings in achalasia are aperistalsis of the esophagus and a high resting lower esophageal sphincter (LES) pressure. A Heller cardiomyotomy, which transects the LES muscle fibers, is curative. After a myotomy, the fibers of the LES are nonfunctional, and gastroesophageal reflux frequently occurs. Therefore, most surgeons also perform a fundoplication of 180–270 degrees to decrease the chance of reflux.

Further Reading

Reber, H. (2011) Pancreaticoduodenectomy (Whipple procedure): techniques. http://www.uptodate.com/online/content/topic.do?topicKey=pancreat/4412&selectedTitle=2~32&source=search_result. (Accessed 7 June 2011)

Schwaitzberg, S. (2010) Surgical management of gastroesophageal reflux in adults. http://www.uptodate.com/online/content/topic.do?topicKey=esophage/4564&selectedTitle=1~21&source=search_result#H21. (Accessed 7 June 2011)

Thompson, A., Padda, S. and Ramirez, F. (2010) Dumping syndrome. http://emedicine.medscape.com/article/173594-overview. (Accessed 7 June 2011)

Weblinks

http://www.merckmanuals.com/professional/sec01/ch006/ch006b.html

http://www.win.niddk.nih.gov/publications/gastric.htm

http://www.nlm.nih.gov/medlineplus/ency/article/002925.htm

http://emedicine.medscape.com/article/173594-overview

Acute Diarrhea

Sagar Garud and Jan-Michael A. Klapproth

CHAPTER 5

Clinical Vignette

A 19-year-old college student presents to the emergency department with a four-day history of diarrhea. He states that he traveled to Cancun a week ago. Within 2 days of arrival, he experienced nausea and the abrupt onset of watery, explosive diarrhea accompanied by a loss of appetite after consuming a meat dish and bottled water from a street vendor. On the third day after arrival, the frequency of bowel movements increased from six to 12 per day, occurring now around the clock. He reports abdominal cramping and fever but denies blood in the stool or vomiting. His past medical history is unremarkable. He takes no prescription or over-the-counter medications. His family history is noncontributory. He is heterosexual and has a single partner. He has an occasional glass of wine and does not smoke cigarettes. On physical examination, the vital signs reveal a blood pressure of 110/70mmHg, pulse rate 96/min, respiratory rate 12/min, and temperature 101.5 °F (38.5 °C). Skin turgor is normal and mucous membranes are moist. Abdominal examination reveals a soft, nontender abdomen with hyperactive bowel sounds. There is no hepatosplenomegaly. Rectal examination shows scant mucus but no stool.

Definition

- Diarrhea is defined as the passage of stools of abnormally loose consistency, usually associated with excessive frequency of defecation (three or more stools per day) and with excessive stool output (>0.2 L per day).
- Acute diarrhea is defined as diarrhea of ≤4 weeks' duration.

Essentials of Gastroenterology, First Edition. Edited by Shanthi V. Sitaraman, Lawrence S. Friedman.
© 2012 John Wiley & Sons, Ltd. Published 2012 by John Wiley & Sons, Ltd.

Epidemiology

- In the US, acute diarrhea accounts for 2–4 million episodes annually, approximately 900 000 hospitalizations, and 6000 deaths per year.

Etiology

- More than 90% of cases of acute diarrhea are caused by infections of the gastrointestinal tract with bacteria, viruses, protozoa, or parasites. Other causes include food allergies and medications. In addition, diseases associated with chronic diarrhea such as inflammatory bowel disease (IBD), celiac disease, and intestinal ischemia may present with an acute onset of diarrhea (see Chapter 6).

Pathogenesis

- Pathogens cause diarrhea by one or more of the following mechanisms:
  - Production of enterotoxin, cytotoxin, or preformed toxin:
    - Enterotoxins induce fluid secretion by activation of intracellular signaling pathways (e.g., adenylate cyclase) without causing damage to the mucosa (e.g., *Vibrio cholerae*).
    - Cytotoxins induce fluid secretion and cause damage to the mucosa (e.g., *Clostridium difficile*).
    - Preformed toxins induce rapid fluid secretion (e.g., *Staphylococcus aureus*).
  - Adherence to the mucosa: some bacteria adhere to the mucosa and elicit fluid secretion without elaborating toxins (e.g., enteroadherent *Escherichia coli* or enteropathogenic *E. coli*).
  - Invasion of the mucosa: some organisms invade the epithelial cells and lamina propria where they elicit an inflammatory response (e.g., *Salmonella* spp., *Shigella* spp.).
- A number of host factors determine the severity of illness once exposure to pathogens has occurred. These include age, personal hygiene, gastric acidity, intestinal motility, enteric microflora, immune status, and expression of intestinal receptors for enterotoxins.

Classification

Acute diarrhea may be classified as watery or inflammatory.

Watery Diarrhea

- Watery diarrhea implies a defect primarily in water and electrolyte absorption.
- Pathogens that cause watery diarrhea usually infect the small intestine. They adhere to the mucosal surface without invading the epithelium or produce enterotoxins that result in minimal or no mucosal inflammation.
- Patients usually present with large-volume, watery stools without blood, pus, or severe abdominal pain.
- Watery diarrhea has the potential to result in profound dehydration.
- Typically, fever and signs of systemic illness are absent.
- Diarrhea may be accompanied by nausea and vomiting.
- Examples of pathogens that cause watery diarrhea include: viruses (rotavirus, norovirus), enterotoxigenic *E. coli*, *Vibrio cholerae*, *Staphylococcus aureus*, *Clostridium perfringens*, *Giardia lamblia*, and *Cryptosporidium* spp.
- Patients who present with watery diarrhea are treated with rehydration and, in general, do not require extensive evaluation to identify the cause.

Inflammatory Diarrhea

- Inflammatory diarrhea results from direct invasion of the intestinal mucosa by pathogens and/or cytotoxins produced by the pathogens that elicit an inflammatory response. The inflammatory response leads to mucosal damage and ulcerations, usually in the colon, resulting in loss of mucus, serum proteins, and blood into the lumen.
- Inflammatory diarrhea is characterized by blood and/or mucus in stool and tenesmus.
- Patients with inflammatory diarrhea usually present with numerous small-volume stools that may be mucoid, grossly bloody, or both.
- Patients usually are febrile and may have signs of systemic illness.
- Patients are less likely to be dehydrated due to the small stool volumes.
- Examples of microbes that cause inflammatory diarrhea include *Shigella* spp., *Campylobacter* spp., enterohemorrhagic *E. coli*, *C. difficile*, *Salmonella* spp., *Yersinia* spp., *and Entamoeba histolytica*.

Pathogens that cause watery diarrhea typically affect the small bowel, and the diarrhea is caused by altered electrolyte secretion or absorption by an enterotoxin elaborated by the organism. In contrast, inflammatory diarrhea is caused by invasive pathogens that usually infect the colon.

Clinical Features

History

* A thorough history is the cornerstone of the diagnosis of acute diarrhea and should include the number of daily bowel movements, their consistency and volume, the duration of illness, the presence of blood, mucus, tenesmus, urgency, nocturnal bowel movements, and associated symptoms such as abdominal pain, nausea, vomiting, and fever (Table 5.1).
* The history should also include recent travel, previous episodes of acute diarrhea, foods consumed, hospitalizations, exposure to pets and livestock, sick contacts, and possible community outbreaks.

Table 5.1 Clues in the history to the cause of acute diarrhea.

History	Associated pathogen
Bloody stools	*Salmonella* spp., *Shigella* spp., *Campylobacter* spp., enterohemorrhagic *E. coli*, *C. difficile*, *E. histolytica*
Rectal pain, tenesmus	*Campylobacter* spp., *Salmonella* spp., *Shigella* spp., *Neisseria gonorrhoeae*, herpes virus, *Chlamydia*, *E. histolytica*
Severe or persistent abdominal pain	*Campylobacter* spp., *Yersinia* spp., *C. perfringens*, *Aeromonas* spp.
Recent antibiotic therapy or chemotherapy	*C. difficile*, *Salmonella* spp.
Travel (Mexico, Africa, Middle or Far East)	Enterotoxigenic *E. coli*
Family or friends affected	*S. aureus*, *Clostridium* spp., *B. cereus*, *Salmonella* spp.
Men who have sex with men	Herpes virus, *Chlamydia*, *Treponema pallidum*, *E. histolytica*, *Shigella* spp., *G. lamblia*, *N. gonorrhoeae*, *Cryptosporidium parvum*
Hospital-acquired	*C. difficile*

Adapted from Hospital Practice, 36, Scheidler MD, Giannella RA. Practical management of acute diarrhea, 49–56., Copyright (2001), with permission from JTE Multimedia.

- A number of medications can cause diarrhea, and a thorough history of prescription, over-the-counter, and herbal medication use should be obtained. Examples of medications associated with diarrhea include antibiotics, antacids, colchicine, laxatives, misoprostol, nonsteroidal anti-inflammatory drugs, and olsalazine.
- Comorbid conditions such as vascular disease, collagen vascular diseases, hyperthyroidism, and human immunodeficiency virus (HIV) infection should be elicited.

Physical Examination
- Physical findings in patients with acute diarrhea are most useful in assessing the severity of diarrhea. Patients should be assessed for fever and signs of dehydration such as hypotension, tachycardia, loss of skin turgor, sunken eyes, and dry conjunctivae and mucous membranes.

Most cases of infectious diarrhea are brief and self-limited, and patients do not seek medical attention. For patients who present to a healthcare provider, a thorough history and physical examination are the cornerstones of diagnosis and of determining the severity and presence of complications and whether diagnostic testing is needed (and, if so, which tests should be used). Diagnostic testing should be kept at a minimum, and treatment should be aimed at rehydration.

Diagnosis
- Most cases of acute diarrhea are self-limited and do not require further diagnostic testing. Indications for further diagnostic testing are outlined in Table 5.2.

Table 5.2 Indications for diagnostic testing in patients with acute diarrhea.

Large-volume diarrhea with dehydration
Severe abdominal pain
>3 days of symptoms
Bloody diarrhea
Fever >101.5°F (38.5°C)
Recent history of international travel
Extreme age (infancy, old age)
Diabetes mellitus
Immunodeficiency state (acquired immunodeficiency syndrome, immunosuppressive medications, chemotherapy)
Malignancy

- Complete blood count: leukocytosis usually indicates a bacterial cause of diarrhea. Anemia may be associated with an invasive organism.
- Serum electrolytes, blood urea nitrogen, and creatinine are useful for assessing dehydration.
- Stool culture for bacteria should be performed in selected patients (see Table 5.2):
  - A stool culture is positive in only 1.5–3% of cases, and the cost is $952–1200 for every positive test.
- Testing of stool for ova and parasites is indicated in immunocompromised patients, homosexual persons, persons who have been in a daycare center, and those who have been on a camping trip or who have travelled to a developing country.
- A stool test for *C. difficile* toxin A and B is indicated in persons with the recent use of antibiotics, IBD, diarrhea developing during hospitalization or subsequent to discharge, and immunocompromised persons.
- Fecal leukocytes are helpful in differentiating inflammatory diarrhea from watery diarrhea. Invasive organisms typically produce large quantities of fecal leukocytes.
- Endoscopy: unprepared flexible sigmoidoscopy or colonoscopy and/or upper endoscopy with duodenal biopsy are indicated in patients with persistent symptoms.

Treatment

Fluid Therapy
- Rehydration and replacement of electrolytes remain mainstays of the treatment of acute diarrhea. Oral rehydration solutions are typically used; however, intravenous fluid replacement may be needed in severe cases.

Diet
- Soft, easily digestible foods are most acceptable to a patient with acute diarrhea.
- Caffeinated products and alcohol should be avoided.
- Milk and milk products should also be avoided because secondary lactase deficiency may occur during an episode of acute diarrhea. In some persons secondary lactase deficiency and intolerance to lactose-containing food may persist for up to 1 year.

Antibiotics
- Fewer than 10% of patients with an acute diarrheal illness benefit from the use of antibiotics (Table 5.3).

Table 5.3 Specific causes of acute diarrhea.

Causative agent	Characteristics	Setting, risk factors	Clinical features	Diagnosis	Treatment
Viruses					
Rotavirus	Most common cause of diarrhea in children <2 years of age	Daycare centers, hospitals	Large-volume, watery diarrhea	Clinical suspicion	Self-limited disease, supportive management. Rotavirus vaccine recommended for all infants
Norovirus	Any age	Outbreaks on cruise ships, at banquets. Consumption of raw oysters	Large-volume, watery diarrhea	Clinical suspicion	Self-limited disease, supportive management

Bacteria

Campylobacter jejuni	Most common cause of acute bacterial diarrhea in the US	Consumption of contaminated poultry, meat, raw milk, eggs	Fever, watery or bloody diarrhea, malaise, abdominal cramps. Complications include Guillain-Barré syndrome, reactive arthritis	Stool culture	Mild–moderate disease is self-limited. For severe disease or symptoms >1 week, a macrolide (erythromycin, azithromycin) is the drug of choice. Alternative drug is a fluoroquinolone
Clostridium difficile	Most common nosocomial infection. Produces cytotoxins	Increasing age, recent antibiotic use, IBD	Fever, abdominal pain, bloody diarrhea	Stool test for toxins A and B	Metronidazole, vancomycin
Enterotoxigenic *Escherichia coli*, enteropathogenic *E. coli*, enteroaggregative *E. coli*	Mediated by enterotoxin or adherence to brush border epithelial cells. Developing countries. Increased risk in children <2 years of age and immunocompromised hosts	Fecal contamination of food, poor hygiene	Watery diarrhea that occurs within 2 days of ingesting contaminated food and resolves within 3 days	Clinical suspicion	Supportive management. A fluoroquinolone, trimethoprim–sulfamethoxazole, azithromycin, or rifaximin for severe disease

(Continued)

Table 5.3 (*Continued*)

Causative agent	Characteristics	Setting, risk factors	Clinical features	Diagnosis	Treatment
Enteroinvasive *Escherichia coli* and enterohemorrhagic *E. coli* (*E.coli* O157:H7)	Invasive, produces cytotoxin	Consumption of contaminated beef, pesto, alfalfa sprouts	Fever, abdominal cramps, tenesmus, rectal prolapse, bloody diarrhea. Complications include toxic megacolon, sepsis, perforation, thrombotic thrombocytopenic purpura, hemolytic-uremic syndrome	Stool culture	Supportive management. Antibiotics and antimotility agents should be avoided
Listeria monocytogenes	Noninvasive or invasive. Resistant to chemical inactivation. Survives even at 4° C. Pregnant women, diabetics, and immunocompromised patients are at increased risk	Consumption of contaminated meat, chocolate milk, unpasteurized cheese	Watery diarrhea, nausea, vomiting, myalgias, arthralgias. Complications include sepsis, meningoencephalitis	Stool culture on selective medium; blood or cerebrospinal fluid cultures	Treatment for severe disease or systemic illness: ampicillin, penicillin G, trimethoprim-sulfamethoxazole.

Salmonella enteritidis, *S. typhimurium,* *S. Heidelberg,* *S. Newport, S. typhii*	Invasive	Consumption of contaminated poultry, egg yolks, fresh produce, ground beef, milk	Enterocolitis: watery or bloody diarrhea, fever, malaise. Complications include sepsis, meningitis, endovascular lesions. Typhoid fever (caused by *S. typhi*): fever, chills, abdominal pain, rose spots	Blood and stool cultures	Enterocolitis: self-limited illness. Antibiotics indicated for severe disease, systemic symptoms, comorbid conditions: a fluoroquinolone, macrolide, or third-generation cephalosporin. Typhoid fever: a fluoroquinolone
Shigella sonnei, *S. flexneri,* *S. dysenteriae,* *S. boydii*	Invasive, produces enterotoxin. Requires <100 organisms to cause infection	Consumption of undercooked food, contaminated water	Fever, abdominal cramps, tenesmus, rectal prolapse, bloody diarrhea. Complications include toxic megacolon, sepsis, perforation, thrombotic thrombocytopenic purpura, hemolytic-uremic syndrome	Stool culture	Antibiotics always recommended: trimethoprim-sulfamethoxazole, a fluoroquinolone, third-generation cephalosporin, rifaximin

(Continued)

Table 5.3 (*Continued*)

Causative agent	Characteristics	Setting, risk factors	Clinical features	Diagnosis	Treatment
Vibrio cholerae	Noninvasive small bowel pathogen that induces cAMP production with subsequent Cl⁻ secretion	Consumption of contaminated water	Massive watery diarrhea	Stool culture	Rehydration
Non-cholera vibrios: *Vibrio vulnificus, V. parahemolyticus*	Patients with chronic liver disease are at highest risk	Consumption of undercooked shellfish	Bloody diarrhea, fever, abdominal cramps	Stool culture	Supportive management
Yersinia enterocolitica, Y. pseudotuberulosis	Uncommon in US; common in Northern Europe	Consumption of contaminated milk products, pork (chitterlings)	Bloody diarrhea, right lower quadrant pain (may mimic appendicitis or Crohn's disease), fever. Complications include reactive arthritis, erythema nodosum, myocarditis, osteomyelitis, nephritis	Stool culture	Antibiotics only for severe cases or complications: a fluoroquinolone, trimethoprim–sulfamethoxazole, or doxycycline plus an aminoglycoside

Parasites

Entameba histolytica	Developing countries	Consumption of contaminated food	Abdominal pain and bloody diarrhea, possibly alternating with constipation. Majority of infected persons are asymptomatic. Complications include liver abscess	Stool examination for trophozoites; serologic testing for antibody in serum by immunofluorescence or hemagglutination	Metronidazole, followed by iodoquinol or paromomycin
Cyclospora cayetanensis	Intracellular pathogen, villous atrophy	Outbreaks due to raspberries from Guatemala, travel to Nepal. Reported in hospital workers in Chicago	Profuse, prolonged diarrhea, nausea, abdominal cramps	Oocysts in stool, blue auto-fluorescence when examined by ultraviolet epifluorescence microscopy	Trimethoprim–sulfamethoxazole
Cryptosporidium parvum	Resistant to chemical inactivation	Immunocompromised hosts	Profuse, prolonged diarrhea	Acid-fast stain, immunofluorescence of stool sample, polymerase chain reaction testing	Paromomycin, nitazoxanide, azithromycin

(Continued)

Table 5.3 (*Continued*)

Causative agent	Characteristics	Setting, risk factors	Clinical features	Diagnosis	Treatment
Giardia lamblia	Chronic infection in patients who are immunodeficient. Recurrent disease in 15%	Found in mountain streams. Men who have sex with men are at increased risk	Explosive fatty diarrhea, abdominal distention	Stool ELISA (30% positive), immunofluorescence, duodenal aspiration	Metronidazole, nitazoxanide, quinacrine
Isospora belli	Intracellular pathogen causing villous atrophy	Immunocompromised hosts. May cause self-limited diarrhea in immunocompetent persons	Acute and chronic diarrhea	Stool microscopy, small bowel biopsy	Trimethoprim–sulfamethoxazole, metronidazole and pyrimethamine for persons with a sulfa allergy
Microsporidia	Intracellular pathogen causing villous atrophy	Opportunistic infection	Watery diarrhea, nausea, malabsorption	Modified trichrome stain of stool sample	Albendazole

cAMP, cyclic adenosine monophosphate; ELISA, enzyme-linked immunosorbent assay; IBD, inflammatory bowel disease

- Infections caused by *Shigella* spp., enteroinvasive *E. coli*, *C. difficile*, *V. cholerae*, *E. histolytica*, *G. lamblia*, and some cases of *Salmonella* infection as well as traveler's diarrhea benefit from antimicrobial treatment (Table 5.3).
- Antibiotics may also benefit patients with prolonged infection caused by *Salmonella*, *Campylobacter*, *Aeromonas*, or *Plesiomonas* spp.
- Empiric treatment with a fluoroquinolone (ciprofloxacin, ofloxacin, norfloxacin) is recommended for patients with traveler's diarrhea, patients with fever and bloody diarrhea, immunocompromised patients, those >65 years of age, and those with diarrhea that lasts >3 days and associated with one or more of the following: abdominal pain, fever, vomiting, myalgias, or headache.

Antidiarrheals and Antimotility Agents

- Antidiarrheal or antimotility agents should be used only in patients who have no fever, fecal leukocytes, or increased peripheral white blood cell count.
- Loperamide, diphenoxylate–atropine, bismuth subsalicylate, tincture of opium, codeine, and paregoric are commonly used agents (see Chapter 6).

Diarrheal Syndromes

Traveler's Diarrhea

- Most frequently caused by enterotoxigenic *E. coli* and to a lesser extent *Shigella* spp., *Campylobacter* spp., *Vibrio* spp., *Salmonella* spp., *Cyclospora cayetanensis*, *G. lamblia*, *Crystosporidium* spp., *E. histolytica*, rotavirus, and norovirus.
- Affects 20–50% of all travelers, predominantly during visits to Latin America, Africa, the Middle East, and Asia.
- Pathogens are usually transmitted through the fecal–oral route. Risk factors include improper disposal of feces, lack of proper hand washing following defecation by food handlers, improper food hygiene, inadequate preservation of food, and consumption of contaminated water.
- Symptoms include the abrupt onset of self-limited watery diarrhea with 4–5 bowel movements per day within 12–72 hours of ingesting food containing the pathogen.
- Diagnosis is based on history.
- Bismuth subsalicylate may be used for prophylaxis. Bismuth should be used with caution if the patient is allergic to aspirin, pregnant, or taking other medications concomitantly.
- Rehydration is the mainstay of treatment. Empiric treatment with a fluoroquinolone (e.g., ciprofloxacin 500 mg twice daily for 3–5 days) is

indicated for patients with three and more loose stools over 8 hours associated with nausea, vomiting, abdominal cramps, fever, or bloody bowel movements.

Food Poisoning
- More than 250 infectious agents have been implicated; the most frequent causes are E. coli O157:H7, *Campylobacter jejuni*, *Salmonella* spp., *Shigella* spp., *Listeria monocytogenes*, *S. aureus*, *Bacillus cereus*, scombroid poisoning, and ciguatera fish poisoning.
- Causes 325 000 hospitalizations and 5000 deaths per year in the US.
- Incubation period is 4–6 hours for *S. aureus* and *Bacillus cereus*, 8–12 hours for *Clostridium perfringens*, and 14 hours for invasive pathogens (e.g., *Salmonella* spp.).
- Symptoms include nausea, vomiting, diarrhea within minutes (scombroid) to 72 hours after consumption of the contaminated food.
- Most cases are self-limited. Rehydration is the mainstay of treatment. Ciprofloxacin (500 mg twice daily for 3–5 days) may be used for severe symptoms (nausea, vomiting, abdominal cramps, fever, or bloody bowel movements). Antibiotics should be considered only in patients in whom E. coli O157:H7 has been ruled out.
- Ciguatera fish poisoning is the most common nonbacterial food-borne disease:
  ○ Dinoflagellates such as *Gambierdiscus toxicus* produce ciguatoxin, which enters the food chain through tropical fish that are later eaten. Symptoms include bradycardia, hypotension, perioral tingling, fever, dysesthesias, myalgias, and arthralgias within 30 minutes to 12 hours of consuming contaminated fish; residual symptoms may linger for years. Ciguatera food poisoning is reported to be associated with chronic fatigue syndrome.
  ○ The diagnosis is made by detecting the toxin in contaminated fish.
- Scombroid poisoning (also called histamine fish poisoning):
  ○ Acute onset of peppery, metallic taste, oral numbness, headache, and occasional diarrhea that begin within minutes of ingesting contaminated fish. Symptoms resolve within 24 hours.

Nosocomial Diarrhea
- C. *difficile* is the main cause of nosocomial diarrhea in developed countries.
- C. *difficile* is an anaerobic, Gram-positive, spore-forming bacillus.
- The prevalence and mortality related to C. *difficile* colitis have increased substantially due to the emergence of a virulent strain of C. *difficile* designated NAP1/027. This strain harbors mutations that confer

antibiotic (fluoroquinolone) resistance, result in increased toxin A and B production, and facilitate sporulation of the bacterium.

- The single most important risk factor for *C. difficile* infection is antimicrobial therapy. Any antimicrobial agent has the potential to cause *C. difficile* infection; antimicrobial agents that are most frequently associated with *C. difficile* infection include amoxicillin or ampicillin, cephalosporins, clindamycin, and fluoroquinolones.
- Other risk factors for *C. difficile* infection include increasing age, hospitalization, chemotherapy, human immunodeficiency virus infection, and IBD.
- *C. difficile* colitis is caused by toxin A and toxin B produced by the organism. These toxins bind to, and are internalized by, colonocytes and elicit an inflammatory response. Several host factors, particularly the immune response to *C. difficile* toxins, determine whether a person remains an asymptomatic carrier or develops colitis.
- The clinical presentation ranges from asymptomatic carriage to life-threatening pseudomembranous colitis. Typical symptoms include fever, abdominal pain, and bloody diarrhea.
- The diagnosis is made by the detection of toxin A and B in a stool sample. Flexible sigmoidoscopy or colonoscopy is usually not required to make the diagnosis but, when performed, may reveal characteristic pseudomembranes (yellow, gray, or white plaques 2–5 mm in diameter). Histologic examination of the colonic mucosa may show focal ulceration associated with the eruption of inflammatory cells and necrotic debris that covers the area of ulceration, a constellation of findings called the "volcano lesion" (see Chapter 26).
- Treatment:
  - Discontinue the precipitating antibiotic if possible. In 20–25% of cases, *C. difficile* infection may resolve without further intervention.
  - Metronidazole, 250–500 mg orally 3–4 times a day for 10–14 days, is the drug of choice for mild–moderate colitis.
  - Vancomycin, 125–500 mg orally four times a day for 10–14 days, may be used in patients with severe colitis, those who are unable to tolerate metronidazole, pregnant women, children <10 years of age, or patients in whom diarrhea does not improve with metronidazole.
  - The response rate to metronidazole or vancomycin is 90–97%.
  - *C. difficile* infection may relapse in up to 20% of patients. Relapse is treated with metronidazole or vancomycin in a tapering schedule. Additional options include probiotics (*Saccharomyces boulardii* or *Lactobacillus* spp.) with and following metronidazole or vancomycin, intravenous immunoglobulin, rifampin, or cholestyramine in combination with vancomycin.

Testing of asymptomatic persons for and treatment of asymptomatic carriers with C. *difficile* toxin are not recommended because treatment may prolong the carrier state.

Some patients may develop irritable bowel syndrome (called postinfection IBS) after an acute infectious diarrheal illness that is characterized by two or more of the following: fever, vomiting, diarrhea, positive stool culture. Postinfection IBS may respond to a trial of probiotics.

Pearls

Most cases of acute diarrhea are a result of an infection; however, a specific organism can be identified in only a minority of cases.

Most episodes of acute diarrhea are self-limited, and investigations should be performed only if the results will influence management and outcome.

A thorough history and physical examination enable the clinician to classify an acute diarrheal illness, assess its severity, and determine whether further investigations are needed.

Antibiotic therapy is not required in most patients with an acute diarrheal disorder. Therapy should be directed mainly to preventing dehydration.

Questions

Questions 1 and 2 relate to the clinical vignette at the beginning of this chapter.

1. The patient's laboratory test results, including a complete blood cell count and comprehensive metabolic profile, are normal. Stool cultures are pending. He receives 1 L of normal saline intravenously in the emergency department. Which of the following should be prescribed next?
   A. Ciprofloxacin
   B. *Lactobacillus*
   C. Amoxicillin
   D. Metronidazole
   E. No drug

2. The patient returns for a follow-up outpatient visit. He states that his symptoms improved initially, but he then developed recurrent symptoms. He reports 4–6 bowel movements each day with blood in at least one to two bowel movements. He has rectal urgency and tenesmus. He has had a 6-lb (2.7-kg) weight loss. He has cramping abdominal pain but denies nausea,

vomiting, or fever. A complete blood count and comprehensive metabolic profile are normal. Stool studies including cultures, examination for ova and parasites, and test for *Clostridium difficile* toxin are negative. Which of the following is the most appropriate next step in the management of this patient?

A. Reassurance
B. Ciprofloxacin
C. Colonoscopy
D. Computed tomography (CT)
E. Metronidazole

3. Match the history with the likely pathogen.

    i. Just returned from a holiday cruise vacation
    ii. Ingestion of chitterlings ("chitlins")
    iii. Recent travel to Mexico
    iv. Ingestion of undercooked hamburger
    v. Ingestion of raw oysters

        A. Enterotoxigenic *E. coli*
        B. *Vibrio vulnificus*
        C. Norovirus
        D. *Yersinia* spp.
        E. *E. coli* O157:H7

4. A 65-year-old man presents with fever, chills, and bloody diarrhea of 3 days' duration. He recently completed a course of ampicillin for otitis media. Laboratory tests show a white blood cell count of $18\,000/mm^3$. Which of the following is the most likely cause of this patient's diarrhea?

A. *E. coli* O157H:7
B. *Clostridium difficile*
C. *Shigella* spp.
D. *Salmonella* spp.
E. *Entamoeba histolytica*

Answers

1. A

The patient's symptoms along with a history of travel to Mexico and consumption of food from a street vendor are consistent with traveler's diarrhea. Traveler's diarrhea is most frequently caused by enterotoxigenic *Escherichia coli* (ETEC) and to lesser extent *Shigella* spp., *Campylobacter* spp., *Vibrio* spp., *Salmonella* spp., *Crystosporidium* spp., and *Entamoeba histolytica*. The patient has nonbloody diarrhea, which makes ETEC the most likely pathogen. Empiric treatment with a fluoroquinolone (e.g., ciprofloxacin

(Continued)

500 mg twice daily for 3–5 days) is indicated for patients with three and more loose stools over 8 hours associated with nausea, vomiting, abdominal cramps, fever, or bloody bowel movements. Metronidazole is used to treat *E. histolytica* infection. Amoxicillin and *Lactobacillus* are not indicated in this patient.

2. C

The patient now has bloody diarrhea and weight loss in the face of negative stool culture. The cause is concerning for a chronic diarrheal illness including inflammatory bowel disease. At this point, colonoscopy is appropriate to diagnose the cause of the diarrhea. Antibiotics are not indicated especially when the stool culture is negative. CT is not indicated.

3.
   i. C
   ii. D
   iii. A
   iv. E
   v. B

4. B

Although any of the listed pathogens can cause bloody diarrhea, given the history of recent ampicillin use, *Clostridium difficile* is the most likely cause of his symptoms.

Further Reading

Marcos, L.A. and DuPont, H.L. (2007) Advances in defining etiology and new therapeutic approaches in acute diarrhea. *Journal of Infection*, 55, 385–393.

Navaneethan, U. and Giannella, R.A. (2008) Mechanisms of infectious diarrhea. *Nature Clinical Practice. Gastroenterology and Hepatology*, 5, 637–647.

Newton, J.M. and Surawicz, C.M. (2011) Infectious gastroenteritis and colitis. In *Diarrhea*, 1st edn (eds S. Guandalini and H. Vaziri), Springer Science + Business Media, New York, pp. 33–59.

Pawlowski, S.W., Warren, C.A. and Guerrant, R. (2009) Diagnosis and treatment of acute or persistent diarrhea. *Gastroenterology*, 136, 1874–1886.

Scheidler, M.D. and Giannella, R.A. (2001) Practical management of acute diarrhea. *Hospital Practice*, 36, 49–56.

Weblinks

http://www.bt.cdc.gov/disasters/disease/diarrheaguidelines.asp
http://www.clevelandclinicmeded.com/medicalpubs/diseasemanagement/gastroenterology/acute-diarrhea/
http://www.fpnotebook.com/gi/diarrhea/actdrh.htm

Chronic Diarrhea

Robin E. Rutherford

CHAPTER 6

Clinical Vignette

A 38-year-old white woman presents with an 8-month history of gradually worsening diarrhea, weight loss, and abdominal discomfort. She describes loose stools three to four times a day. She denies blood in the stool, urgency, tenesmus, or nocturnal bowel movements. There is no history of travel or recent use of antibiotics. Her past medical history is remarkable for osteoporosis, for which she takes alendronate. Her parents are alive and healthy; her mother has had "intestinal problems." One of her three siblings also has similar complaints but has never seen a physician. She is married, has no children, and is a homemaker. Review of systems is remarkable for infertility, depression, and easy bruisability. Physical examination reveals a blood pressure of 109/70 mmHg, pulse rate 67/min, and body mass index 18. She is afebrile. The remainder of the examination is unremarkable. Rectal examination reveals brown stool that is negative for occult blood. Routine laboratory tests show a normal white blood cell count, hemoglobin level of 11.1 g/dL, mean corpuscular volume 75 fL, and normal platelet count. A comprehensive metabolic panel is notable for slightly elevated alanine aminotransferase and aspartate aminotransferase levels and a normal serum albumin level. Iron saturation is 6%. Stool culture for enteric pathogens and stool examination for ova and parasites are negative.

General

- Diarrhea is defined as the passage of stools of abnormally loose consistency, usually associated with excessive frequency of defecation

---

Essentials of Gastroenterology, First Edition. Edited by Shanthi V. Sitaraman, Lawrence S. Friedman.
© 2012 John Wiley & Sons, Ltd. Published 2012 by John Wiley & Sons, Ltd.

Table 6.1 Daily fluid intake, secretion, and absorption along the gastrointestinal tract (in liters).

	Intake or secretion	Absorption
Oral intake	1–2	–
Salivary glands	0.5	–
Stomach	1–2	–
Pancreas/bile	2	–
Jejunum		6
Ileum	2–3	2.5
Colon	–	1.4

(three or more stools per day) and with excessive stool output (>0.2 L per day) (see Chapter 5).

- Chronic diarrhea is defined as diarrhea that lasts more than 4 weeks.
- The prevalence of chronic diarrhea in the US is 5%.
- With the exception of a few infections (e.g., *Aeromonas* spp., *Yersinia* spp.), chronic diarrhea is usually not caused by an infectious agent in immunocompetent persons.

Classification and Pathophysiology

- The small intestine and colon absorb 99% of the combination of oral fluid intake and endogenous secretions from the salivary glands, stomach, liver, and pancreas, totaling 9–10 L/day (Table 6.1). Diarrhea ensues when the normal physiologic secretion or absorption process is deranged.
- Normal stool is comprised of 75% water and 25% solid, and stool output is 100–150 g/day.
- Chronic diarrhea may be classified based on stool volume (small or large volume), stool characteristics (watery, fatty, or inflammatory), or pathophysiology (osmotic or secretory). In this chapter, we will use the classification based on stool characteristics because this classification is clinically useful in that it takes into account the patient's history and simple laboratory tests and thereby focuses the differential diagnosis (Table 6.2) and allows efficient diagnosis.
  - **Inflammatory diarrhea** implies damage to gastrointestinal mucosa due to infection or inflammation, which leads to a passive loss of protein-rich fluids and a decreased ability to absorb fluids and electrolytes. Stools typically contain frank or occult blood and

Table 6.2 Causes of diarrhea according to clinical presentation.

Type of diarrhea	Causes
Inflammatory diarrhea	Inflammatory bowel disease (Crohn's disease, ulcerative colitis) Infectious diseases (*Giardia lamblia, Aeromonas* spp., *Pleisomonas* spp.) Ischemic colitis Microscopic colitis (lymphocytic and collagenous colitis) Radiation enteritis

Watery diarrhea	*Osmotic*
	Carbohydrate malabsorption (lactase deficiency, pancreatic insufficiency)
	Ingestion of poorly absorbed sugars (sorbitol, lactulose)
	Ingestion of laxatives that contain magnesium, phosphate, sulfate, or lactulose
	
	Secretory
	Bile acid malabsorption (following surgical resection of the terminal ileum or after cholecystectomy)
	Endocrine causes
	  Hyperthyroidism
	  Addison's disease
	Medications (antacids, antibiotics, antiretroviral medications, chemotherapeutic agents, mineral supplements, nonsteroidal anti-inflammatory drugs, proton pump inhibitors, quinidine, vitamins)
	Neoplasms
	  Carcinoid syndrome
	  Colon cancer
	  Gastrinoma
	  Lymphoma
	  Pheochromocytoma
	  Somatostatinoma
	  Vasoactive intestinal peptide (VIP)oma
	
	Dysmotility
	Diabetic autonomic neuropathy
	Irritable bowel syndrome
	Postsympathatectomy
	Postvagotomy

(Continued)

Table 6.2 (*Continued*)

Type of diarrhea	Causes
Fatty diarrhea	*Maldigestion* Atrophic gastritis Chronic pancreatitis Bile acid deficiency (surgical resection of the terminal ileum, cirrhosis, primary sclerosing cholangitis, primary biliary cirrhosis) *Malabsorption* Amyloidosis Celiac disease Chronic mesenteric ischemia Heart failure Constrictive pericarditis *Giardia* infection Lymphangectasia Mastocytosis Short bowel syndrome Small intestinal bacterial overgrowth Whipple disease

leukocytes. Features of osmotic, secretory, and fatty diarrhea may also be present.

○ **Watery diarrhea** implies that there is no structural damage to the intestinal mucosa. Watery diarrhea may be:
  ▪ **Osmotic**: results from ingestion of a poorly absorbed substance. Diarrhea stops when the offending agent is stopped.
  ▪ **Secretory**: results from a defect primarily in water absorption as a result of increased secretion or reduced absorption of electrolytes. Diarrhea continues even if there is no oral intake, and the stools are isotonic with plasma (see later).
  ▪ **Dysmotility-related**: diarrhea is typically intermittent and may alternate with periods of constipation. The most common cause of dysmotility-related diarrhea is irritable bowel syndrome (see Chapter 7).
○ **Fatty diarrhea** (also called steatorrhea) implies the presence of excess fat in stools. Fatty diarrhea results from malaborption or maldigestion of fat and other nutrients. Stools may float in the toilet bowl due to the presence of excess lipid and are especially foul smelling. The most common cause of fatty diarrhea is celiac disease.

Clinical Features

History

- The clinical history helps distinguish inflammatory, watery, and fatty diarrhea and is one of the most important aspects in the evaluation of a patient with chronic diarrhea.
- The history should include a description of the onset (abrupt, gradual, lifelong), pattern (intermittent, continuous), and duration of symptoms.
- Epidemiologic factors such as travel, exposures to foods, source of water, and sick contacts should be identified.
- Patients should be questioned regarding fecal incontinence; patients may mistake incontinence for diarrhea.
- Associated symptoms such as abdominal pain, fever, weight loss, muscle weakness, and visual disturbances should be elicited.
- Aggravating factors such as diet, medication, and stress should be elicited.
- A thorough medication history including prescription, over-the-counter, and herbal medications should be obtained. Use of laxatives should be elicited.
- The past medical history including surgical history or radiation therapy should be obtained.
- The family history should include lactose intolerance, celiac disease, inflammatory bowel disease (IBD), and cystic fibrosis.
- A history of alcohol and tobacco use should be obtained.
- Previous evaluations and therapeutic trials should be reviewed.

> A thorough history is required to (1) differentiate "organic" from "functional" causes (see Chapter 7), (2) establish the type of diarrhea – inflammatory, watery, or fatty, and (3) narrow the differential diagnosis. Symptoms suggestive of an organic disease include a history of diarrhea of less than 3 months' duration, nocturnal symptoms, daily symptoms, and significant weight loss.

Physical Examination

- The physical examination is normal in the majority of patients.
- Certain signs may give a clue to the cause of diarrhea:
  - dermatitis herpetiformis: celiac disease;
  - angular cheilitis: malabsorption, IBD;
  - erythema nodosum or pyoderma gangrenosum: IBD;
  - edema: protein-losing enteropathy;
  - oral ulcerations: IBD;
  - hyperpigmentation: Whipple disease, Addison's disease;

- wheezing: cystic fibrosis, carcinoid syndrome;
- arthritis and arthralgias: *Campylobacter jejuni* infection, common variable immunodeficiency, Whipple disease;
- fistulas or perianal abscess: Crohn's disease;
- decreased rectal sphincter tone: fecal incontinence.

Differential Diagnosis

> The differential diagnosis should be narrowed based on the history and physical examination. Laboratory tests, endoscopy, and radiographic studies should be chosen selectively to confirm the suspected diagnosis (Table 6.3).

Diagnosis

Stool Tests

- Fecal occult blood testing: a positive result is suggestive of inflammation or an invasive infectious etiology.
- Fecal leukocytes: suggestive of intestinal inflammation, ischemia, infection.
  - Techniques: Wright stain and microscopic examination, lactoferrin agglutination test.
- Fecal fat testing is performed when maldigestion or malabsorption is suspected.
  - Qualitative: a random stool sample is examined under the microscope to visualize fat globules after staining with Sudan III. Visible fat globules indicate maldigestion or malabsorption.
  - Quantitative: patients are asked to consume a diet containing 100 g of fat/day, and stool is collected for 72 hours. A stool fat concentration >8% of measured fat intake over the 3-day period or >7 g/24 hours is consistent with malabsorption or maldigestion. A stool fat of 7–10 g/24 hours generally indicates malabsorption due to mucosal disease, whereas a stool fat >14 g/24 hours indicates maldigestion due to pancreatic insufficiency or bile salt deficiency.
- Fecal osmotic gap: this test is used to differentiate osmotic from secretory diarrhea. Stool sodium and potassium concentrations and osmolality are measured. Stool is isotonic with plasma; a low osmolality is suggestive of factitious diarrhea (stool mixed with water or dilute urine). Fecal osmotic gap = $290 - 2([Na^+] + [K^+])$ mOsm/kg:
  - osmotic diarrhea: osmotic gap >100 mOsm/kg;
  - secretory diarrhea: osmotic gap <50 mOsm/kg.

Table 6.3 Clinical features and diagnostic work-up of chronic diarrhea.

Type of diarrhea	Clinical history	Laboratory tests	Imaging tests	Endoscopy
Inflammatory	Small volume, frank or occult blood in stool, rectal urgency, tenesmus, abdominal pain, travel, exposure to potentially unclean water	Complete blood count (anemia, leukocytosis); stool occult blood and leukocytes; stool culture, examination for ova and parasites, *Giardia* antigen	Not indicated	Flexible sigmoidoscopy or colonoscopy
Osmotic	Postprandial diarrhea, laxative use, ingestion of sugar-free food (e.g., sorbitol), secondary gain from illness, weight loss	Serum electrolytes (hypokalemia, hyponatremia), stool osmotic gap (>100 mOsm/kg)	Lactose-hydrogen breath test may be considered	Not indicated
Secretory	Typically large-volume watery diarrhea, nocturnal diarrhea, no improvement with fasting, history of recent surgery (e.g., terminal ileal resection, cholecystectomy), use of certain medications	Comprehensive metabolic panel (hypokalemia, hyponatremia); stool osmotic gap (<50 mOsm/kg)	Computed tomography of the abdomen (neoplasms)	Not indicated

(Continued)

Table 6.3 (*Continued*)

Type of diarrhea	Clinical history	Laboratory tests	Imaging tests	Endoscopy
Dysmotility	Intermittent small-volume watery diarrhea, no weight loss	Complete blood count (normal), comprehensive metabolic panel (normal)	Not indicated	Not indicated unless patient is at least 45 years of age
Fatty	Foul-smelling, sticky stool with oil droplets or food particles, weight loss, abdominal pain, history of alcohol and/or tobacco use, diabetes mellitus, prior surgical resection of bowel	Complete blood count (anemia), comprehensive metabolic panel (hypoalbuminemia), vitamin B12 (low) and folate (high) levels (small intestinal bacterial overgrowth), tissue transglutaminase and endomysial antibodies (celiac disease), stool fat determination	Computed tomography of the abdomen (chronic pancreatitis, neoplasm), magnetic resonance imaging or angiography, mesenteric angiography (mesenteric ischemia)	Upper endoscopy, small bowel biopsy and aspirate

> The most common causes of osmotic diarrhea include ingestion of exogenous magnesium, consumption of poorly absorbable carbohydrates (e.g., sorbitol, lactulose), and carbohydrate malabsorption (e.g., lactose intolerance).

- Stool pH:
  - pH <5.3: suggestive of carbohydrate malabsorption;
  - pH 6.0–7.5: seen in generalized malabsorptive states.
- *Clostridium difficile* toxin A and B.
- Culture: chronic diarrhea due to bacteria in immunocompetent adults is rare; bacteria such as *Aeromonas* spp. or *Pleisiomonas* spp. have been associated with chronic diarrhea in this population. A stool culture should be performed in all immunocompromised persons with chronic diarrhea (see Chapter 5).
- Ova and parasites: a fresh stool specimen should be examined for ova and parasites when indicated (e.g, history of camping, swimming in mountain streams, travel to developing countries, immunocompromise). An enzyme-linked immunosorbent assay for *Giardia lamblia* has a higher sensitivity than microscopic examination of a stool specimen.
- Fecal elastase: levels <200 µg/g are indicative of pancreatic insufficiency.
- Fecal alpha-1 antitrypsin level or clearance: indicated when protein-losing enteropathy is suspected; an increased level or clearance is indicative of protein-losing enteropathy.

Blood Tests
- Complete blood count:
  - anemia may indicate gastrointestinal blood loss due to inflammation or celiac disease;
  - leukocytosis suggests infection or ischemia.
- White blood count and differential cell count:
  - eosinophilia suggests diarrhea due to a parasite or medication;
  - lymphocytosis and eosinophilia may be seen in adrenal insufficiency.
- Comprehensive metabolic panel:
  - electrolyte abnormalities: chronic diarrhea may cause hypokalemia, hypomagnesemia, or hyponatremia.
- Erythrocyte sedimentation rate (ESR) and C-reactive protein (CRP):
  - ESR or CRP are nonspecific markers of inflammation and may be useful as surrogate tests for inflammatory diarrhea such as IBD (see Chapter 8).

- Thyroid function tests may be obtained if hyperthyroidism is suspected.
- Immunoglobulin (Ig) A and IgG tissue transglutaminase antibodies and endomysial antibodies are highly sensitive and specific for celiac disease.

> Endocrine tumors of the pancreas are rare causes of chronic diarrhea. The prevalence of functional tumors of the pancreas is approximately 10/million. Chronic diarrhea occurs as part of a symptom complex, and its frequency varies depending on the tumor type: 100% in patients with a vasoactive intestinal peptide (VIP)oma, 60–65% in those with a gastrinoma, and 15% in those with a glucagonoma. The diagnosis is made by measuring hormone levels in the serum. Therefore, an extensive work-up for endocrine tumors should only be performed after common diagnoses are ruled out.

Urine Tests
- 5-hydroxyindole acetic acid (5-H1AA), histamine, or vanillylmandelic acid levels are indicated if carcinoid syndrome or pheochromocytoma is suspected.

> Screening blood tests in a person with chronic diarrhea should include a complete blood count, comprehensive metabolic panel, ESR, CRP, vitamin B12 and folate levels, and thyroid function tests. These blood tests have high specificity but low sensitivity for the presence of organic disease.

Endoscopy
Endoscopic examination of the colon by flexible sigmoidoscopy or colonoscopy is indicated in persons who present with inflammatory diarrhea or if a neoplasm is suspected. Although flexible sigmoidoscopy may be sufficient to make a diagnosis, some conditions require colonoscopy for examination of the proximal colon and terminal ileum (see later). Random mucosal biopsies should be obtained even if the visualized mucosa is normal because some diagnoses can only be made by histologic examination.
- Diagnoses made by mucosal biopsy of the colon:
  - lymphocytic colitis, collagenous colitis, amyloidosis, granulomatous infections, schistosomiasis.
- Diagnoses made by endoscopic examination of the proximal colon:
  - infections: *Campylobacter* spp., cytomegalovirus;
  - inflammation: Crohn's disease;
  - neoplasms.

Esophagogastroduodenoscopy (EGD, upper endoscopy) is indicated when intestinal malabsorption is suspected.
- Upper endoscopy with small bowel biopsy:
  - inflammation: Crohn's disease, eosinophilic gastroenteritis, abetalipoprotenemia, amyloidosis, mastocytosis;
  - infection: Whipple disease, mycobacteria, *Giardia lamblia*;
  - neoplasm: intestinal lymphoma.
- Small bowel aspirate:
  - quantitative bacterial culture of a small bowel aspirate is the gold standard for the diagnosis of small intestinal bacterial overgrowth ($>10^5$ bacteria/mL).

Imaging
Imaging evaluation is of limited utility in the work-up of chronic diarrhea.
- Small bowel follow through is indicated when the following conditions are suspected:
  - small intestinal diverticulosis (with bacterial overgrowth);
  - ileal stricture (Crohn's disease);
  - extensive bowel surgery (to define postsurgical anatomy);
  - entero-enteric or enterocolonic fistula (Crohn's disease).
- Mesenteric angiography or magnetic resonance angiography is indicated when mesenteric ischemia is suspected.
- Computed tomography or magnetic resonance imaging is indicated to evaluate for chronic pancreatitis and neoplasms.

Lactose Hydrogen Breath Test
- Lactose hydrogen breath testing is used to diagnose lactose intolerance and small intestinal bacterial overgrowth.
- The patient ingests 20–25 g of lactose, and blood is collected at 15, 30, 60, 120, and 180 minutes. A rise of breath hydrogen by 20 ppm at 120 or 180 minutes over the previous value indicates lactose malabsorption.
- An early rise in breath hydrogen of 20 ppm over the previous value at 30 or 60 minutes is suggestive of small intestinal bacterial overgrowth.

In persons less than 45 years of age with symptoms typical of functional bowel disease (see Chapter 7), a normal physical examination, and normal screening blood test results, no further investigation is necessary. In persons 45 years of age or older, colonoscopy may yield a diagnosis in up to 30% of persons.

Treatment

- The treatment of chronic diarrhea depends on the cause. A few examples are given below:
  - celiac disease: gluten-free diet;
  - lactose intolerance: avoidance of lactose-containing food (e.g., milk products, ice cream) and use of lactase supplements;
  - mesenteric ischemia: supportive measures;
  - IBD: topical and systemic anti-inflammatory medications (see Chapter 8);
  - eosinophilic gastroenteritis: dietary elimination and glucocorticoids;
  - pancreatic insufficiency: pancreatic enzyme supplements and gastric acid suppression;
  - small intestinal bacterial overgrowth: antibiotics.
- General antidiarrheal agents:
  - nonspecific antidiarrheal agents (Table 6.4) are frequently used to reduce the frequency and volume of bowel movements and abdominal cramps.

Table 6.4 Antidiarrheal agents.

Medication class	Agent	Representative dose*
Luminally acting		
Fiber supplements	Psyllium (Metamucil, Fiberall)	10–20 g daily
Bile-acid binding agents	Cholestyramine Colestipol	1–4 g four times daily
Systemically acting		
α-Adrenergic agonists	Clonidine	0.1–0.3 g three times daily
Somatostatin analogs	Octreotide	25–250 mg subcutaneously three times daily
Opiates	Loperamide (Imodium)	2–4 mg four times daily
	Diphenoxylate with atropine (Lomotil)	2.5–5 mg four times daily
	Codeine	15–30 mg four times daily
	Tincture of opium	2–20 drops four times daily

*Taken orally unless otherwise indicated.

Pearls

Stools may look normal in the presence of excess fat.

Patients with carbohydrate malabsorption (e.g., lactose intolerance) often present with watery diarrhea, flatulence, and bloating, typically occurring within 90 minutes after a meal.

Abdominal pain is uncommon in patients with chronic diarrhea, except in those with irritable bowel syndrome, chronic pancreatitis, Crohn's disease, or mesenteric ischemia.

The most common cause of fatty diarrhea is celiac disease. Tissue transglu-minase and endomysial antibodies should be obtained in patients who present with fatty diarrhea. The clinical presentation of celiac disease can be subtle, and a history of childhood illness, celiac disease in the family, iron-deficiency anemia, growth retardation, diabetes mellitus, osteopenia, and mild liver bio-chemical test abnormalities should be elicited.

Symptomatic treatment with an antidiarrheal agent is often necessary in a patient with chronic diarrhea because specific treatment may not be available.

Questions

Question 1 relates to the clinical vignette at the beginning of this chapter.

1. What is the next step in the management of this patient?
   A. Colonoscopy
   B. Computed tomography (CT) of the abdomen
   C. Tissue transglutaminase antibodies
   D. Serum immunoglobulins
   E. Stool test for fecal fat

2. A 28-year-old Asian woman presents with a 6-month history of intermittent bloating, diarrhea, and flatulence. She denies blood in the stool, nocturnal bowel movements, or weight loss. Her past medical history is unremark-able. She takes no prescription, herbal, or over-the-counter medications. She recently moved to the US. Physical examination is unremarkable. Laboratory tests including a complete blood count, comprehensive metabolic panel, and stool cultures, examination for ova and parasites, *Clostridium difficile* toxin, occult blood test, and Sudan stain are normal. Which of the following would be most helpful in determining the cause of her diarrhea?

(Continued)

A. Colonoscopy
B. Sigmoidoscopy
C. Computed tomography (CT) of the abdomen
D. Trial of abstinence from milk products
E. Transglutaminase antibodies

Questions 3 and 4 relate to the case presented below.

A 63-year-old man complains of a 6-month history of progressively worsening diarrhea and abdominal pain. His symptoms usually occur after a meal. His stools are foul smelling, sticky, and hard to flush due to the presence of oil droplets on the stool. The abdominal pain is mild, diffuse, and cramping in nature. He reports a 15-lb (7-kg) weight loss but denies nausea, vomiting, reflux symptoms, fever, or chills. His past medical history is notable for hypertension, type 2 diabetes mellitus, retinopathy, and mild chronic kidney disease. He smokes one pack of cigarettes and drinks a six-pack of beer daily. Physical examination is notable for mild muscle wasting. The remainder of the examination is normal. Laboratory tests show a normal complete blood count and comprehensive metabolic panel except for a serum creatinine level of 2 mg/dL (unchanged from previous values). A fecal occult blood test is negative. A Sudan stain of the stool is highly positive. A stool lactoferrin test is negative.

3. Which of the following is/are possible cause(s) of the patient's diarrhea?
    A. Chronic pancreatitis
    B. Chronic mesenteric ischemia
    C. Small intestinal bacterial overgrowth
    D. A or B
    E. A, B, or C

4. Which of the following is the next appropriate diagnostic step?
    A. Computed tomography (CT) of abdomen
    B. Colonoscopy
    C. Small-bowel follow through
    D. 72-hour stool collection for fat
    E. Stool sodium potassium concentrations and osmolality

5. A 66-year-old woman presents with a 2-year history of progressively worsening watery diarrhea. She describes 6–8 small-volume watery bowel movements a day. She denies blood in the stool, mucus, rectal urgency, tenesmus, nocturnal bowel movements, abdominal pain, or weight loss. She is afraid to leave the house because of her symptoms. She denies recent travel or antibiotic use. Her past medical history is remarkable for osteoarthritis for which she takes ibuprofen. She does not drink alcohol or smoke cigarettes. Physical examination is unremarkable. Laboratory tests including a complete blood count, comprehensive metabolic panel, tissue transglutaminase antibodies, and thyroid stimulating hormone level are normal.

Stool studies including culture, examination for ova and parasites, *Clostridium difficile* toxin, Sudan stain for fat, and occult blood test are negative. Which of the following diagnostic tests is indicated?

A. Colonoscopy with biopsy
B. Barium enema
C. Computed tomography (CT) of the abdomen
D. Upper endoscopy with small bowel biopsy
E. Small-bowel follow through

Answers

1. C

The patient presents with chronic diarrhea associated with weight loss, osteoporosis, anemia, infertility, and easy bruisability suggestive of intestinal malabsorption. Because she is a white woman, suspicion for celiac disease is high in the differential diagnosis of malabsorption. Celiac disease is the most common cause of malabsorption in adults, with a prevalence of 0.5–1/100 in the US. There is a female predominance, and the disease is associated with human leukocyte antigen (HLA)-DQ2 or HLA-DQ8. Iron-deficiency anemia is a common presenting symptom in adults with celiac disease. Detection of transglutaminase (or endomysial) antibodies is diagnostic of celiac disease with a sensitivity and specificity of 98% and 100%, respectively. A stool test for fecal fat will confirm malabsorption but will not indicate a specific diagnosis. CT should be considered if celiac disease is ruled out to evaluate the patient for other causes of steatorrhea such as chronic pancreatitis. Some patients with celiac disease may have IgA deficiency and falsely negative IgA transglutaminase antibodies; serum immunoglobulins may be obtained to look for IgA deficiency.

2. D

Lactose intolerance is seen most commonly in Asians and African Americans; >90% of Asians and African Americans have decreased activity of intestinal lactase. The patient's symptoms including diarrhea associated with bloating and flatulence in the absence of nocturnal symptoms, blood in the stool, and weight loss are consistent with the diagnosis of lactose intolerance. The diagnosis can be established with a hydrogen breath test that measures exhaled hydrogen gas following ingesting of a standard dose of lactose. However, improvement in symptoms with avoidance of lactose-containing foods or use of lactase supplements with dairy products is sufficient to make a diagnosis of lactose intolerance. Because the patient has no evidence of inflammatory diarrhea, colonoscopy or sigmoidoscopy is not indicated. Computed tomography is not indicated in this patient. Celiac disease is

(Continued)

uncommon in Asians, and testing for transglutaminase antibodies should not be necessary if the patient responds to a therapeutic trial of a lactose-free diet.

3. E

The presence of fat droplets in the stool implies steatorrhea, as confirmed by a Sudan stain. Weight loss along with steatorrhea is suggestive of maldigestion (as may occur with chronic pancreatitis or small bowel bacterial overgrowth) or malabsorption (as occurs with chronic mesenteric ischemia). The history of alcohol use is a risk factor for chronic pancreatitis. Type 2 diabetes mellitus with end-organ complications, hypertension, and smoking are risk factors for vascular disease, and mesenteric ischemia is a consideration. Diabetes mellitus is also associated with intestinal dysmotility and small intestinal bacterial overgrowth.

4. A

CT of the abdomen may detect chronic pancreatitis, mesenteric ischemia, or a neoplasm. If the test is unrevealing, a trial of antibiotics for small intestinal bacterial overgrowth may be considered. Alternatively, an upper endoscopy with small bowel aspirate for bacterial culture and mucosal biopsy or mesenteric angiography may be considered. Colonoscopy and small-bowel follow through have a low yield as diagnostic tests in a patient with steatorrhea. Stool determination of sodium and potassium concentrations and osmolality may help differentiate secretory from osmotic diarrhea and is not indicated in this patient, who has steatorrhea. A Sudan stain for fecal fat is positive, and a quantitative stool fat determination is not needed.

5. A

Microscopic colitis should be considered in a middle-aged woman who presents with watery diarrhea in the face of normal laboratory test and stool study results. The female:male ratio of collagenous colitis is 9:1, and the disorder typically occurs in women over 50 years of age. The mucosa usually appears normal on colonoscopy. The diagnosis is made by histologic examination of colonic mucosal biopsies, which reveal collagen deposition in the lamina propria.

Further Reading

American Gastroenterological Association Medical Position Statement. (1999) Guidelines for the evaluation and management of chronic diarrhea. *Gastroenterology*, 116, 1461–1463.

Schiller, L.R. and Sellin, J.H. (2010) Diarrhea, in *Sleisenger and Fordtran's Gastrointestinal and Liver Disease: Pathophysiology/Diagnosis/Management*, 9th edn (eds M. Feldman, L.S. Friedman and L.J. Brandt), Saunders Elsevier, Philadelphia, pp. 211–232.

Thomas, P.D., Forbes, A. and Green, J. (2003) Guidelines for the investigation of chronic diarrhea. *Gut*, 52, s5:1–15.

Weblinks

http://www.fpnotebook.com/gi/diarrhea/ChrncDrh.htm
http://www.acg.gi.org/patients/gihealth/diarrheal.asp

Irritable Bowel Syndrome

Shanthi Srinivasan

CHAPTER 7

Clinical Vignette

A 28-year-old woman is seen in the office for intermittent abdominal pain for the past several years. The pain occurs approximately once or twice a week and is diffuse, cramping in nature, and worse after she eats. The pain is relieved by a bowel movement. She has alternating episodes of mild diarrhea and mild constipation. Her diarrheal episodes are characterized by watery stool that usually occurs after she eats, and the constipation is characterized by hard, lumpy stools and a sense of incomplete evacuation. There is no associated urgency or tenesmus, and she has no nocturnal bowel movements. She has noted some mucus in the stool and mild bloating but has not noted any blood in the stools. She denies nausea, vomiting, or weight loss. Her past medical and surgical history is unremarkable. She does not take any prescription or over-the-counter medications. Her family history is unremarkable. She works as a nurse and describes her work as stressful. She drinks a glass of wine with dinner and smokes one half of a pack of cigarettes per day. She has no history of illicit drug use. Physical examination reveals a blood pressure of 130/70 mmHg, pulse rate 70/min, temperature 98.6 °F (37 °C), and body mass index 22. The remainder of the examination including an abdominal examination is unremarkable. Rectal examination reveals hard stool that is brown and negative for occult blood. Sphincter tone and squeeze pressure are normal. Routine laboratory tests show a normal complete blood count, blood glucose, and comprehensive metabolic panel.

Essentials of Gastroenterology, First Edition. Edited by Shanthi V. Sitaraman, Lawrence S. Friedman.
© 2012 John Wiley & Sons, Ltd. Published 2012 by John Wiley & Sons, Ltd.

General

- Irritable bowel syndrome (IBS) is a functional gastrointestinal disorder characterized by abdominal pain and altered bowel habits that occur in the absence of biochemical or structural abnormalities.
- Based on the predominant symptom, IBS is classified as diarrhea predominant (IBS-D), constipation predominant (IBS-C), and mixed (IBS-M).
- Lifetime prevalence of IBS is 7–10% worldwide. It is the most frequent gastrointestinal disorder seen by gastroenterologists. IBS is more common in women, persons younger than 50 years of age, and lower socioeconomic groups.

Pathophysiology

- The pathophysiology of IBS is poorly understood. Altered gastrointestinal motility, visceral hypersensitivity, emotional stress, small instestinal bacterial overgrowth, microscopic mucosal inflammation, and altered fecal microflora have been implicated.
- Heightened visceral pain sensitivity is a characteristic feature of patients with IBS. Patients typically perceive the sensation of a balloon distended in the rectum or small bowel at significantly lower volumes than control subjects.
- 5-hydroxytryptamine (5-HT, or serotonin) receptors have been shown to play an important role in diarrhea as well as pain perception. This has led to the development of $5\text{-}HT_3$ antagonists as a therapy for diarrhea-predominant IBS (see later).
- Patients with IBS have a higher frequency of panic disorder, major depression, anxiety disorder, and hypochondriasis compared with the general population. Patients who seek medical attention for IBS are more likely to have been victims of physical or sexual abuse.

Risk factors for developing IBS include a past history of gastrointestinal infection, abdominal surgery, and psychologic stress; postinfection IBS (i.e., IBS following gastroenteritis) has been recognized with increasing frequency.

Clinical Evaluation

- The Rome III criteria for the diagnosis of IBS (Table 7.1) specify that patients have recurrent abdominal pain or discomfort at least 3 days per month during the previous 3 months that is associated with two or more of the following:

Table 7.1 Rome III criteria for the diagnosis of IBS*.

At least 3 months of recurrent abdominal pain or discomfort (at least 3 days per month) associated with two or more of the following:
Relief by defecation Onset associated with a change in frequency of stool Onset associated with a change in form (appearance) of stool
*Criteria should be met for the previous 3 months with symptom onset ≥6 months prior to diagnosis.

- ○ relief by defecation;
- ○ onset associated with a change in stool frequency;
- ○ onset associated with a change in stool form or appearance.
- Other symptoms that support a diagnosis of IBS include altered stool frequency, altered stool form, altered stool passage (straining and/or urgency), mucus in the stool, and abdominal bloating.
- A thorough history and physical examination including a rectal examination should be performed.
- Routine laboratory testing should include a complete blood count, comprehensive metabolic panel, thyroid stimulating hormone, and stool for ova and parasites. Testing for serum tissue transglutaminase antibodies to evaluate for celiac disease is recommended in patients suspected of IBS, especially those with possible IBS-D or IBS-M.
- Colonoscopy or barium enema to evaluate for colon cancer, stricture, ischemia, inflammatory bowel disease, or other structural causes is recommended for persons over 50 years of age and for younger persons with "alarm" symptoms, such as anemia or substantial weight loss. For patients with IBS-D or IBS-M, colonic mucosal biopsies should be obtained to evaluate for microscopic colitis.

Treatment

- The primary goal of treatment for IBS is relief of symptoms. Therefore, treatment should be individualized based on the predominant symptom (pain, constipation, diarrhea). Table 7.2 provides a guide to the treatment of IBS.
- Pharmacotherapy is directed at the underlying pathophysiology of altered gastrointestinal motility. Use of low-dose antidepressants such as tricyclic antidepressants and selective serotonin reuptake

Table 7.2 Treatment options for IBS. All medications are administered orally.

Category	Agent	Suggested dose
Dietary modification	Increase soluble fiber intake Avoid foods that may cause bloating such as lactose, fructose, and beans Avoid caffeine or alcohol	20 g/day
Antispasmodic agents	Dicyclomine	20 mg four times a day as needed
	Hyoscamine	0.125–0.25 mg every 4 hours as needed
Antiflatulence agents	Simethicone	250–500 mg as needed

Motility agents
  a. Diarrhea predominant
  b. Constipation predominant
(see also Chapter 9)
	Imodium
	
	Polyethylene glycol
	Magnesium hydroxide
	
	Lubiprostone
		2 mg two to three times a day as needed
		17–26 g/day
		5–15 mL one to four times a day as needed
		8 µg twice a day

Antibiotics	Rifaximin	400 mg twice a day
Tricyclic antidepressants	Amitriptyline Doxepin Imipramine Desipramine Nortriptyline Trimipramine	12.5–150 mg/day 25–150 mg/day 10–50 mg/day 25–100 mg/day 10–75 mg/day 25–150 mg/day
Selective serotonin reuptake inhibitors	Fluoxetine (Prozac) Citalopram (Celexa)	20–40 mg/day 20–60 mg/day
Psychotherapy	Counseling by a psychologist or psychiatrist	–

(Continued)

Table 7.2 (*Continued*)

Category	Agent	Suggested dose
Alternative therapies	Probiotics*	–
	Peppermint oil	0.2–0.4 mL in enteric-coated capsules
	Hypnosis	–
	Cognitive behavioral therapy	–
	Yoga	–
	Acupuncture	–

*e.g., *Lactobacillus plantarum, Bifidobacteria infantis.*

inhibitors may decrease visceral hypersensitivity. In some patients, a trial of an antibiotic such as rifaximin to treat presumed small intestinal bacterial overgrowth may reduce bloating, flatulence, and diarrhea. Some patients may benefit from behavioral therapy such as counseling and cognitive psychotherapy by a psychologist or psychiatrist.

- One of the mainstays of therapy is a good doctor–patient relationship, patient reassurance and education, and maintaining continuity of care. It is recommended that initially the patient be seen in clinic every 6–8 weeks.

Patients with a shorter duration of symptoms, no previous surgeries, or postinfection IBS, and those with a good doctor–patient relationship, respond the best to treatment.

Pearls

The pathophysiology of IBS is complex and involves altered central and intrinsic neuronal sensitivity to pain perception.

A thorough history, physical examination, and simple laboratory testing are of utmost importance in diagnosing IBS.

The primary goal of treatment is relief of symptoms; therefore, treatment should be individualized, based on the predominant symptom of abdominal pain, constipation, or diarrhea.

The mainstays of therapy are a good doctor–patient relationship, patient reassurance and education, and maintaining continuity of care.

Questions

Questions 1 and 2 relate to the clinical vignette at the beginning of this chapter.

1. The most likely diagnosis in this patient is
   A. Colon cancer
   B. Irritable bowel syndrome
   C. Inflammatory bowel disease
   D. Intestinal obstruction
2. The initial approach to treatment of this patient's condition is
   A. Increased dietary fiber and fluid intake
   B. Osmotic laxative
   C. Stimulant laxative
   D. Rectal enemas
3. The Rome III criteria for the diagnosis of IBS include recurrent abdominal pain or discomfort for at least 3 days per month in the past 3 months with symptom onset at least 6 months prior to diagnosis. An additional principal criterion is which of the following?
   A. Abdominal distension, incomplete evacuation, or passage of mucus
   B. Change in the frequency of stool, change in the form of stool, or abdominal pain relieved by defecation
   C. Abdominal pain relieved by defecation, presence of bloating, or a major psychiatric illness
   D. Weight loss, blood in stool, or nocturnal bowel movements
4. The risk factor most strongly associated with IBS is which of the following?
   A. Depression
   B. Food intolerance
   C. Bacterial gastroenteritis
   D. Hypochondria
   E. Oral glucocorticoid use
5. Which of the following best describes irritable bowel syndrome?
   A. A functional gastrointestinal disorder most commonly seen in women less than 50 years of age
   B. A functional gastrointestinal disorder associated with abdominal pain that is continuous and not relieved with defecation
   C. A functional gastrointestinal disorder that exclusively affects the gastrointestinal tract
   D. A functional gastrointestinal disorder that is rarely associated with altered pain perception
   E. A degenerative disorder of the enteric nervous system

(Continued)

Answers

1. B

The patient meets the Rome III diagnostic criteria for irritable bowel syndrome. She has chronic abdominal pain that is worse when she eats and relieved by a bowel movement. She has no alarm symptoms such as weight loss or anemia. Her physical examination, laboratory test, and colonoscopy results are normal. Hence, the diagnoses of colon cancer, inflammatory bowel disease, and intestinal obstruction are unlikely.

2. A

In a stepwise approach to treat IBS, the patient should be educated regarding her condition, and dietary fiber and fluid intake should be increased. If symptoms are persistent despite dietary and lifestyle modifications, pharmacotherapy can be used to treat the predominant symptom of constipation, or diarrhea. IBS symptoms may be triggered by stress. Hence, psychologic therapy or stress management may be considered if symptoms do not improve with dietary and lifestyle modifications.

3. B

4. C

Studies have shown the correlation between gastrointestinal infections and the occurrence of IBS to be strongest. Depression is prevalent among IBS patients, but a causal association has not been demonstrated.

5. A

Further Reading

Brandt, L.J., Chey, W.D., Foxx-Orenstein, A.E., *et al.* (2009) An evidence-based systematic review on the management of irritable bowel syndrome. *American Journal of Gastroenterology*, 104, S1–S35.

Talley, N.J. (2010) Irritable bowel syndrome, in *Sleisenger and Fordtran's Gastrointestinal and Liver Disease: Pathophysiology/Diagnosis/Management*, 9th edn (eds M. Feldman, L.S. Friedman and L.J. Brandt), Saunders Elsevier, Philadelphia, pp. 2091–2104.

Weblinks

http://www.merckmanuals.com/professional/sec02/ch021666/ch021666a.
html?qt=irritable%20bowel%20syndrome&alt=sh

http://www.nlm.nih.gov/medlineplus/irritablebowelsyndrome.html

http://www.gastrojournal.org/article/S0016-5085(02)00480-8/fulltext

http://www.gastrojournal.org/article/S0016-5085(02)00481-X/fulltext

Inflammatory Bowel Disease

Jan-Michael A. Klapproth

CHAPTER 8

Clinical Vignette

A 22-year-old female college student on the track team is questioned by her coach regarding a lack of performance during a recent track meet. The student admits to a 6-lb (2.7-kg) weight loss over the previous 6 months accompanied by a lack of appetite and amenorrhea. She also reports persistent, nonradiating, right lower quadrant pain that she describes as cramping and dull in nature. She has one to two bowel movements per day. The stools are watery in consistency, but she reports no rectal bleeding. The concerned coach sends her to the Student Health Service, and laboratory tests are remarkable for a hematocrit value of 21% and mean corpuscular volume 75 fL.

General

- Inflammatory bowel disease (IBD) is comprised of two major chronic intestinal diseases, **Crohn's disease** (CD) and **ulcerative colitis** (UC). The distinguishing features of CD and UC are outlined in Table 8.1.
- Approximately 1.4 million persons are affected with IBD in the US.

Epidemiology

- Age of onset: IBD can occur at any age, and the mean age of onset appears to be increasing. IBD has a bimodal age distribution: the first peak is at 15–30 years, and the second peak is after age 60 years; 10–15% of patients are diagnosed before age 18.
- Geographic distribution: there is a north–south gradient with the highest incidence rates in the US and United Kingdom and the lowest in Croatia and Africa.

Essentials of Gastroenterology, First Edition. Edited by Shanthi V. Sitaraman, Lawrence S. Friedman.
© 2012 John Wiley & Sons, Ltd. Published 2012 by John Wiley & Sons, Ltd.

Table 8.1 Distinguishing features of ulcerative colitis and Crohn's disease.

	Ulcerative colitis	Crohn's disease
Age of onset (years)	15–30	15–30
Male:female	1:1	1:1
Disease location	Colon only: Entire colon (pancolitis): 45–50% Rectum and sigmoid (proctosigmoiditis): 15–35% Left colon: 35-40%	Any portion of the GI tract*: Small bowel alone: 30% Colon alone: 30% Ileocolonic: 40%
Distribution	Continuous inflammation that extends proximally from the anorectal junction. Rectum is almost invariably involved	Skip lesions Rectal sparing
Depth of inflammation	Mucosa/submucosa	Transmural
Ulcerations	Small, superficial	Deep, serpiginous
Terminal ileal involvement	Typically not involved; backwash ileitis may be present in 15–20% of patients with pancolitis	Commonly involved; ulcerations, strictures, or fistulas
Extraintestinal disease	Yes	Yes
Strictures/fistulas	No	Yes
Postoperative recurrence†	No	Yes
Serology	pANCA: 60–65% ASCA: 5%	pANCA: 20–25% ASCA: 40–76%

*90% of patients <20 years of age have small bowel involvement compared with 60% of those >40 years of age.

†Colectomy for ulcerative colitis, resection for Crohn's disease.

ASCA, *anti-Saccharomyces cerevisae* antibodies; pANCA, perinuclear antineutrophil cytoplasmic antibodies; GI, gastrointestinal.

- Race: the incidence of IBD is highest in Caucasians in general and Ashkenazi Jews in particular and lowest in Hispanics, African Americans, and Asian Americans.

Etiology

The etiology of IBD is largely unknown. IBD is thought to result from an inappropriate or aberrant inflammatory response to intestinal microbes in a genetically susceptible host.

Genetic Factors
- First-degree relatives of affected persons have a 4–20-fold increased risk of developing IBD.
- A positive family history of IBD is seen in 25% of patients with CD and 20% of patients with UC.
- Mutations in multiple genes involved in bacterial antigen presentation and the innate immune response have been associated with IBD. A few important genes are as follows:
  - autophagy-related 16-like 1 (*ATG16L1*): protective of or increased risk for CD, depending on a single nucleotide polymorphism;
  - nucleotide-binding oligomerization domain containing 2 (*NOD-2*), also called caspase recruitment domain family, member 15 (CARD15): three mutations in leucine-rich repeats increase the risk for CD;
  - immunity-related GTPase (*IRGM*): increased risk for CD;
  - interleukin-23 receptor (*IL-23R*): increased risk for CD.

Environmental Factors
- Social status:
  - upper middle class is associated with a higher risk of developing IBD;
  - male bricklayers, unskilled laborers, security personnel, and women working in the cleaning and maintenance business have lower risks of developing IBD.
- Smoking: protective for UC but increased risk for CD. Patients with CD who smoke have more severe disease, require more medications to control the disease, and have an increased rate of recurrent disease activity.
- Appendectomy reduces the risk of developing UC; unclear role in CD.
- Breastfeeding appears to be protective for IBD.
- Nonsteroidal anti-inflammatory drugs (NSAIDs) have been implicated in exacerbations and as potential precipitants of new cases of IBD.

Immune Factors and Microbes

- The intestinal epithelium acts as a barrier between the luminal contents and the mucosal immune system. Loss of intestinal barrier function is thought to precede the development of inflammation in patients with IBD. A defective intestinal barrier has been reported in first-degree relatives of patients with CD.
- Intestinal microbes are documented to play an important role in the inflammatory response. Although no single bacterial strain has been identified conclusively as playing a causal role in IBD, depletion and reduced diversity of members of the mucosa-associated phyla *Firmicutes* and *Bacteroidetes* have been documented in patients with IBD compared with control subjects. In addition, bacteria that can adhere to and invade the intestinal mucosa such as *Escherichia coli* have been implicated.
- The histologic hallmark of active inflammatory bowel disease is a prominent infiltration of innate immune cells (polymorphonuclear neutrophils, macrophages, dendritic cells, and natural killer T cells) and adaptive immune cells (B cells and T cells) into the lamina propria. Immune activation in the mucosa leads to elevated levels of several cytokines and chemokines, such as tumor necrosis factor alpha (TNF-α), interleukin-1β, interferon-γ, and the interleukin-23–T helper (Th)17 pathway. Although the precise molecular pathway is unknown, a defective innate and adaptive immune response has been implicated in the pathogenesis of IBD.

Clinical Features

- Characteristic symptoms of IBD include chronic diarrhea and abdominal pain. Constitutional symptoms such as fatigue, fever, and weight loss are frequently present.
- The onset of symptoms is usually insidious.
- Typical symptoms of UC include left lower quadrant pain, and rectal urgency, tenesmus, bleeding, mucoid discharge, and bloody diarrhea.
- Depending on the segment of bowel involved, patients with CD may present with right lower quadrant pain associated with diarrhea, obstructive symptoms (nausea, vomiting, abdominal distention), fever, and weight loss.
- A thorough history should be obtained to exclude other causes of diarrhea (see Chapter 5).
- Physical examination helps to assess the clinical status of a patient with IBD (for signs of dehydration, anemia, and muscle wasting). In patients with CD, an abdominal mass, abdominal tenderness, or perianal fissures, fistulas, and abscesses may be present. In addition,

a dermatologic examination may reveal erythema nodosum, pyoderma gangerenosum, or aphthous ulcers (see Chapter 28).

Extraintestinal Manifestations

- Extraintestinal manifestations of IBD may be related to bowel activity, have an independent course, or be related to intestinal malabsorption in the case of CD.
  - Related to bowel activity: peripheral arthritis, erythema nodosum, episcleritis, aphthous stomatitis, pyoderma gangrenosum (see Chapter 28).
  - Independent course: ankylosing spondylitis, sacroileitis, uveitits, primary sclerosing cholangitis (see Chapter 15).
  - Related to malabsorption: anemia, cholelithiasis, nephrolithiasis, metabolic bone disease.

Diagnosis

The diagnosis of UC or CD is based on a combination of the clinical presentation and results of laboratory, imaging, and endoscopic studies. No single test is considered diagnostic of CD or UC.

Laboratory Features

- Laboratory tests are useful in assessing the severity of disease.
- A complete blood count may reveal leukocytosis, anemia, or thrombocytosis.
- A comprehensive metabolic panel may reveal electrolyte abnormalities related to fluid loss and hypoalbuminemia related to intestinal malabsorption.
- Markers of inflammation:
  - Serum C-reactive protein level and erythrocyte sedimentation rate:
    - these markers are neither sensitive nor specific for IBD but may be useful to assess disease activity in individual patients;
    - levels correlate with clinical, endoscopic, and radiologic measures of disease activity;
    - elevations predict relapse;
    - elevations may identify patients likely to progress to colectomy for severe UC.
  - Fecal lactoferrin and calprotectin levels:
    - not routinely used in practice;
    - levels correlate with disease activity;
    - elevations predict relapse.

- Stool culture for bacterial pathogens and stool examination for ova and parasites should be performed in patients during their initial presentation.
- The incidence of *Clostridium difficile* colitis is increased in patients with IBD. Stool samples for *C. difficile* toxin should be obtained during acute flares of IBD, whether or not there is a history of antibiotic use or recent hospitalization.
- Serologic markers:
  ○ A serology panel including perinuclear antineutrophil cytoplasmic antibodies (pANCA), anti-*Saccharomyces cerevisae* antibodies (ASCA), anti-CBir1, anti-I2, and anti-outer membrane porin from *E. coli* (OmpC) antibodies is available to help diagnose IBD.
  ○ "Atypical" ANCA yielding a perinuclear staining pattern (pANCA) with alcohol-fixed neutrophils are found in 60–65% of patients with UC; pANCA are also detectable in 20–25% of patients with CD (with colonic involvement).
  ○ ASCA, anti-Bir, and anti-OmpC are detected primarily in patients with CD; ASCA are detectable in 46–70% of patients with CD and 5% of those with UC.
  ○ Anti-CBir1 expression is associated independently with small-bowel, penetrating, and fibrostenosing CD.

> The serologic tests lack sensitivity to diagnose IBD and are not recommended for routine use. There does not seem to be a correlation between pANCA or ASCA titers and disease activity, duration of illness, extent of disease, extraintestinal manifestations, or need for surgical or medical treatment in patients with IBD.

Imaging Studies (see Chapter 27)
- Small bowel follow through and enteroclysis:
  ○ these tests are no longer used as first-line diagnostic tests;
  ○ small bowel imaging may be helpful for the detection of small bowel strictures ("string sign" indicates a long-segment stricture) and fistulas;
  ○ mucosal edema alternating with ulcerations is described on imaging tests as a cobblestone pattern.
- Computed tomography (CT):
  ○ useful in the detection of extraluminal disease and complications of CD such as perforation and abscess;
  ○ the sensitivity is 80–88% for diagnosis of suspected CD.

- Magnetic resonance imaging (MRI) and MR enterography:
  - MRI and MR enterography are used to assess inflammatory processes in the bowel wall, submucosal inflammation, and fibrosis as well as complications such as abscess or fistula;
  - MR enterography is highly sensitive and specific for the diagnosis of small bowel ulceration, strictures, and fistulas with a specificity approaching 100% and sensitivity of 80–100%.

Endoscopy
- Indications:
  - Establishing a diagnosis of IBD: endoscopic examination with biopsies for microscopic examination is considered an integral part of the initial evaluation of possible IBD and for assessing the severity of the disease and instituting appropriate medical therapy.
    - Colonoscopy with intubation of the terminal ileum is recommended.
    - Depending on the symptoms, upper endoscopy (esophagogastroduodenoscopy, EGD) may be considered. Endoscopic features that distinguish CD from UC are illustrated in Figure 8.1).
    - Microscopic examination of the mucosa (see Chapter 26) typically shows crypt abscesses, crypt distortion, and increased cellularity in the lamina propria. These findings do not distinguish IBD from infectious colitis.

> The presence of noncaseating granulomas on histologic examination, present in 20–40% of patients with suspected CD, is specific for the diagnosis of CD.

  - Colon cancer surveillance with colonoscopy is indicated in patients with pancolonic UC or CD of at least 8 years' duration. Four-quadrant mucosal biopsies should be obtained every 10 cm starting in the terminal ileum as the colonoscope is withdrawn, for a minimum of 32 biopsies, and all suspicious lesions should also be biopsied. This approach has a 90% sensitivity for detecting dysplasia.
- Wireless capsule endoscopy (WCE):
  - 30% of patients with CD have small bowel disease alone, and WCE has a higher diagnostic yield for small bowel CD than endoscopic and radiologic studies.

Differential Diagnosis

- Acute infectious colitis (e.g., caused by *Salmonella* spp., *Shigella* spp., *C. difficile*, *Campylobacter* spp., cytomegalovirus, amebiasis, intestinal tuberculosis)

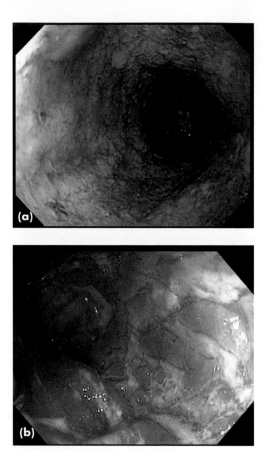

Figure 8.1 Endoscopic views of mild to moderately active ulcerative colitis (UC) characterized by mucosal friability, hemorrhage, granularity, mucus, and edema that are present in a continuous fashion (a) and colonic Crohn's disease (CD) characterized by deep, serpiginous ulcerations, and normal intervening mucosa (b).

- Behçet's disease
- Diverticulitis
- Drugs and toxins (e.g., chemotherapy, gold, pencillamine)
- Ischemic colitis
- Microscopic colitis (collagenous colitis and lymphocytic colitis)
- Neutropenic colitis (typhlitis)
- Nonsteroidal anti-inflammatory drug-induced mucosal damage
- Radiation colitis.

Treatment

• The goals of treatment are to induce and maintain remission and to improve the patient's quality of life.
• The choice of medical therapy depends on the extent, location, and severity of the disease and the presence or absence of fistulas.
• Several scoring systems are available to assess disease activity in CD and UC. These scoring systems (e.g., the Crohn's Disease Activity Index) are typically used for clinical studies. In daily practice, the severity of IBD is assessed on the basis of the patient's symptoms, signs, and laboratory test results.
• Medical therapy varies between UC and CD, with significant overlap between the two (Table 8.2).
• Certain drugs are used for induction of remission (IOR) and others for maintenance of remission (MOR). Some agents may be used for both IOR and MOR (Table 8.2).

Surgical options are generally reserved for patients who are refractory to medical therapy or have fulminant disease (such as toxic megacolon), a complication (such as perforation), dysplasia, or malignancy.

Mesalamine (5-Aminosalicylic Acid, 5-ASA)
• Mesalamine and sulfasalazine (sulfapyridine bound to 5-ASA), collectively referred to as aminosalicylates, are considered first-line agents for mild–moderate UC. They are minimally effective in CD.
• The therapeutic effect of aminosalicylates depends on the local concentration at the inflamed mucosa.
• Various 5-ASA preparations have been developed to increase local concentration: balsalazide (5-ASA conjugated to an inactive compound; Colazol®), olsalazine (5-ASA dimer; Dipentum®), Asacol® and Lialda® (mesalamine with delayed-release coating), Pentasa® (5-ASA encapsulated in ethylcellulose microgranules that release 35% of the drug in the small bowel), 5-ASA enemas (Rowasa®) and suppositories (Canasa®).
• Side effects of mesalamine include hair loss, headache, and abdominal pain. Rarely, mesalamine may be associated with interstitial nephritis.
• Side effects of sulfasalazine (attributed to the sulfa moiety) include nausea, dyspepsia, headache, interference with intestinal folic acid absorption, and occasionally hemolytic anemia, agranulocytosis, hepatitis, or pneumonitis. Patients taking sulfasalazine should be given folic acid 1 mg daily.
• Olsalazine can be associated with diarrhea.

Table 8.2 Commonly used medications for the treatment of UC and CD.

Class of drug	Medication	Dose	Indication	IOR/MOR
5-ASA	Mesalamine: oral 5-ASA (various formulations)	2–4.8 g/day	Mild–severe UC, mild–moderate CD	IOR and MOR
	Sulfasalazine (5-ASA bound to sulfapyridine)	1–4 g/day	Mild–severe UC	IOR and MOR
	Mesalamine: topical (enema or suppository)	1–4 g/day	Mild–moderate left-sided UC	IOR and MOR
Glucocorticoids	Oral: prednisone	Varies with the formulation. Typically, starting dose is 40 mg/day, tapered over 1 month	Moderate–severe UC, moderate–severe small bowel or colonic CD	IOR
	Oral (high first-pass metabolism): budesonide	9 mg/day	Mild–moderate small bowel and colonic CD	IOR and MOR (6 months)
	Intravenous	Typically, methylprednisolone 40 mg/day	Moderate–severe UC or CD	IOR
	Enema: hydrocortisone	100 mg/day	Moderate–severe left-sided UC	IOR

Class	Drug	Dose/schedule	Indication	Use
Immunomodulators	Azathioprine	2–4 mg/day orally	UC, CD	MOR
	6-Mercaptopurine	1.5–2.5 mg/day orally	UC, CD	MOR
	Methotrexate	15–25 mg weekly, intramuscularly, subcutaneously, or orally	Small bowel CD	IOR and MOR
	Cyclosporine	4 mg/kg/day titrated to therapeutic blood levels	Severe UC	IOR and MOR with transition to azathioprine or 6-mercaptopurine
Biologics	**Anti-TNF-α agents**			
	Infliximab	5 mg/kg intravenously 0, 2, 6 and then every 8 weeks	CD – small bowel, colon, or fistula; severe UC	IOR and MOR
	Adalimumab	Variable dose and schedule, 40–160 mg subcutaneously	Moderate–severe CD	IOR and MOR
	Certolizumab pegol	400 mg 0, 2, 4 weeks and then 200 mg every 4 weeks subcutaneously	Moderate–severe CD	IOR and MOR
	α4 integrin antibody			
	Natalizumab	300 mg every 4 weeks intravenously	Moderate–severe CD refractory to anti-TNF agents	IOR and MOR
Antibiotics	Metronidazole	10–20 mg/kg/day orally	Perianal CD	IOR
	Ciprofloxacin	500 mg twice a day orally	Used in conjunction with metronidazole for perianal CD	IOR

ASA, aminosalicylic acid; CD, Crohn's disease; IOR, induction of remission; MOR, maintenance of remission; TNF, tumor necrosis factor; UC, ulcerative colitis.

Glucocorticoids

- Glucocorticoids are used to treat mild to severe UC and CD to induce remission.
- They are available in oral (prednisone, prednisolone, budesonide), intravenous (hydrocortisone, methylprednisolone), and enema (hydrocortisone) formulations.
- Budesonide is a glucocorticoid with high (>90%) first-pass liver metabolism; as a result, budesonide is considered to have considerably fewer side effects than conventional glucocorticoids. It has a slow onset of action.
- Budesonide is used to treat mild–moderate terminal ileal and ileocolonic CD.
- Side effects of glucocorticoids include acne, hypertension, hirsutism, cataracts, striae, hyperglycemia, hyperlipidemia, insomnia, hyperactivity, acute psychotic episodes, adrenal suppression, and weight gain.

Immunomodulators

- Methotrexate:
  - Methotrexate is used primarily for the treatment of patients with glucocorticoid-refractory or glucocorticoid-dependent CD. It is not effective in UC.
  - Side effects include stomatitis, nausea, diarrhea, hair loss, leukopenia, and hypersensitivity pneumonitis.
  - Folic acid 1–2 mg a day orally should be administered.
  - Methotrexate is contraindicated in women who are pregnant or considering pregnancy.
  - Routine toxicity monitoring should include a complete blood count, liver biochemical tests, and serum creatinine level every 4–8 weeks.
- Azathioprine and 6-mercaptopurine (6-MP):
  - Azathioprine is a prodrug that is converted to 6-MP through a nonenzymatic reaction.
  - These drugs are used to maintain remission in UC and CD.
  - They have a slow onset of action.
  - Side effects:
    - dose-dependent: hepatitis, bone marrow suppression;
    - dose-independent (idiosyncratic): acute pancreatitis, nausea, vomiting, diarrhea, flu-like symptoms.
  - The patient's thiopurine methlytransferase level or genotype should be determined prior to initiation of therapy to guide proper dosing of the medication.
  - A complete blood count and liver biochemical test levels should be monitored during therapy.

Biologic Agents

- Anti-tumor necrosis factor (TNF) alpha agents:
  - ○ Available anti-TNF agents include infliximab (Remicade), adalimumab (Humira), and certolizumab pegol (Cimzia), a polyethyleneglycosylated Fab' fragment of a humanized anti-TNF antibody. Infliximab is a chimeric monoclonal antibody against TNF; adalimumab and certolizumab are human immunoglobulin G1 (IgG1) monoclonal antibodies against TNF.
  - ○ Anti-TNF agents bind to and neutralize TNF. Although the precise mechanism of action is unknown, they inhibit T cell proliferation and induce apoptosis.
  - ○ In UC, these agents are used for glucocorticoid-refractory moderate–severe disease.
  - ○ In CD, these agents are used for luminal and fistulizing disease.
  - ○ They also may be used for extraintestinal manifestations of IBD.
  - ○ Side effects include sepsis, reactivation of tuberculosis, fungal infections, and hepatosplenic T cell lymphoma. Infusion reactions, which include chest pain, shortness of breath, rash, and hypotension, are more common with infliximab than with other anti-TNF agents. Delayed hypersensitivity is an uncommon complication that can occur 2–12 days after an infusion of an anti-TNF agent.
  - ○ A negative tuberculin skin test (or chest X-ray) is mandatory prior to initiation of anti-TNF therapy.
  - ○ Hepatitis B virus infection also should be ruled out prior to anti-TNF therapy.
- Natalizumab:
  - ○ Natalizumab is a humanized monoclonal antibody against α4 integrin that inhibits leukocyte adhesion and migration into inflamed tissue.
  - ○ The agent is used for moderate–severe CD with evidence of active inflammation refractory to prior treatment, including anti-TNF therapy.
  - ○ Natalizumab is usually well tolerated in patients with CD. Rare but serious side effects include progressive multifocal leukoencephalopathy and hepatic toxicity.

Antibiotics

Antibiotics are used alone or in combination for treatment of mild–moderate left-sided colonic and fistulizing CD.

- Metronidazole:
  - ○ side effects include nausea, peripheral neuropathy, metallic taste, and a disulfiram effect.

- Ciprofloxacin. Efficacy is similar to that for metronidazole for the treatment of colonic disease with a more favorable side-effect profile:
  - side effects include nausea, diarrhea, skin rashes, tendinitis, and Achilles tendon rupture.

Surgery

- Surgery is indicated for the treatment of medication-refractory, worsening disease and complications, including severe medication side effects, fistulas, toxic megacolon, and obstruction.
- Options in UC: total or subtotal colectomy with end-ileostomy, ileal pouch-anal anastomosis, ileo-anal anstomosis.
- Options in CD (74% of all patients will require surgery): fistulectomy, segmental resection, diverting ileostomy for distal disease.

Complications

- Toxic megacolon:
  - Toxic megacolon is a complication of severe UC. It is defined as acute colonic dilatation with a transverse colon diameter of >6 cm (on radiologic examination) in a patient with a severe attack of colitis.
  - It occurs in 5% of patients with severe UC.
  - Precipitating factors for toxic megacolon include hypokalemia, antimotility agents, narcotics, and colonoscopy during a severe UC flare.
  - Medical management includes correcting electrolyte imbalances, empiric antibiotics, discontinuation of antimotility agents and narcotics, intravenous cyclosporine or infliximab, and, in some cases, subtotal colectomy.
- Dysplasia and colorectal cancer:
  - Patients with long-standing UC or colonic CD are at increased risk of colorectal cancer.
  - The most important risk factors include the duration and extent of colitis. Pancolitis is associated with the highest risk. Distal rectosigmoid colitis is not associated with an increased risk above that seen in persons without colitis. Other risk factors include primary sclerosing cholangitis, a family history of colon cancer, younger age at diagnosis of disease, and more severe inflammation.
  - The risk of colorectal cancer is estimated to be 7–10% after 20 years of colitis and as high as 30% after 35 years.

○ Annual or biennial colonoscopy with biopsies is recommended for patients who have colitis extending beyond the rectum and who have had disease for at least 8 years.
• Additional complications in patients with CD include small intestinal bacterial overgrowth, choledocholithiasis, amyloidosis, metabolic bone disease including osteoporosis, fistulas, nephrolithiasis (due to dehydration or oxalate malabsorption), malabsorption, and nutritional deficiencies including deficiencies of fat-soluble vitamins, iron, folate, and vitamin B12.

Prognosis

• CD: 75% relapse rate over the course of 5 years:
  ○ if the disease is inactive, there is an 80% chance of being relapse free at 1 year;
  ○ the rate of relapse is not affected by the segment of bowel involved, age of the patient, or severity of disease.
• UC: the behavior of the disease is affected by the extent, progression, and associated systemic symptoms:
  ○ the overall colectomy rate is 24% at 10 years and 30% at 25 years;
  ○ approximately 80% of patients have a disease course characterized by intermittent flares interposed between variable periods of remission. More than 50% of patients have mild disease at the time of initial presentation.

Pearls

Up to 10% of patients with CD present with proctitis.

Persistently elevated serum alkaline phosphatase levels may be seen in about 3% of patients with UC (or occasionally Crohn's colitis) and should prompt further investigation to exclude primary sclerosing cholangitis (see Chapter 15).

A colonic stricture in a patient with UC should be considered malignant until proven otherwise.

The incidence of C. *difficile* colitis is increased in patients with IBD. Stool samples for C. *difficile* toxin should be obtained during acute flares of IBD, whether or not there is a history of antibiotic use or recent hospitalization.

Questions

Question 1 relates to the clinical vignette at the beginning of this chapter.

1. Which of the following is the most likely to reveal the diagnosis?
   A. Colonoscopy
   B. Computed tomography (CT) of the abdomen and pelvis
   C. Stool culture and examinations for ova and parasites and *Clostridium difficile* toxin
   D. Small bowel follow through
   E. Esophagogastroduodenoscopy (EGD)

2. A 56-year-old man with long-standing Crohn's disease (CD) of the cecum and terminal ileum, confirmed by colonoscopy 3 months ago, presents for the third time in a year with a flare characterized by right lower quadrant pain, loss of appetite, and loose stools. Physical examination reveals normal vital signs and right lower quadrant tenderness without rebound tenderness. Besides a slightly elevated white blood count, the blood work is unremarkable. He is placed on therapy with prednisone 40 mg daily, which is tapered over the course of 2 months, but he becomes symptomatic again at a dose of 20 mg per day. What is the next appropriate step?
   A. Reassurance
   B. Computed tomography
   C. Colonoscopy
   D. Thiopurine methyltransferase (TPMT) level or genotype
   E. Magnetic resonance (MR) enterography

3. A 43-year-old woman with a 10-year history of ulcerative colitis (UC) presents for an annual health examination. Which of the following test(s) would you recommend?
   A. Serum alkaline phosphatase level
   B. Colonoscopy
   C. Complete blood count
   D. All of the above

4. A 23-year-old man with a history of terminal ileal Crohn's disease presents with nausea, vomiting, and abdominal pain of 2 days' duration. Magnetic resonance enterography reveals a fibrotic stricture approximately 8 inches (20 cm) in length with proximal dilatation of the small bowel. There is no evidence of an intra-abdominal abscess or fistula. Which of the following is the best treatment option for this patient?
   A. Glucocorticoids
   B. Infliximab
   C. Mesalamine
   D. Metronidazole
   E. Surgical resection

5. A 33-year-old man with a history of ulcerative colitis (UC) presents to the emergency department with a severe flare of UC. Due to work-related activities over the previous 3 weeks, he has not been taking his prescribed medications regularly. On admission, the patient is pale and diaphoretic with a pulse of 120/min, blood pressure 90/55 mmHg, and temperature 101 °F (38.3 °C). The white blood cell count is 18 000/mm^3, hematocrit value 15%, and hemoglobin level 6 g/dL. An intravenous line is started, and fluids and packed red blood cells are administered. Which of the following tests should be ordered next?
   A. Colonoscopy
   B. Flexible sigmoidoscopy
   C. Plain X-ray of the abdomen
   D. Barium enema
   E. Small bowel follow through

Answers

1. A
   The symptoms (right lower quadrant pain, weight loss, and diarrhea) and laboratory test results (iron-deficiency anemia) are consistent with a diagnosis of Crohn's disease (CD). Colonoscopy is a reasonable option to confirm the diagnosis. CT may also be obtained. Because infectious diarrhea is much more common than IBD, it must be ruled out by stool studies prior to embarking on other tests. A small bowel follow through and EGD are not indicated in this patient.

2. D
   The patient has symptoms consistent with a flare of long-standing CD but has become glucocorticoid dependent. Vital signs, physical examination, laboratory test results, and recent endoscopy are all consistent with mild–moderate disease. The next step is to prescribe a glucocorticoid-sparing drug, specifically azathioprine or 6-mercaptopurine. Before initiation of this therapy, however, a TPMT level or genotype should be obtained to determine the appropriate dosing. Patients with a low (10% of persons) or absent (0.3% of persons) activity of TPMT are at increased risk for bone marrow toxicity.

3. D
   Long-standing UC is associated with an increased risk of colorectal cancer. Therefore, surveillance colonoscopy should be obtained annually or biennially after 8 years of disease. Five percent of patients with UC may develop primary sclerosing cholangitis, and liver biochemical tests that include a serum alkaline phosphatase level are recommended. A complete blood

(Continued)

count should also be obtained annually to evaluate the patient for anemia.

4. E

This patient's symptoms are consistent with small bowel obstruction secondary to a stricture. Surgical resection of the strictured terminal ileum with primary anastomosis of the small bowel to the colon is the best option for this patient. Medical therapy is not indicated for fibrotic strictures.

5. C

The patient's clinical presentation is concerning for toxic megacolon, a life-threatening complication of severe UC. A colonic diameter of >6 cm on a plain abdominal X-ray (or computed tomography) is suggestive of toxic megacolon. All the other tests listed above are contraindicated in a patient suspected of having toxic megacolon.

Further Reading

Abraham, C. and Cho, J.H. (2009) Inflammatory bowel disease. *New England Journal of Medicine*, 361, 2066–2078.

Osterman, M.T. and Lichtenstein, G.R. (2010) Ulcerative colitis, in *Sleisenger and Fordtran's Gastrointestinal and Liver Disease: Pathophysiology/Diagnosis/Management*, 9th edn (eds M. Feldman, L.S. Friedman and L.J. Brandt), Saunders Elsevier, Philadelphia, pp. 1975–2012.

Regueiro, M. and Barrie, A.M. (2009) Challenges in inflammatory bowel disease. *Gastroenterology Clinics of North America*, 38, 577–774.

Sands, B.E. and Siegel, C.A. (2010) Crohn's disease, in *Sleisenger and Fordtran's Gastrointestinal and Liver Disease: Pathophysiology/Diagnosis/Management*, 9th edn (eds M. Feldman, L.S. Friedman and L.J. Brandt), Saunders Elsevier, Philadelphia, pp. 1941–1973.

Schirbel, A. and Fiocchi, C.J. (2010) Inflammatory bowel disease: established and evolving considerations on its etiopathogenesis and therapy. *Digestive Diseases*, 11, 266–276.

Weblinks

http://www.clevelandclinicmeded.com/medicalpubs/diseasemanagement/gastroenterology/inflammatory-bowel-disease

http://www.acg.gi.org/physicians/guidelines/CrohnsDiseaseinAdults2009.pdf

http://emedicine.medscape.com/article/179037-overview

http://www.gastrojournal.org/article/S0016-5085(06)00074-6/fulltext

Constipation

Shanthi Srinivasan

CHAPTER 9

Clinical Vignette

A 52-year-old woman is seen in the office for difficulty with bowel movements for the past 7–8 years. She reports having two bowel movements per week. Her stools are hard and lumpy. She denies experiencing nausea or vomiting. She has no nocturnal pain, early satiety, abdominal cramps, diarrhea, rectal bleeding, or weight loss. A screening colonoscopy at age 50 was unremarkable. Her past medical and surgical history is unremarkable. She does not take any prescription or over-the-counter medications. Her parents are alive and well. Her two siblings are healthy. Her paternal grandfather died of colon cancer at age 80. She works as a computer analyst. She is married with two children who were both delivered vaginally. She drinks a glass of wine with dinner and does not smoke. She has no history of illicit drug use. Physical examination reveals a blood pressure of 130/70 mmHg, pulse rate 70/min, and body mass index 25; she is afebrile. The remainder of the examination, including an abdominal examination, is unremarkable. Her thyroid is not enlarged. Rectal examination reveals normal sphincter tone, squeeze pressure, and hard stool that is brown and negative for occult blood. Routine laboratory tests show a normal complete blood count and normal levels of blood glucose, serum electrolytes, creatinine, and calcium.

General

- Constipation affects approximately 15% of the general population but can affect up to 50% of persons over 65 years old. It is twice as common in women as in men.

Essentials of Gastroenterology, First Edition. Edited by Shanthi V. Sitaraman, Lawrence S. Friedman.
© 2012 John Wiley & Sons, Ltd. Published 2012 by John Wiley & Sons, Ltd.

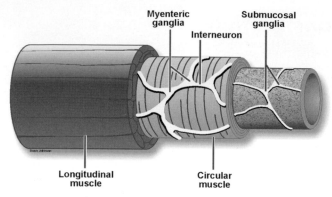

Figure 9.1 Diagram of the colon showing the myenteric plexus located between the circular and longitudinal muscles and the submucosal (Meissner's) plexus located in the submucosa.

- Constipation is defined as at least two of the following symptoms for a period of 12 weeks, which need not be consecutive, during the preceding 6 months:
  - ○ infrequent bowel movements (less than three bowel movements per week);
  - ○ straining during >25% of bowel movements;
  - ○ lumpy or hard stools;
  - ○ sensation of incomplete bowel evacuation;
  - ○ sensation of anorectal obstruction or blockade;
  - ○ use of manual maneuvers to facilitate defecation (e.g., digital evacuation, support of the pelvic floor).

Physiology

Colonic Motility
- Coordinated contraction of the colonic muscle is essential to propel colonic contents towards the anus. Peristalsis involves contraction of the colon proximal to an area of distention and relaxation of the colon distal to the area of distention.
- Colonic motility is regulated by intrinsic and extrinsic neuronal innervation. The enteric nervous system is the intrinsic nervous system of the gastrointestinal tract (Figure 9.1) that plays a central role in colonic motility. It is formed by the myenteric plexus, which lies between the circular and longitudinal muscle, and the Meissner's plexus, which is located in the submucosa.
- The major extrinsic innervation of the colon includes the sympathetic and the parasympathetic nerves. Sympathetic innervation is through

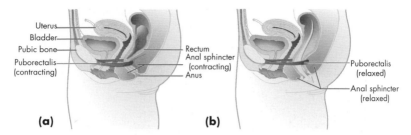

Figure 9.2 Diagram showing the process of defecation. Under normal circumstances (a), the puborectalis is contracted, resulting in an acute anorectal angle. During defecation (b) there is relaxation of the puborectalis with widening of the anorectal angle, thus facilitating the passage of stool.

the lumbar colonic nerves that synapse onto the postganglionic neurons in the spinal cord. Sympathetic input results in reduced colonic motility, intestinal secretion, and contraction of the internal anal sphincter. Parasympathetic innervation is through the vagus and pelvic nerves and results in increased colonic contractility and fluid secretion.

Defecation

- The presence of stool in the rectum results in the urge to defecate, and if the social circumstances are appropriate, the process of defecation is initiated. The process of defecation (Figure 9.2) involves relaxation of the puborectalis muscle and the internal anal sphincter, accompanied by increased abdominal pressure. Rectal distention results in relaxation of the internal anal sphincter and descent of stool into the anal canal. The relaxation of the puborectalis muscle causes a straightening of the anorectal angle and reduction in outflow resistance. Voluntary relaxation of the external anal sphincter then results in expulsion of stool.

Etiology

- Constipation can be divided into primary (functional) or secondary.
- Primary, or functional, constipation can be "simple" constipation associated with insufficient dietary fiber, inadequate fluid intake or decreased physical activity (and reversible by lifestyle modification) or due to irritable bowel syndrome (associated with abdominal pain or distension, see Chapter 7), slow transit/colonic inertia (characterized by infrequent bowel movements), or pelvic outlet obstruction/ pelvic dyssynergia (characterized by excessive straining). The most common type of constipation is "simple" constipation.

Table 9.1 Secondary causes of constipation.

Category	Causes
Structural lesions	Colon cancer, colonic stricture, proctitis, anal fissure
Metabolic abnormalities/ endocrine diseases	Hypercalcemia, hypothyroidism, diabetes mellitus, heavy metal intoxication
Neurologic disorders	Hirschsprung's disease, Chagas disease, pseudo-obstruction, autonomic neuropathy, multiple sclerosis, Parkinson's disease, muscular and myotonic dystrophy, spinal cord lesions (sacral nerves transection or injury to lumbosacral spine, meningomyelocele, spinal anesthesia)
Medications	Anticholinergics, antispasmodics, antidepressants, antipsychotics, cations such as iron and aluminium, opiates, calcium channel blockers, ganglion blockers, vinca alkaloids, 5-hydroxytryptamine$_3$ antagonists

• Secondary causes of constipation (Table 9.1) include structural lesions in the colon, metabolic abnormalities, endocrine diseases, neuromuscular disorders, and medications.

Risk factors for developing constipation include advanced age, female gender, physical inactivity, low income and educational status, and depression.

Clinical Evaluation

• **History**. A complete history should be obtained. Onset and duration of the complaint should be determined. A recent change in bowel habit is of concern, especially in adults. The medication history should include all medications, including those taken over the counter. Typical symptoms include infrequent bowel movements, hard stools, prolonged and excessive straining, and a need for perineal or vaginal pressure or for direct digital manipulation to defecate. Other symptoms may include a sensation of incomplete evacuation, abdominal

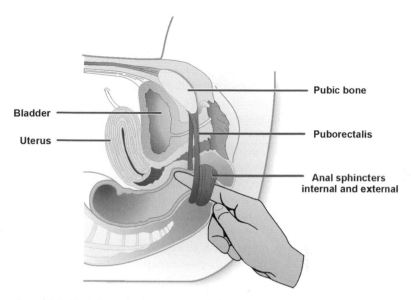

Figure 9.3 Digital rectal examination and the structures that are palpated, including the internal and external anal sphincters and the puborectalis muscle.

bloating, abdominal pain, and malaise. The presence of pain or bleeding with defecation should be noted.

- **Physical examination.** The physical examination should include a detailed rectal examination (Figure 9.3). This includes inspection of the anus for fissures, hemorrhoids, scars, or fistulas. Pelvic floor function should be evaluated by asking the patient to bear down and examining the descent of the perineum. The normal descent of the perineum is 1–3 cm. The digital rectal examination should be performed to determine the resting sphincter tone as well as the presence of a stricture, mass, or stool impaction. The appropriate relaxation of the puborectalis (felt posteriorly) and reduction in anal sphincter tone in response to the initiation of defecation is determined by asking the patient to bear down during the digital rectal examination (Figure 9.3). It should be noted whether the patient finds the examination to be exquisitely painful. The patient should also be asked to squeeze against the examining finger to assess the contractility of the external anal sphincter. In female patients, one should look for a rectocele or prolapsed rectum.
- **Laboratory tests** should include a complete blood count, serum thyroid stimulating hormone (TSH) level, and a comprehensive metabolic profile.

- **Colonoscopy** (or in some cases **flexible sigmoidoscopy**) or **air contrast barium enema** is done to look for structural lesions such as colon cancer or colonic stricture. This is important in patients with "alarm symptoms" (recent worsening of constipation, blood in the stools, weight loss, anorexia, nausea, or vomiting) or as a screening procedure in patients older than age 50.
- **Physiologic tests** to assess colonic motility (measurement of the colonic transit time) and anal sphincter pressure and function (anorectal manometry) are usually performed in patients with refractory constipation. In patients who exhibit excessive straining or prolonged or unsatisfactory defecation, with or without anal digitation, it is best to begin with anorectal manometry to assess for a problem in the process of defection (defecatory disorder). If defecation is normal, a colonic transit time can be measured.
  - *Colon transit study.* This test determines the colonic transit time, which is measured using radiopaque markers. The patient ingests a gelatin capsule that contains 24 small radiopaque rings (Sitz Mark). A plain X-ray of the abdomen is taken 5 days after ingestion of the capsule. The normal colonic transit time is less than 72 hours. If 80% or more ($\geq$19) of the markers are expelled within 5 days, the colonic transit time is considered normal. Slow colonic transit is indicated by the retention of 20% or more ($\geq$5) of the markers in the colon. Scattered distribution of the markers is consistent with colonic inertia, whereas collection of markers in the pelvis is consistent with pelvic outlet obstruction (Figure 9.4). A wireless capsule has also been developed that can assess colonic transit time.

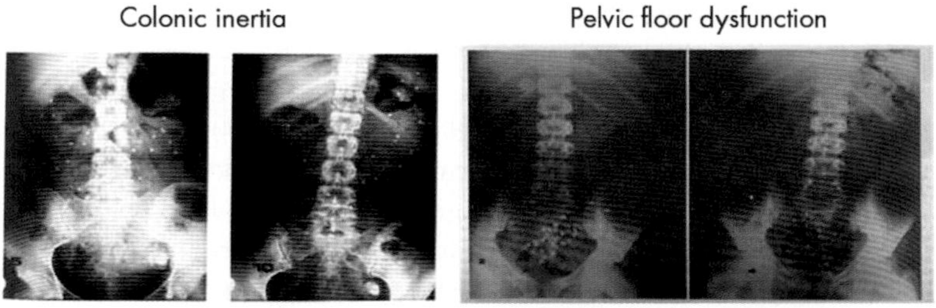

Colonic inertia   Pelvic floor dysfunction

Figure 9.4 Colonic transit study showing plain X-rays of the abdomen taken on day 5 after ingestion of a capsule containing 24 radiopaque markers. The two films on the left from a patient with colonic inertia show markers that are evenly distributed throughout the colon. The two films on the right from a patient with pelvic floor dysfunction show retention of the markers in the pelvic area (distal colon).

○ *Anorectal manometry.* This technique is used to measure internal and external anal sphincter pressures as well as the anorectal inhibitory reflex. The resting anal canal pressure indicates the tonic activity of the internal and external anal sphincter pressures. The anal pressure measured during maximal voluntary anal contraction indicates the external anal sphincter pressure. The anorectal inhibitory reflex is assessed by the ability of the internal anal sphincter to relax in response to a balloon distended in the rectum. The anorectal inhibitory reflex is reduced in megarectum and its absence is pathognomonic of Hirschsprung's disease (congenital aganglionosis, usually in a short segment of sigmoid colon).

○ *Other methods of assessing the defecatory process.* With defecography, barium is instilled in the rectum and the patient is asked to defecate on a commode while X-rays are taken. This technique can allow the evaluation of the anorectal angle and detect anatomic abnormalities such as a prolapsed rectum. Increasingly, dynamic magnetic resonance imaging (MRI) has replaced standard barium defecography. In addition, endoscopic ultrasonography of the internal and external anal sphincters can be used to detect tears or scarring of the sphincters.

Treatment

• The first step in the treatment of constipation is to address the underlying cause, such as a structural lesion, metabolic abnormality, or use of a constipation-inducing medication.

• For primary (functional) constipation, the first line of therapy is diet and lifestyle modification:

○ Patients should be encouraged to drink at least 2 L (eight glasses) of fluid per day and ingest 20–35 g of fiber per day, preferably in the form of fruits and vegetables.

○ If adequate fruit and vegetable intake is not possible, a fiber supplement (bulk-producing laxative) is recommended (Table 9.2). It is important to introduce an increasing amount of fiber gradually.

○ Other lifestyle modifications include regular exercise, weight loss, and reserving enough time to have a bowel movement. In addition, patients should be advised not to ignore the urge to have a bowel movement.

• Once fiber and fluid intake is optimized, persistent constipation can be treated with an osmotic laxative such as polyethylene glycol. The dose of osmotic laxative should be adjusted to achieve stools of soft consistency. Stimulant laxatives are used when an osmotic laxative does not produce the desired effect. Lubiprostone is a recently

Table 9.2 Laxatives.

Category	Medications	Dosage
Bulk-producing agents	Psyllium (Metamucil)	Titrate to 20 g/day
	Methyllcellulose (Citrucel)	Titrate to 20 g/day
	Polycarbophil (FiberCon)	Titrate to 20 g/day
Osmotic laxatives		
a. Saline laxatives	Magnesium hydroxide	15–30 mL/day
	Magnesium citrate	15–30 mL/day
	Sodium phosphate	10–25 mL with 350 mL of water
b. Poorly absorbed sugars and other compounds	Lactulose	15–30 mL/day
	Sorbitol	15–30 mL/day
	Polyethyelene glycol (e.g., Miralax)	17–36 gm/day
Stool softener	Docusate sodium	100 mg/day
Emollient	Mineral oil	5–15 mL orally every night
Stimulant laxatives	Anthraquinones	
	Cascara	325 mg/day
	Senna	187 mg/day
	Castor oil	15–30 mL/day
	Diphenylmethane derivative (Dulcolax)	5–10 mg/daily
Rectal enemas and suppositories	Phosphate enema	120 mL/day
	Mineral oil enema	100 mL/day
	Tap water enema	500 mL/day
	Soap suds enema	1500 mL/day
	Glycerin suppository	10 mg/day
	Bisacodyl suppository	1–2 2.4 gm suppositories/day
Chloride channel activator	Lubiprostone	24 µg twice a day

approved laxative that stimulates chloride and water secretion into the intestinal lumen. Table 9.2 lists the agents used in the treatment of constipation.

- In hospitalized and bed-bound patients, periodic enemas can be given to prevent fecal impaction.
- **Colonic inertia**. In patients with colonic inertia, a combination of diet, exercise and medication is the first line of therapy. Usually these patients require osmotic and stimulant laxatives in addition to enemas. Colonic resection with anastomosis of the ileum to the rectum (ileorectostomy) is reserved for patients with severe constipation that is refractory to medical treatment.
- **Pelvic floor dysfunction**. Surgical repair of a functionally significant rectocele or a prolapsed rectum can lead to resolution of constipation. Usually one should demonstrate improvement in defecation when pressure is placed on the posterior wall of the vagina during defecation before proceeding with repair of a rectocele. Biofeedback training is useful in patients with paradoxical puborectalis contraction to retrain muscles involved in the process of defecation. During biofeedback therapy, patients receive visual and auditory feedback on the functioning of the pelvic floor and anal canal muscles. Using these cues, the patient can learn to relax the pelvic floor muscles during straining, thus facilitating evacuation of the rectum.

Pearls

Constipation is classified as either simple (functional) or secondary to diseases of the colon, metabolic disorders, neurologic disorders, or medications.

Diagnostic testing for patients with constipation should include a complete blood count and serum TSH, glucose, calcium, and creatinine levels. In addition, a colonoscopy to rule out diseases is important, especially in patients with "alarm" symptoms such as unintentional weight loss, gastrointestinal bleeding, or iron-deficiency anemia.

Treatment of constipation should be individualized according to the etiology.

Questions

Questions 1 and 2 relate to the clinical vignette at the beginning of this chapter.

1. Which of the following is indicated at this time?
   A. Colonoscopy
   B. Defecography
   C. Anorectal manometry
   D. Capsule endoscopy
   E. No additional diagnostic test

2. The initial approach to the treatment of constipation in this patient is which of the following?
   A. Increase dietary fiber and fluid
   B. An osmotic laxative
   C. A stimulant laxative
   D. A rectal phosphate enema

3. Defecation is associated with which one of the following?
   A. Contraction of the external anal sphincter
   B. Contraction of the puborectalis muscle
   C. Widening of the anorectal angle
   D. Ascent of the pelvic floor

4. A 42-year-old woman presents with constipation that persists despite diet and lifestyle modification. Digital rectal examination shows a large rectocele. Vaginal examination confirms prolapse of the rectum anteriorly into the vagina. A colonic transit study shows markers in the rectosigmoid region 5 days after ingestion. Anal manometry shows normal internal and external anal sphincter function. A trial of laxatives does not improve symptoms. Which of the following is the best treatment option for this patient?
   A. Increase fluid intake to 16 glasses of water per day
   B. Increase the fiber in her diet to 100 g per day
   C. Surgical removal of the entire colon
   D. Surgical repair of the rectocele

5. All of the following conditions can result in constipation EXCEPT which of the following?
   A. Anal fissure
   B. Excessive fluid intake
   C. Colon cancer
   D. Colonic stricture
   E. Proctitis

Answers

1. E
2. A
   This patient has constipation (less than three bowel movements a week and hard, lumpy stool). Her bloating is likely related to constipation. These

symptoms do not fit into the criteria for irritable bowel syndrome (see Chapter 7). Her history, physical examination, prior colonoscopy, and routine blood work do not suggest secondary causes of constipation. Therefore, she has primary constipation, which is best treated by diet and lifestyle modifications. Oral laxatives or a rectal enema (or both) are indicated if her symptoms fail to respond to diet and lifestyle modifications. Additional tests (colonic transit study, anorectal manometry, and defecography) to evaluate for colonic inertia or anorectal dysfunction should be reserved for refractory constipation.

3. C

The process of defecation involves relaxation (not contraction) of the external and internal anal sphincter and the puborectalis muscle. This results in widening of the anorectal angle, descent (not ascent) of the perineum, and facilitation of the passage of stool.

4. D

This patient has already tried dietary and lifestyle modification with a poor response. A colonic transit test shows accumulation of markers in the anorectal area, indicating pelvic floor dysfunction associated with a large rectocele. The rectocele is likely secondary to anorectal dysfunction. Repair of the rectocele, in some patients, will improve defecation. Biofeedback therapy may be considered in conjunction with rectocele repair to prevent a recurrent rectocele.

5. B

Proctitis, anal fissures, colonic stricture, and colon cancer cause constipation due to inflammation or obstruction. Reduced fluid intake can be associated with constipation.

Further Reading

Lembo, A. and Camilleri, M. (2003) Chronic constipation. *New England Journal of Medicine*, 349, 1360–1368.

Lembo, A.J. and Ullman, S.P. (2010) Constipation, in *Sleisenger and Fordtran's Gastrointestinal and Liver Disease: Pathophysiology/Diagnosis/Management*, 9th edn (eds M. Feldman, L.S. Friedman and L.J. Brandt), Saunders Elsevier, Philadelphia, pp. 259–278.

Wald, A. (2010) A 27-year-old woman with constipation: diagnosis and treatment. *Clinical Gastroenterology and Hepatology*, 8, 838–842.

Weblinks

http://www.mayoclinic.com/health/constipation/DS00063
http://www.merckmanuals.com/professional/sec02/ch008/ch008b.html

Colorectal Neoplasms

Muhammad Fuad Azrak and Vincent W. Yang

CHAPTER 10

Clinical Vignette

A 65-year-old man is seen in the office for increasing fatigue over the past 6 months. He denies abdominal pain, early satiety, nausea, vomiting, or rectal bleeding. His appetite is normal, but he reports an unintentional weight loss of 10 lb (4.5 kg) in the past 6 months. He has never had a colonoscopy. His past medical and surgical history is unremarkable except for hypertension. He takes amlodipine, 2.5 mg once a day. He does not take any over-the-counter medications. His family history is unremarkable. He is a schoolteacher, is married, and has one son, who is healthy. He occasionally drinks one or two glasses of wine and does not smoke cigarettes. He has no history of illicit drug use. Physical examination reveals a blood pressure of 135/85 mmHg, pulse rate 72/min, and body mass index 33. He is afebrile. The remainder of the examination including an abdominal examination is unremarkable. Rectal examination reveals brown stool. Routine laboratory tests show hemoglobin of 7.9 g/dL, mean corpuscular volume 65 fL, iron saturation 3%, and ferritin 7 ng/mL.

General

- The frequency of colorectal cancer (CRC) varies remarkably among different populations and regions. Incidence rates are highest in developed countries of North America and in Australia and New Zealand.
- Lifetime risk of developing CRC in the US is approximately 6%.
- The number of new cases of CRC was estimated to be approximately 147 000 in 2009.

Essentials of Gastroenterology, First Edition. Edited by Shanthi V. Sitaraman, Lawrence S. Friedman.
© 2012 John Wiley & Sons, Ltd. Published 2012 by John Wiley & Sons, Ltd.

- CRC is the second leading cause of cancer-related deaths in the US, accounting for approximately 9% of all cancer deaths.
- CRC incidence and death rates have been declining slowly in both sexes since 1998, as a result of increased screening for CRC.

Definitions

Polyp refers to a discrete mass of tissue that protrudes into the lumen of the bowel. A polyp can be nonadenomatous, adenomatous (premalignant), or malignant (Table 10.1).

- Colorectal neoplasia: this term refers to either CRC or premalignant adenomas.
- More than 95% of CRCs are adenocarcinomas (Figure 10.1); therefore, the term CRC refers to adenocarcinoma of the colon or rectum unless otherwise specified. Other types of cancers in the colon are lymphoma, carcinoid, leiomyosarcoma, and metastatic lesions.
- By definition, all colorectal adenomas are dysplastic. Adenomatous epithelium is characterized by hypercellularity of colonic crypts

Table 10.1 Classification of colonic polyps.

Based on appearance	Sessile (flat) Pedunculated (attached to the colonic wall by a stalk)

Based on histology	Neoplastic:
	• Adenoma (benign):
	  ○ Serrated (mixed hyperplastic and adenoma)
	  ○ Tubular (most common)
	  ○ Tubulovillous
	  ○ Villous
	• Carcinoma (malignant):
	  ○ Noninvasive:
	    • Carcinoma-in-situ (confined to the epithelium)
	    • Intramucosal (extends to lamina propria)
	  ○ Invasive: extends to the submucosa and beyond
	
	Non-neoplastic:
	• Hyperplastic, inflammatory, lymphoid, or hamartomatous

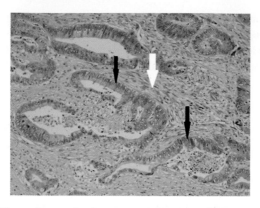

Figure 10.1 Photomicrograph of invasive moderately differentiated colorectal adenocarcinoma. Shown here are the characteristic glandular formation and the characteristic central necrosis (black arrows). There is also stromal desmoplasia with increased fibroblasts surrounding the malignant glands (white arrow). Hematoxylin and eosin, 10x. (Courtesy of Stephen Lau, MD, Emory University, Atlanta, GA, USA.)

with cells that possess variable amounts of mucin and hyperchromatic elongated nuclei.
- Advanced adenomas: this term indicates adenomas that have an increased potential of progressing to malignancy. These are tubular adenomas ≥1 cm in size, villous or tubulovillous adenomas, and adenomas with high-grade dysplasia (HGD).
- Because of the lack of lymphatics in the lamina propria in the colonic mucosa, malignant glands that are confined to the colonic mucosa do not have metastatic potential. Therefore, some pathologists refer to carcinoma-in-situ and intramucosal carcinoma as HGD. Labeling non-invasive carcinoma as HGD removes confusion about the need for further intervention or work-up if the lesion is removed completely by endoscopic polypectomy.

Molecular Features of CRC

- Most CRCs are considered to develop from adenomas. Transition from normal epithelium to adenoma and carcinoma is associated with acquired molecular alterations that occur in a stepwise fashion and involve multiple genes involved in the regulation of cell growth and/ or differentiation.
- A major consequence of molecular alterations is genomic instability.

- Genomic instability can be divided into two categories:
  - Chromosomal instability (CIN) is found in 80–85% of CRCs. For example, adenomatous polyposis coli (*APC*), a tumor suppressor gene, is mutated in 70% of colorectal cancers. In contrast, *K-ras* is the most frequently activated oncogene.
  - Microsatellites instability (MSI) refers to changes in tandem repeated DNA sequences secondary to mutations in the DNA mismatch repair (MMR) genes. MSI is found in approximately 15% of sporadic colorectal cancers. The most commonly involved genes are *MLH1* and *MSH2*.
- Epigenetic alterations:
  - Epigenetics refers to post-transcriptional silencing of specific genes by a variety of mechanisms such as methylation. CRCs that have a high frequency of methylation of some CpG (cytosine-phosphodiesterase bond-guanine) islands are referred to as CpG island methylator phenotype (CIMP) tumors. These epigenetic alterations in the promoter for the MMR genes can silence their transcription and subsequent protein expression.
  - Activating mutations in the *BRAF* gene occur almost exclusively in sporadic CRCs with high degree of MSI and CIMP. This group of CRCs is considered to have developed from serrated polyps.

Risk Factors

- Age: 90% of CRCs occur in persons aged 50 years or older
- Prior personal history of colorectal adenoma or CRC
- Family history of CRC
- Inflammatory bowel disease
- Obesity
- Potential environmental factors:
  - high-fat and low-fiber consumption;
  - alcohol;
  - low dietary selenium;
  - environmental carcinogens and mutagens (from colonic bacteria and charbroiled meats);
  - smoking.

No underlying etiology can be identified in the majority of persons (approximately 75%) with CRC. These cancers are considered "sporadic" CRCs, and the affected population is termed "average risk."

- Ten to thirty percent of colorectal cancers occur in persons with a family history of a polyp or CRC.
- A small percentage of CRCs occur as part of an inherited syndrome. Approximately 5% are associated with **Lynch syndrome**, also called hereditary nonpolyposis colorectal cancer (HNPCC), and 1% are associated with familial adenomatous polyposis (FAP). Less than 0.1% are associated with other rare colorectal cancer syndromes.

Clinical Features

- Most patients with early CRC are asymptomatic. When symptoms are present, they are nonspecific.
- Clinical manifestations are often related to tumor size and location. Forty-five percent of CRCs occur in the proximal colon (cecum to splenic flexure). Common symptoms and signs of proximal neoplasms include ill-defined abdominal pain, weight loss, and occult bleeding. Fifty-five percent of CRCs occur in the distal colon (descending colon to rectum), and symptoms include altered bowel habits, decreased stool caliber, and hematochezia.
- Tumors that are circumferential and large may cause symptoms of bowel obstruction. Patients may present with fatigue (due to anemia from chronic occult blood loss), weight loss, or loss of appetite.
- Up to 5% of patients with colorectal cancer will have a synchronous malignant lesion in the colon or rectum at the time of diagnosis.
- *Streptococcus bovis* bacteremia and *Clostridium septicum* sepsis are due to underlying colonic malignancies in 10–25% of cases.

Diagnosis and Staging

- Colonoscopy is the test of choice to establish a diagnosis when CRC is suspected. It provides visual inspection of the colonic mucosa and the ability to obtain tissue biopsies. If a patient is diagnosed with CRC but preoperative obstruction prevents a complete colonoscopy (to the cecum), then a colonoscopy should be done within 3–6 months after surgery to diagnose any synchronous lesion.
- Computed tomography (CT) of the abdomen and pelvis (Figure 10.2) and chest radiographs are obtained for staging purposes prior to surgery.
- In rectal cancer, endoscopic ultrasonography (EUS) is performed to evaluate the depth of tumor invasion and the status of regional lymph nodes. EUS detects regional lymph node metastasis accurately as compared with CT.

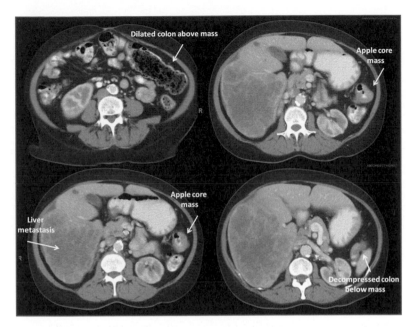

Figure 10.2 Computed tomography in a person with colonic adenocarcinoma. The mass, which has an "apple-core" appearance, is obstructing the descending colon with resulting dilatation of the colon proximal to the mass. Extensive metastasis in the liver is also seen. (Courtesy of Sherif Nour, MD, Emory University, Atlanta, GA, USA.)

- Carcinoembryonic antigen (CEA) is a tumor marker for CRC but has low sensitivity and specificity, which has limited its use in screening and diagnosis. Elevated serum CEA levels preoperatively may have some prognostic value in advanced colorectal cancer. Patients with stage III disease have a median time to recurrence of 13 months if CEA preoperative levels are >5 ng/mL, and 28 months if <5 mg/mL. CEA is used mainly to monitor for recurrent CRC following surgical resection of CRC.

Prognosis

- The American Joint Commission on Cancer (AJCC) system (utilizing the TNM [Tumor Node Metastasis] classification) is commonly used for staging (Table 10.2).
- Stage I has a favorable prognosis with a 5-year survival rate of 93%. Stage IV CRC (distant metastases) is associated with a 5-year survival rate of 8%.

Table 10.2 Colorectal cancer staging.

Stage*	TNM classification
0	Tis N0 M0
I	T1 or T2 N0 M0
II	T3 or T4 N0 M0
III	T1-T4 N1-N2 M0
VI	Any T Any N M1

*This is a simplified staging system. Stage II, III, IV can be further subcategorized.
Primary tumor (T): Tis, carcinoma in situ; T1, tumor invades submucosa; T2, tumor invades muscularis propria; T3, tumor invades through the muscularis popria into the subserosa; T4 tumor invades through the entire colorectal wall to the surface of the visceral peritoneum or directly invades other structures.
Regional lymph nodes (N): N0, no regional lymph node metastasis; N1, metastasis in 1–3 regional lymph nodes; N2, metastasis in 4 or more regional lymph nodes.
Distant metastasis (M): M0, no distant metastasis, M1 distant metastasis.

Treatment

Surgery is the mainstay of treatment of CRC if no metastatic disease is identified. In selected cases, surgery is performed to resect isolated liver or lung metastases.

- Colon cancer:
  - Surgical excision (usually segmental resection) is recommended for patients without evidence of metastasis (stages I to III) who are medically fit for surgery. Subtotal colectomy is performed in patients who have multiple neoplasms. Proctocolectomy is reserved for patients with familial cancer syndromes (see below).
  - Postoperative chemotherapy is recommended for patients with stage III cancer and some patients with stage II cancers.
- Rectal cancer:
  - Anterior resection with colorectal anastomosis for middle and upper rectal cancers.
  - Abdominoperineal resection with a permanent colostomy for lower rectal cancers.
  - Preoperative chemotherapy with radiotherapy for cancers that are T3 and higher or N1 and higher.
  - Postoperative chemotherapy for stage II or stage III cancers.

Inherited CRC Syndromes

- Inherited CRC syndromes account for a small percentage of all CRCs. Often, affected patients also have an increased risk of cancers in organs other than the colon.
- **Familial adenomatous polyposis (FAP):**
  - FAP is caused by a germline mutation in the *APC* gene and inherited in an autosomal dominant manner.
  - The estimated incidence is ~1 in 8000 live births.
  - FAP is characterized by multiple (100s–1000s) adenomas in the colon, first appearing around 15 years of age.
  - Almost 100% of patients will have colon cancer at a mean age of approximately 40 years if prophylactic colectomy is not performed before then.
  - Patients may have extracolonic manifestations, which include duodenal adenomas and mandibular osteomas.
  - Gardner's syndrome is a variant of FAP. In addition to the typical findings of FAP, affected patients have osteomas of the skull and long bones, desmoid tumors, epidermoid cysts, and congenital hypertrophy of the retinal pigmented epithelium.
  - Attenuated FAP is also caused by mutations in the *APC* gene. It is associated with fewer colonic adenomas (<100), older age of CRC onset (age of ~55), lower cancer penetrance, and greater proximal colonic involvement than in classic FAP.
- **Lynch syndrome:**
  - Also known as hereditary nonpolyposis colon cancer (HNPCC), Lynch syndrome is caused by germline mutations in one of the DNA mismatch repair (MMR) genes, leading to MSI. It is inherited in an autosomal dominant manner.
  - The incidence is 1 in 1000 live births.
  - Seventy percent of the affected persons will develop CRC if surveillance colonoscopy and polypectomy are not performed.
  - The adenoma–carcinoma sequence progresses much more rapidly in Lynch syndrome than in sporadic colon cancer. CRC can occur within 2–3 years after a negative colonoscopy.
  - The mean age of onset of CRC is 46 years.
  - There is an increased risk of extracolonic malignancies, including endometrial, gastric, small bowel, renal pelvic, ureteral, and ovarian neoplasms.
  - The Amsterdam II criteria identify high-risk persons for genetic testing ("3-2-1" rule): ≥3 relatives with Lynch syndrome-related cancers, with at least one of them being a first-degree relative of the other two; ≥2 successive generations affected, ≥1 person with a

---

Table 10.3 Revised Bethesda guidelines for testing colorectal cancers for microsatellite instability.

CRC from persons should be tested for MSI in the following situations:
1. CRC diagnosed in a patient who is less than 50 years of age
2. Presence of synchronous or metachronous colorectal or other HNPCC-related tumors, regardless of age
3. CRC with MSI-H* histology diagnosed in a patient who is less than 60 years of age
4. CRC diagnosed in one or more first-degree relatives with HNPCC-related tumors, with one of the persons being diagnosed before age 50 years
5. CRC diagnosed in two or more first- or second-degree relatives with HNPCC-related tumors, regardless of age

---

*MSI-H, microsatellite instability-high refers to changes in two or more of the five National Cancer Institute-recommended panels of microsatellite markers.

Lynch syndrome-related cancer diagnosed before age 50. FAP should be excluded in cases with CRC.
○ The revised Bethesda guidelines for testing colorectal tumors for MSI (Table 10.3) are more inclusive than the Amsterdam II criteria.
○ Genetic testing for mutations in the MMR genes is performed to confirm the diagnosis.
• Muir–Torre syndrome:
○ Affected persons have sebaceous gland tumors and visceral malignancies.
○ It is inherited in an autosomal dominant manner and is associated with defective DNA MMR genes and may represent a variant of Lynch syndrome.
• MutYH-associated polyposis (MAP):
○ MAP is an autosomal recessive syndrome caused by biallelic mutations in the *MYH* gene, which is a DNA base excision repair enzyme.
○ The clinical phenotype (colonic polyp burden) is similar to that of attenuated or classic FAP.
• Turcot's syndrome:
○ Turcot's syndrome is characterized by the development of central nervous system tumors in association with FAP (often medulloblastoma) or Lynch syndrome (often gliobastoma multiforme).
• Peutz–Jeghers syndrome (PJS):
○ PJS is characterized by multiple hamartomatous polyps throughout the gastrointestinal tract. It is inherited in an autosomal dominant manner.

- ○ Up to 60% of cases are attributable to germline mutations in the *LKB1* gene.
- ○ The hamartomatous polyps involve the epithelium, lamina propria, and mucularis mucosa.
- ○ The development of CRC is rare; however, foci of adenomatous changes or carcinoma may develop in the hamartomatous polyps.
- ○ Other features are pigmented lesions around the mouth, hands, and feet. Affected persons have an increased risk of extracolonic malignancy involving the small intestine, pancreas, esophagus, ovaries or sex cords, testis, and breast.
- Juvenile polyposis syndrome (JPS)
  - ○ JPS is characterized by the presence of 10 or more juvenile mucous retention polyps in the colon or elsewhere in the gastrointestinal tract.
  - ○ It is inherited in an autosomal dominant manner, and germline mutations in *PTEN* and *SMAD4* have been implicated in the etiology.
  - ○ Affected patients may have symptoms of colonic obstruction or bleeding during childhood. Their risk of CRC is not well defined.

Prevention

Average-Risk Population

- Multiple CRC screening guidelines have been developed, including those by the American Cancer Society in conjunction with gastroenterologic and radiologic societies (joint society guidelines), US Preventive Services Task Force (USPSTF), and the American College of Gastroenterology (ACG), all published in 2008–2009 (Table 10.4).
- ○ All guidelines recommend CRC screening beginning at age 50.
- ○ The USPSTF guidelines do not recommend routine screening of adults aged 76–85 years and do not recommend any screening for adults older than 85 years.
- ○ All the guidelines provide multiple screening options. Colonoscopy every 10 years is included in all guidelines.
- ○ The joint society guidelines favor "cancer prevention" screening tests (evaluation of the colon by colonoscopy or radiologic imaging that can diagnose polyps) over "cancer detection" screening tests (fecal occult blood and stool DNA tests).
- ○ The American College of Physicians recommends colonoscopy as the preferred screening method.

Table 10.4 Screening tests for colorectal cancer in average-risk persons.

Category	Test
Accepted screening tests	• Annual FOBT*, three cards on three specimens ○ Guaiac-based FOBT: detects peroxidase activity of hemoglobin (diet restriction is needed) ○ FIT: detects human hemoglobin (diet restriction is not necessary) • Sigmoidoscopy every 5 years (+ FOBT every 3 years, per USFSTF) • Colonoscopy every 10 years
Screening tests not widely performed or accepted	• CT colonography (virtual colonoscopy) every 5 years • Fecal DNA testing: detects DNA mutations known to be associated with CRC; interval of testing is uncertain • Barium enema every 5 years

*Only highly sensitive FOBTs are accepted for use in screening by all guidelines.
CRC, colorectal cancer; CT, computed tomography; FIT, fecal immunochemical test; FOBT, fecal occult blood test; USPSTF, United States Preventive Services Task Force.

High-Risk Populations

- Colonoscopy is the preferred screening method for persons who are at increased risk of CRC, such as those with inflammatory bowel disease, a personal or family history of colonic neoplasms, or hereditary colorectal cancer syndromes.
- The starting age for screening and screening intervals depend on the specific condition.
- For persons who have a family history of CRC or adenomatous polyps in a first-degree relative before age 60 or in two or more first-degree relatives at any age, screening with colonoscopy should begin at age 40 or 10 years before the age at which the youngest family member was diagnosed. The screening interval is every 5 years. For persons with a first-degree relative diagnosed with CRC at age 60 or older or with two second-degree relatives with cancer, screening should begin at age 40. The screening interval is every 10 years, and screening modalities beside colonoscopy can be used.
- Others:
  ○ Lynch syndrome: colonoscopy every 1–2 years, beginning at age 20.

- Peutz–Jeghers syndrome: first colonoscopy in the second decade; subsequent screening interval is based on the findings.
- Inflammatory bowel disease: colonoscopy with surveillance biopsies every 1–2 years beginning 8–10 years after the onset of symptoms.
- Post-polypectomy surveillance:
  - Advanced adenoma (see above) or three or more adenomas: repeat colonoscopy in 3 years.
  - One or two small tubular adenomas (<1 cm): repeat colonoscopy in 5–10 years.
- Post-colorectal cancer resection surveillance:
  - Repeat colonoscopy 1 year after curative resection. If the examination is normal, then the interval before the next examination should be 3 years, and then 5 years thereafter if the examinations remain negative for adenomas.
  - Serum CEA determinations at regular intervals may be cost-effective for detecting recurrent cancers. National Comprehensive Cancer Network (NCCN) recommends CEA testing every 3 months in the first 2 years and every 6 months for another 3 years.

Pearls

CRC should be considered when a patient, especially one older than 40 years of age, presents with hypochromic microcytic anemia or rectal bleeding.

Screening for CRC should begin at age 50 in average-risk persons and at an earlier age in high-risk populations.

Colonoscopy is universally accepted as one of the modalities of CRC screening in the average-risk population. It is the preferred screening modality in high-risk populations and the preferred diagnostic test in patients with any symptom or sign suggestive of CRC.

Questions

Questions 1 and 2 relate to the clinical vignette at the beginning of this chapter.

1. The next step in the management of this patient should be which of the following?
   A. Fecal occult blood test (FOBT) and, if positive, colonoscopy
   B. Upper endoscopy
   C. Colonoscopy
   D. Computed tomography (CT) of the abdomen and pelvis with oral and intravenous contrast
   E. Oral iron supplementations and repeat complete blood count in 8 weeks

(Continued)

2. Colonoscopy revealed a 5-cm mass in the ascending colon and an additional 2-cm mass in the descending colon. Biopsies of both masses were consistent with invasive adenocarcinoma. Chest X-rays and CT of the abdomen and pelvis did not reveal lymphadenopathy or metastasis. The next step in the management of this patient is which of the following?
   A. Right hemicolectomy and endoscopic resection of the colon cancer in the descending colon
   B. Subtotal colectomy
   C. Preoperative chemotherapy with radiotherapy, followed by subtotal colectomy
   D. Chemotherapy
3. A 74-year-old man undergoes colonoscopy because of intermittent rectal bleeding and is found to have a 3-cm pedunculated polypoid mass in the sigmoid colon. The mass is ulcerated. A polypectomy is performed. The pathology report shows high-grade dysplasia; no tumor cells are seen in the polyp stalk. What is the appropriate management of this patient?
   A. CT of the abdomen and pelvis
   B. Positron emission tomography (PET)
   C. Subtotal colectomy
   D. Repeat colonoscopy in 3 years
4. Germline mutations in one of the DNA mismatch repair (MMR) genes can lead to which of the following familial cancer syndromes?
   A. Peutz–Jeghers syndrome (PJS)
   B. Lynch syndrome
   C. Familial adenomatous polyposis (FAP)
   D. Gardner's syndrome
Questions 5 and 6 pertain to the case below.
   A 65-year-old man is seen for a routine physical examination by a new primary care provider. He has no gastrointestinal complaints and states that a flexible sigmoidoscopy done approximately 5 years ago was normal.
5. Which one of the following tests is **not recommended** as a screening tool for colorectal cancer in this patient?
   A. Digital rectal examination and fecal occult blood test (FOBT) performed in the office
   B. A series of three FOBTs
   C. Flexible sigmoidoscopy
   D. Colonoscopy
6. The new physician performs a digital rectal examination, and a fecal occult blood test (FOBT) done on the stool sample using Hemoccult II guaiac test is positive. Which one of the following tests should be recommended?

A. A series of three FOBTs using a highly sensitive guaiac test such as Hemoccult SENSA
B. A fecal immunochemical test
C. Flexible sigmoidoscopy
D. Colonoscopy

Answers

1. C
The patient has iron-deficiency anemia in the setting of unintentional weight loss. Occult bleeding from the gastrointestinal (GI) tract, especially from the colon, is the most likely etiology. The patient has not had a prior colonoscopy. In the setting of unexplained iron-deficiency anemia, FOBT is not necessary because the patient will require colonoscopy even if the FOBT is negative. Upper endoscopy should be performed if colonoscopy does not reveal a source of blood loss or if the patient has upper GI symptoms such as nausea, vomiting, early satiety, or epigastric pain. CT should not be done routinely for evaluation of iron-deficiency anemia. CT could be helpful if the patient has signs of colonic obstruction or severe abdominal pain. CT may be helpful to evaluate for metastasis if the patient is found to have CRC on colonoscopy. Empiric treatment with oral iron is inappropriate in this setting.

2. B
The patient has invasive adenocarcinomas of the left and right colon. The most appropriate management is a subtotal colectomy. Endoscopic resection is not recommended for invasive adenocarcinoma. Preoperative chemotherapy with radiotherapy is used to treat locally advanced rectal cancer. Stage II and III rectal cancers and stage III colon cancers also require postoperative chemotherapy.

3. D
Malignant polyps in the colon and rectum do not metastasize if cancer is confined to the mucosa. Polypectomy is adequate treatment for a polyp with high-grade dysplasia. This polyp is considered an advanced neoplasm, and the patient should undergo a repeat colonoscopy in 3 years. CT and PET are not indicated because there is no risk of metastasis if dysplasia in the polyp is confined to the mucosa. Subtotal colectomy is not indicated because the polyp has been completely resected endoscopically.

4. B
PJS is caused by germline mutations in the *LKB1* gene. Germline mutations of one of the MMR genes lead to Lynch syndrome. FAP is caused by

germline mutations in the *APC* gene. Gardner's syndrome is a variant of FAP and is also caused by mutations in the *APC* gene.

5. A

FOBT done on a stool sample (obtained by digital rectal examination) has low sensitivity. Only 4.9% of advanced adenomas and 9% of cancers are detected by this method. Because the accuracy of FOBT done in the office setting is so low, it is not endorsed as a method of CRC screening. The other options are acceptable.

6. D

Colonoscopy is the best test to further evaluate a positive FOBT result. The other choices would not be appropriate. Hemoccult II and Hemoccult SENSA are commonly used types of guaiac-based FOBTs. Hemoccult SENSA detects lower levels of peroxidase activity of heme than are detected by Hemoccult II. Current CRC screening guidelines recommend use of the more sensitive FOBT tests, such as Hemoccult SENSA. A fecal immuno-chemical test, or FIT, is another acceptable option for CRC screening. It detects human hemoglobin, so diet restriction is not necessary. However, because the Hemoccult II test is positive, the next step should be colonoscopy.

Further Reading

Bresalier, RS. (2010) Colorectal cancer, in *Sleisenger and Fordtran's Gastrointestinal and Liver Disease: Pathophysiology/Diagnosis/Management*, 9th edn (eds M. Feldman, L.S. Friedman and L.J. Brandt), Saunders Elsevier, Philadelphia, pp. 2191–2238.

Levin, B., Lieberman, D.A., McFarland, B., *et al.* (2008) Screening and surveillance for the early detection of colorectal cancer and adenomatous polyps, 2008: a joint guideline from the American Cancer Society, the US Multi-Society Task Force on Colorectal Cancer, and the American College of Radiology. *Gastroenterology*, 134, 1570–1595.

US Preventive Services Task Force. (2008) Screening for colorectal cancer: US Preventive Services Task Force recommendation statement. *Annals of Internal Medicine*, 149, 627–637.

Weblinks

http://www.merckmanuals.com/professional/sec02/ch021/
  ch021h.html?qt=colon%20cancer&alt=sh

http://www.ncbi.nlm.nih.gov/pubmedhealth/PMH0001308/

http://www.gastrojournal.org/article/S0016-5085%2808%2900232-1/fulltext

Liver

Frank A. Anania

Liver Anatomy and Histopathology

Frank A. Anania

CHAPTER 11

Clinical Vignette 1

A 21-year-old woman with abdominal pain is found on an imaging study to have a large hemangioma in the left lobe of the liver. She wishes to become pregnant, but because estrogen may induce the hemangioma to grow, the obstetrician recommends that she undergo resection of the hemangioma. A partial left lobectomy is performed, and she recovers uneventfully. Follow-up computed tomography 1 month later shows a normal liver size and contour.

Clinical Vignette 2

A 4-year-old boy requires liver transplantation for biliary atresia. One of his parents is identified as a donor. The surgeon explains that he will remove 55–70% of the liver from the parent's right lobe and transplant it into the child and that both the parent's and the child's livers will regenerate to full size in 4–6 weeks.

Embryonic Development

- Week 4: the liver bud or hepatic diverticulum is formed from an outgrowth of the endodermal epithelial lining of the foregut. The epithelial liver cords (hepatocytes) and primordia of the biliary system (epithelial lining of the biliary tree and gallbladder) develop from the hepatic diverticulum.
- Week 5: the hepatocytes arrange into a series of branching and anastomosing cords in the mesenchyme of the septum transversum. These

Essentials of Gastroenterology, First Edition. Edited by Shanthi V. Sitaraman, Lawrence S. Friedman.

cords subsequently intermingle with the vitelline and umbilical veins to form hepatic sinusoids. The hematopoietic cells, Kupffer cells, and connective tissue of the liver are also derived from the septum transversum.

- Week 6: hematopoiesis starts in the liver and gradually subsides during the last 2 months of fetal life. This is a key fetal function that is absent in postfetal life.
- Week 7: the liver accounts for 10% by weight of the fetus.
- Week 12: bile formation begins. At the time of birth, the liver accounts for 5% of the weight of the newborn.
- The major blood supply to the fetal liver is from the umbilical vein.

> The endoderm and mesoderm are both involved in liver development. The endoderm gives rise to hepatocytes and cholangiocytes, which line the biliary tree. The mesoderm contributes to the sinusoids and forms the stroma, liver capsule, hematopoietic tissue (including Kupffer cells), connective tissue, and smooth muscle of the biliary tract.

Liver Regeneration

- In adults, the liver is the only internal organ that can regenerate. The liver regenerates by hepatocyte hyperplasia (proliferation of cells resulting in increased number of cells). Hyperplasia is different from hypertrophy in that the adaptive cell change in hypertrophy is an increase in the size of cells, whereas hyperplasia involves an increase in the number of cells.
- Hyperplasia restores exactly the same cell mass that was removed so that the liver regenerates to its original size. This principle applies to live donor liver transplantation and hepatic resection.

Anatomy

- The liver can be divided anatomically into lobes or segments based on morphologic or functional features, respectively. The four lobes of the liver are **right**, **left**, **caudate**, and **quadrate**, based on the relationship to the falciform ligament and morphologic features. The eight segments of the liver are designated 1 to 8. Each segment has its own vascular inflow, outflow, and biliary drainage. The importance of the functional anatomy of the liver lies in the planning of anatomic resection for transplantation or tumor resection.
- The liver has a dual blood supply, which includes the portal vein and the hepatic artery. The **portal vein** provides 75% of the liver's blood

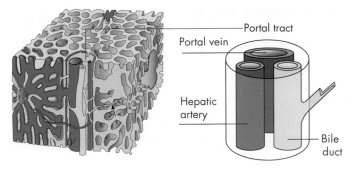

Figure 11.1 Schematic representation of the microscopic anatomy of the normal human liver. The liver consists of a system of anastomosing hepatic plates and sinusoidal spaces. A network of bile duct radicles opens into the portal bile ducts (green). An intralobular artery (red), deriving from a portal branch of the hepatic artery, bypasses the parenchyma and communicates directly with the sinusoids (blue). The portal vein (blue) drains through the sinusoids into the central vein. (Adapted with permission from Dancygier, H. (2010) Springer Images: *Microscopic Anatomy*. Springer, New York.)

supply and carries venous blood rich in nutrients drained from the spleen, gastrointestinal tract, and associated organs. The **hepatic artery** supplies arterial blood, accounting for the remainder of the liver's blood flow. Oxygen is provided from both sources: approximately half of the oxygen demand of the liver is met by the portal vein, and the other half is met by the hepatic artery. The hepatic artery is the major source of oxygen to the bile ducts.

- The **hepatic lobule** is the functional unit of the liver (Figure 11.1). In the center of the lobule is the central vein. At the periphery of the lobule are the portal tracts (or portal triads), which consist of a portal venule, bile duct, and hepatic arteriole. Connecting the portal tracts with the central vein are sheets or cords of hepatocytes lined by sinusoids on one side and biliary canaliculi on the other. Blood flows from the hepatic arteriole and portal venule in the portal tract toward the central vein. Bile is secreted by the hepatocytes into the canaliculi and flows towards the portal tract to drain into the bile ducts (Figure 11.1).

- Functionally, the liver can be divided into acini. Each **acinus** has three zones, based on oxygen and nutrient supply. The periportal zone 1 encircles the portal tracts, where the oxygenated blood from hepatic arteries and nutrient-rich blood from the portal vein enter. The centrilobular zone 3 is located around central veins, where oxygenation is poor. Zone 2 is located between zones 1 and 3 (Figure 11.2).

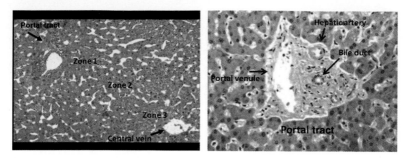

Figure 11.2 Microscopic structure of the liver (Left ×40, Right ×100). (Photomicrographs courtesy of Charles W. Sewell, MD, Department of Pathology, Emory University, Atlanta, GA, USA.)

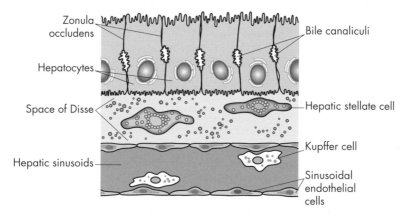

Figure 11.3 Schematic representation of the microscopic anatomy of the liver.

Zone 3 is most susceptible to states of low blood flow such as hypotension or heart failure. Therefore, zone 3 is most susceptible to necrosis of the liver in such conditions.

Major Cell Types

Major cell types are illustrated in Figure 11.3.

Hepatocyte

• Hepatocytes are the chief functional cells of the liver and constitute 60–80% of liver mass. They are polarized epithelial cells with distinct apical and basolateral surfaces separated by an intercellular junctional complex (zonula occludens or tight junction).

- Hepatocytes perform numerous metabolic and synthetic functions, including gluconeogenesis, glycogenolysis, and production of cholesterol and bile salts, clotting factors (except factor VIII), and albumin, and possess enzymatic machinery to metabolize, detoxify, and inactivate exogenous chemicals.

Kupffer Cell

- Kupffer cells are specialized macrophages that reside in the hepatic sinusoids.
- They are members of the reticuloendothelial system.
- Kupffer cells provide the major defense of the liver. Some important functions of the Kupffer cell are antigen presentation, phagocytosis of bacterial products, synthesis and secretion of key cytokines and macromolecules, and host defense against microbes.

Sinusoidal Endothelial Cell

- Sinusoidal endothelial cells (SECs) line the sinusoidal wall. Along with the Kupffer cells, the SECs constitute the reticuloendothelial system. They are fenestrated and are separated from hepatocytes by the space of Disse (also called the perisinusoidal space).
- In cirrhosis, the fenestrations become occluded with extracellular matrix.

Hepatic Stellate Cell

- Hepatic stellate cells (HSCs) are found in the space of Disse. In normal liver, they store vitamin A and do not divide.
- When the liver is injured, these cells undergo mitosis and secrete extracellular matrix (e.g., collagen). The amount of stored vitamin A decreases progressively in liver injury.
- HSCs are the cells primarily responsible for the development of hepatic fibrosis.

Pearls

Liver regenerates by hepatocyte hyperplasia, which restores exactly the same cell mass as the original liver.

The main blood supply to the liver is provided by the portal vein. Oxygenated blood is provided by both the portal vein and the hepatic artery. However, the hepatic artery is the major source of oxygen to the bile duct.

Hepatic stellate cells play a central role in the development of hepatic fibrosis.

Questions

The following questions relate to clinical vignettes 1 and 2 at the beginning of this chapter.

1. The liver regenerates by which of the following mechanisms?
   A. Hypertrophy
   B. Hyperplasia
   C. Metaplasia
   D. Dysplasia

2. In the photomicrograph of the liver below (Figure 11.4), the areas containing the blue double-ended arrows are which of the following?
   A. Portal tracts
   B. Hepatocytes
   C. Zonula occludens
   D. Sinusoids
   E. Kupffer cells

3. In Figure 11.5, match each number with the name of the structure:
   A. Space of Disse
   B. Portal blood
   C. Kupffer cell
   D. Bile canaliculi
   E. Zonula occludens

4. Which of the following cell types is associated with facilitating hepatic fibrosis?
   A. Hepatic stellate cell
   B. Hepatocyte
   C. Kupffer cell
   D. Sinusoidal endothelial cell

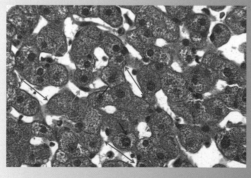

Figure 11.4 See Question 2. (Photomicrograph courtesy of Charles W. Sewell, MD, Department of Pathology, Emory University, Atlanta, GA, USA.)

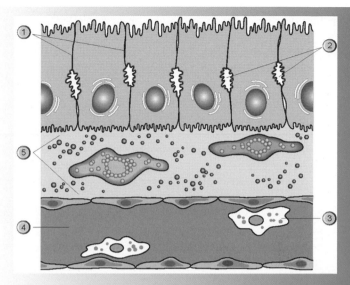

Figure 11.5 See Question 3.

5. Which of the following statements regarding oxygen tension and blood flow in the hepatic lobule is correct?
   A. Oxygen tension is highest near the central vein; blood flows from the portal tract to the central vein
   B. Oxygen tension is lowest near the central vein; blood flows from the portal tract to the central vein
   C. Oxygen tension is lowest near the central vein; blood flows from the central vein to the portal tract
   D. Oxygen tension is highest near the central vein; blood flows from the central vein to the portal tract
   E. None of the above statements is correct
6. Which of the following pairs of cells and products synthesized or stored is correct?
   A. Hepatic stellate cell: vitamin A
   B. Hepatocyte: alkaline phosphatase
   C. Cholangiocyte: glycogen
   D. Kupffer cell: cholesterol
   E. Sinusoidal endothelial cell: vitamin E

(*Continued*)

7. A patient develops hepatic artery thrombosis following liver transplantation. Which of the following structures is most likely to be damaged as a result of the thrombus?
   A. Hepatocytes in zone 3
   B. Central veins
   C. Hepatic stellate cells
   D. Bile ducts
   E. Sinusoidal endothelial cells

8. Which of the following statements regarding embryologic development of the liver is correct?
   A. The fetal liver is derived from elements of both the endoderm and the mesoderm.
   B. The fetal liver does not have hematopoietic function.
   C. Bile flow begins around week 6 of fetal life.
   D. The transverse septum is primarily responsible for the development of hepatocytes and biliary tract.
   E. Hepatic sinusoids are derived from the hepatic diverticulum.

9. Drug X was recently withdrawn from the market by the US Food and Drug Administration due to its association with acute liver failure. A toxic intermediate of the drug accumulates when high doses of the drug are administered and the toxic intermediate destroys the hepatocyte cell membrane, thereby leading to cell death. Cells located in areas of low oxygen tension are most susceptible to injury by the drug. Which cells are most likely to die first?
   A. Hepatocytes closest to the central veins (zone 3).
   B. Hepatocytes closest to the portal tracts (zone 1).
   C. Hepatocytes in zone 2.
   D. All hepatocytes are equally susceptible to injury.

Answers

1. B

   The liver regenerates by hyperplasia (proliferation of cells, including hepatocytes, resulting in an increase in the number of cells). Hyperplasia restores the same cell mass that was removed so that the liver regenerates to its original size. This principle applies following hepatic resection, including live liver donation.

2. D

   The blue double-ended arrows are in sinusoids, the yellow arrows point to the zonula occludens (intercellular junctions), the red arrows point to hepatocytes, and the green arrows point to Kupffer cells.

3. A5; B4; C3; D2; E1
4. A
5. B
6. A
7. D
   The principal supply of oxygen to the bile ducts is the hepatic artery, not the portal vein.
8. A
9. A

Further Reading

Boron, W.F. and Boulpaep, E.L. (eds) (2003) *Medical Physiology: A Cellular and Molecular Approach*, 2nd edn. Saunders Elsevier, New York.

Boyer, T.D., Wright, T.L. and Manns, M.P. (eds) (2006) *Zakim and Boyer's Hepatology: A Textbook of Liver Disease*, 5th edn, Saunders Elsevier, New York.

Dancygier, H. (2010) Microscopic anatomy, in *Clinical Hepatology: Principles and Practice of Hepatobiliary Diseases*, (ed. H. Dancygier), Springer, New York, pp. 15–51.

Eruschenko, V.P. (ed) (2005) *DiFiore's Atlas of Histology with Functional Correlates*, 10th edn, Lippincott, Williams & Wilkins, Philadelphia.

Weblinks

http://facstaff.gpc.edu/~ssadri/1612%20for%20website/Chapter23B.pdf
http://www.hepatitis.org.uk/s-crina/liver-fs2.htm
http://www.anatomyatlases.org/MicroscopicAnatomy/Section10/Plate10215.shtml

Liver Biochemical Tests

Nader Dbouk and Samir Parekh

CHAPTER 12

Clinical Vignette

A 46-year-old man is seen in the office for his annual health check-up. He is asymptomatic. His past medical history is remarkable for an appendectomy at age 16. He does not take prescription, over-the-counter, or herbal medications. He has no history of illicit drug use. His family history is unremarkable. He drinks a glass of red wine with dinner and does not smoke cigarettes. He is married and has two children. On physical examination the vital signs are normal. He is overweight with a body mass index of 29. The remainder of the examination is unremarkable. Routine laboratory tests including a complete blood count and a complete metabolic panel are normal except for a serum alanine aminotransferase (ALT) level of 140 U/L and aspartate aminotransferase (AST) of 110 U/L.

General

- An estimated 1–4% of persons in the US who are asymptomatic have mildly elevated liver biochemical test levels (also called "liver enzymes" or "liver function tests," although some of the tests do not measure liver function).

Patterns of Liver Biochemical Test Level Elevations

- The standard liver biochemical tests used in assessing hepatobiliary disease include serum bilirubin (see Chapter 24), aminotransferases, and alkaline phosphatase (ALP). Common laboratory tests used to

Essentials of Gastroenterology, First Edition. Edited by Shanthi V. Sitaraman, Lawrence S. Friedman.
© 2012 John Wiley & Sons, Ltd. Published 2012 by John Wiley & Sons, Ltd.

Table 12.1 Patterns of liver injury.

	Hepatocellular	Cholestatic	
		Intrahepatic	Extrahepatic
Aminotransferases	+++	0 – +	0 – +
Alkaline phosphatase	0 – +	+++	++ – +++
Bilirubin	0 – ++	0 – ++	+++

assess synthetic function of the liver include the prothrombin time and albumin.

• Depending on the predominant liver biochemical test abnormality, two patterns of liver injury can be recognized: hepatocellular and cholestatic (Table 12.1). In **hepatocellular** injury there is a predominant increase in serum aminotransferase levels compared with ALP or bilirubin. In **cholestatic** disease, the cause may be intrahepatic or extrahepatic (see Chapter 24). Intrahepatic cholestasis is typically associated with an isolated or predominant elevation of the serum ALP level, compared with serum aminotransferase levels; the serum bilirubin level may be normal or elevated. Extrahepatic cholestasis (biliary obstruction) is associated with a predominant increase in the ALP level as well as the serum bilirubin level compared with serum aminotransferase levels.

Impaired synthetic function in the setting of elevated liver biochemical test levels generally indicates hepatic decompensation, and patients should undergo an expedited evaluation to identify the underlying cause of liver disease.

Aminotransferases

• Aspartate aminotransferase (AST, or serum glutamic oxaloacetic transaminase [SGOT]), and alanine aminotransferase (ALT, or serum glutamic pyruvic transaminase [SGPT]) catalyze the transfer of amino acids from aspartate and alanine to ketoglutaric acid to form oxaloacetate and pyruvate, respectively, during gluconeogenesis.

• ALT is localized predominantly in the cytoplasm of hepatocytes and is more specific to the liver than AST. AST is present in the cytoplasm and mitochondria of hepatocytes and is also present in various extra-hepatic sites, including skeletal muscle, myocardium, kidneys, pancreas, lungs, brain cells, and red blood cells, and is therefore a less specific marker of liver injury than ALT.

- An isolated AST elevation can be seen in various nonhepatic conditions including myocardial ischemia, muscle disorders such as polymyositis, rhabdomyolysis, muscular dystrophy, and strenuous physical exertion. On the other hand, an isolated elevation in the ALT level generally indicates liver injury.
- A transient rise in the ALT level may follow a large, fatty meal or use of acetaminophen 4 g per day for several days.

> Elevated serum aminotransferase levels indicate hepatocellular injury. Levels of 1000 U/L or more are typical of acute viral hepatitis. ALT is more specific than AST for hepatocellular injury. The level of AST or ALT elevation does not correlate with the severity of liver injury.

- The normal range of aminotransferase levels in serum varies among laboratories, but generally accepted values are ≤30 U/L for men and ≤19 U/L for women.
- Mild elevations in serum aminotransferase levels (two to five times the upper limit of normal, or ≤150 U/L) can be seen in 1–4% of seemingly healthy persons in the US.
  - Common causes of mildly elevated serum aminotransferase include:
    - nonalcoholic fatty liver disease (NAFLD);
    - chronic hepatitis B or C;
    - alcholic liver disease;
    - medications and toxins (Table 12.2);
    - hemochromatosis;
    - cytomegalovirus (CMV) or Epstein–Barr virus (EBV) infection.
  - Less common causes include:
    - autoimmune hepatitis;
    - Wilson disease;
    - alpha-1 antitrypsin deficiency.
  - Systemic diseases that can cause mildly elevated serum aminotransferase levels include:
    - celiac disease;
    - congestive hepatopathy secondary to passive venous congestion in patients with right-sided heart failure;
    - hyperthyroidism.

Table 12.2 Some medications, herbal preparations, and substances of abuse that can result in elevated serum aminotransferase levels.

Prescription medications
Antibiotics: ciprofloxacin, isoniazid, ketoconazole, pencillins, rifampin, trimethoprim–sulfamethoxazole
Antidepressants: bupropion, fluoxetine, paroxetine, sertraline
Antiepileptics: carbamezipine, phenytoin, valproic acid
Highly active antiretroviral therapy drugs
3-Hydroxy-3-methylglutaryl-coenzyme A (HMG-CoA) reductase inhibitors (statins)
Oral hypoglycemics: acarbose, glipizide
Proton pump inhibitors: omeprazole, pantoprazole
Others: amiodarone, angiotensin converting enzyme inhibitors, methotrexate, vitamin A

Over-the-counter medications
Acetaminophen
Nonsteroidal anti-inflammatory drugs (NSAIDs)

Substances of abuse
Anabolic steroids, cocaine, ecstasy, glues, solvents, phencyclidine (angel dust)

Herbal preparations
Chaparral leaf, Chinese herbs (ephedra), gentian, germander, Jin bu huan, kava, shark cartilage, senna, skullcap

Approach to the Patient with Elevated Serum Aminotransferase Levels

- The first step in the evaluation of a patient with mildly elevated serum aminotransferase levels is to obtain a careful history and perform a thorough physical examination (Figure 12.1).
  - The history should focus on identifying risk factors for liver disease, including excessive alcohol use or substance abuse; use of medications, including prescription drugs, over-the-counter agents, and herbal supplements (Table 12.2); prior blood transfusions, tattoos, and promiscuous or unprotected sexual activity; a family history of liver disease; and a history of autoimmune disorders or celiac disease.
  - The physical examination should focus on identifying signs of liver disease such as ascites, splenomegaly, and jaundice as well as dermatologic manifestations of liver disease such as spider angiomas,

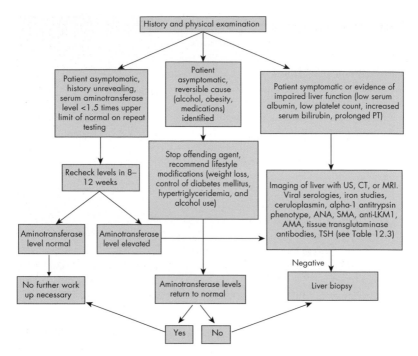

Figure 12.1 Algorithm for the evaluation of patients with mildly elevated serum aminotransferase levels. (AMA, antimitochondrial antibodies; ANA, antinuclear antibodies; CT, computed tomography; LKM1, liver-kidney microsome type 1; MRI, magnetic resonance imaging; PT, prothrombin time; SMA, smooth muscle antibodies; TSH, thyroid stimulating hormone; US, ultrasonography.)

palmar erythema, and palpable purpura, often of the lower extremities, which may be associated with cryoglobulinemia in patients with chronic hepatitis C and occasionally B. A careful neurologic examination should also be performed to detect signs of Wilson disease or hepatic encephalopathy (see Chapter 15).

- If the history, physical examination, and tests of liver function or portal hypertension (e.g., prolonged prothrombin time, low serum albumin, low platelet count) indicate decompensated liver disease, expedited evaluation to identify the cause of liver disease should be performed.
- If potential hepatotoxins (medications, alcohol) are identified in the history and the patient is asymptomatic, the offending agent should be stopped and the liver biochemical tests repeated in 6–8 weeks.
- If the history is unrevealing, further laboratory testing to identify common causes of chronic liver disease including chronic hepatitis B

Table 12.3 Ancillary tests in the evaluation of persons with elevated serum aminotransferase levels.

Viral serologies for hepatitis B and C: HBsAg and antibody to HCV

Autoimmune markers: ANA, SMA, and anti-LKM1

AMA

Serum iron, iron saturation, ferritin, *HFE* gene mutation

Serum ceruloplasmin level, 24-hour urine copper level, slit-lamp examination

Alpha-1 antitrypsin phenotype (protease inhibitor type)

Other tests: endomysial antibodies, tissue transglutaminase antibodies, immunoglobulin levels, TSH

AMA, antimitochondrial antibodies; ANA, antinuclear antibodies; HBsAg, hepatitis B surface antigen; HCV, hepatitis C virus; LKM1, liver-kidney microsome type 1; SMA, smooth muscle antibodies; TSH, thyroid stimulating hormone.

and C and hemochromatosis, and, if necessary, autoimmune hepatitis, Wilson disease, alpha-1 antitrypsin deficiency, celiac disease, and thyroid disease, should be performed (Table 12.3). A creatine kinase level should be considered, particularly if the AST level is elevated predominantly.

- If the biochemical and serologic tests associated with various liver diseases are normal or negative and the patient is asymptomatic and has no evidence of hepatic decompensation, a liver biopsy may be considered. Alternatively, lifestyle modifications, including weight loss and control of diabetes mellitus, hypertriglyceridemia, and alcohol use, should be recommended if NAFLD is suspected, and the liver biochemical test levels should be followed regularly.

The AST:ALT ratio may provide a clue to the underlying diagnosis. An AST:ALT ratio ≥2 is suggestive of alcoholic liver disease particularly when there is a concomitant increase in the gamma-glutamyl transpeptidase (GGTP) level. On the other hand, an AST:ALT ratio <1 is often seen in NAFLD or chronic viral hepatitis, but the ratio may rise to >1 when cirrhosis develops.

- Marked elevation in AST and ALT levels (>3000 U/L) can be seen in patients with the following conditions:
  - ischemic (or hypoxic) hepatitis (shock liver), a condition often seen in critically ill patients in the intensive care unit. The ALT level may

be >5000 U/L; the lactate dehydrogenase (LDH) level is also typically high, with an ALT:LDH ratio <1.5, in contrast to viral hepatitis;
   ○ toxicity caused by certain medications, especially acetaminophen (values often >2000 U/L);
   ○ rarely, autoimmune hepatitis or viral hepatitis.
- Marked elevations in serum aminotransferase levels should prompt an expedited evaluation to identify the underlying cause of hepatocellular injury.

> NAFLD is the most common cause of asymptomatic, mildly elevated aminotransferase levels in the US and accounts for as many as 67% of cases.

Alkaline Phosphatase

- ALP is a catalytic enzyme of uncertain function; it is distributed widely in tissues.
- The liver and bones are the major sources of serum ALP activity. ALP is also present in the placenta, small intestine, kidneys, and leukocytes as well as some neoplasms. In the liver ALP is found in the canalicular membrane of hepatocytes.
- Electrophoretic isoenzyme analysis allows fractionation of ALP to determine the tissue origin of an isolated elevation of ALP in serum.
- Alternatively, GGTP or 5′ nucleotidase (5′NT) levels can be measured to verify the hepatobilary (vs. bone) origin of ALP.
   ○ GGTP is a microsomal enzyme that is found in hepatocytes and biliary epithelium as well as various extrahepatic organs, including the pancreas, heart, lungs, kidneys, spleen, and brain, but not bone; it is not elevated in pregnancy.
   ○ Alcohol increases serum GGTP levels. Several medications including phenytoin, barbiturates, and some of the highly active antiretroviral therapy drugs also increase serum GGTP levels.
   ○ 5′NT is a sensitive test for underlying liver disease and is not elevated in bone disease.

> Low serum ALP levels are characteristic of Wilson disease, especially in patients with fulminant hepatitis and hemolysis.

Approach to the Patient with an Elevated Serum Alkaline Phosphatase Level

- ALP may be elevated in liver disease or in nonhepatic diseases (Table 12.4).

Table 12.4 Common causes of an elevated serum alkaline phosphatase (ALP) level.

Physiologic causes
Adolescence (bone ALP)
Advanced age, particularly in postmenopausal women
Fatty meal (intestinal ALP)
Pregnancy (usually in the 3rd trimester, placental ALP)

Liver disease
Bile duct obstruction (choledocholithiasis, cholangiocarcinoma, pancreatic adenocarcinoma)
Drug-induced cholestasis
Infiltrative liver diseases (granulomatous hepatitis, sarcoidosis, amyloidosis, metastatic cancer, some primary liver tumors such as hepatocellular carcinoma)
Primary biliary cirrhosis
Primary sclerosing cholangitis
Primary familial intrahepatic cholestasis and benign recurrent intrahepatic cholestasis

Bone disease
Paget's disease
Bone metastasis

- Serum ALP levels can be elevated after a fatty meal due to increased influx of intestinal ALP and should therefore be measured in the fasting state.
- A two- to threefold rise in serum ALP levels (with normal serum aminotransferase levels) can be seen in physiologic conditions such as pregnancy as well as in adolescents, presumably due to increased bone growth. A gradual rise in serum ALP levels is also seen with increasing age, particularly in women.
- Many drugs can cause a predominant rise in serum ALP levels, with or without elevations in other liver enzymes (see Table 12.3).
- The first step in the evaluation of a patient with an isolated and asymptomatic elevation in the ALP level is to identify the tissue of origin. This is done most precisely by fractionation of ALP. Alternatively, a serum GGTP or 5'NT level can be measured.
- Hepatobiliary disease may be associated with isolated elevation of the ALP or elevation of the ALP that is out of proportion to the elevation in serum aminotransferase levels.
- As with elevated serum aminotransferase levels, a thorough history that includes prescription, over-the-counter, and herbal medication

use should be obtained, and a careful physical examination should be performed.

- If the history is unrevealing for an offending agent, the patient should be evaluated for a cholestatic disorder (see Chapter 24). Abdominal imaging with ultrasonography or CT should be performed to look for extrahepatic causes of cholestasis. If the imaging studies show no dilatation of intra- or extrahepatic bile ducts, the patient should be evaluated for intrahepatic causes of cholestasis. The most common causes of intrahepatic cholestasis include primary biliary cirrhosis (PBC) and granulomatous disease (e.g., sarcoidosis).
- Intrahepatic cholestasis is typically associated with an isolated elevation in the serum ALP early in the course. PBC is diagnosed by detection of antimitochondrial antibodies (AMA) in serum (Chapter 15). An elevated angiotensin converting enzyme (ACE) level is seen in patients with sarcoidosis.
- Further evaluation of the patient with cholestasis is summarized in Figure 12.2 and discussed in more detail in Chapter 24.

Albumin

- The majority of proteins circulating in plasma are synthesized by the liver; levels reflect the synthetic capability of the liver.
- Albumin accounts for 10% of hepatic protein synthesis and 75% of protein in the serum; it accounts for 75% of plasma colloid oncotic pressure.
- Albumin has a half-life of about 15 days, and its concentration in blood depends on the synthetic rate (normal = 12 g/day) and plasma volume.
- Hypoalbuminemia:
  ○ may result from expanded plasma volume or decreased albumin synthesis;
  ○ is frequently associated with ascites and expansion of the extravascular albumin pool at the expense of the intravascular pool;
  ○ is common in chronic liver disease and an indicator of severity; it is less common in acute liver disease.
- Therapeutic administration of albumin:
  ○ The benefit of intravenous albumin administration in critically ill patients with hypoalbuminemia is uncertain; it has been reported to reduce the risk of hepatorenal syndrome and mortality in patients with cirrhosis and spontaneous bacterial peritonitis (see Chapter 16).
  ○ An albumin-containing dialysate is used in the molecular adsorbent recirculating system (MARS) in patients with hepatic failure, because of the ability of albumin to bind toxins.

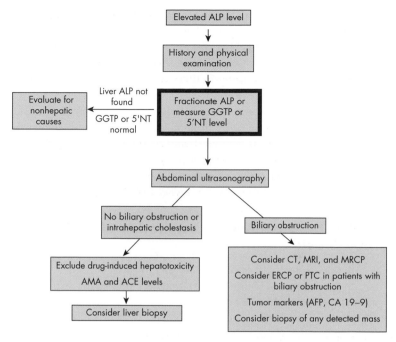

Figure 12.2 Algorithm for the evaluation of patients with an elevated serum alkaline phosphatase level. (AMA, antimitochondrial antibodies; ACE, angiotensin converting enzyme; AFP, alpha fetoprotein; CA, cancer antigen; CT, computed tomography; ERCP, endoscopic retrograde cholangiopancreatography; GGTP, gamma-glutamyl transpeptidase; MRI, magnetic resonance imaging; MRCP, magnetic resonance cholangiopancreatography; 5'NT, 5'nucleotidase; PTC, percutaneous transhepatic cholangiography.)

Immunoglobulins

- Serum levels of immunoglobulins are often increased in chronic liver disease.
- The pattern of elevation may suggest the etiology of underlying liver disease:
  - ○ elevated IgG: autoimmune hepatitis;
  - ○ elevated IgM: primary biliary cirrhosis;
  - ○ elevated IgA: alcoholic liver disease.

Coagulation Factors

- Most (not factor VIII) are synthesized by the liver.
- The half-lives of these factors are much shorter than that of albumin.

- The prothrombin time is useful in assessing the severity and prognosis of acute liver disease but correlates poorly with bleeding risk in patients with liver disease because of counterbalancing disturbances in anticoagulant activity (e.g., protein S and C).
- Prolongation of the prothrombin time in cholestatic liver disease may result from vitamin K deficiency.
- The international normalized ratio (INR) of prothrombin time is calibrated based on blood samples from normal controls and patients who are therapeutically anticoagulated, and results from different laboratories may not be consistent in patients with liver disease. Calibration based on normal controls and patients with liver disease gives more consistent results in patients with liver disease.

Tests for the Noninvasive Estimation of Liver Fibrosis

- Serum ALT (sensitivity of only 61–71%).
- Serum hyaluronic acid (and other markers of hepatic extracellular matrix metabolism): under study.
- FibroSure (FibroTest): panel of blood tests that includes α_2-macroglobulin, haptoglobin, GGTP, total bilirubin, and apolipoprotein A1 (the addition of ALT is used to estimate the degree of hepatic inflammation). The negative predictive value of FibroSure for excluding significant fibrosis is 91%; a high score is accurate for predicting cirrhosis; intermediate scores are less reliable.
- Transient elastography (FibroScan): uses ultrasound to measure the elasticity of the liver; magnetic resonance elastography assesses fibrosis by magnetic resonance imaging. These methods are not yet widely available.

Pearls

The most common cause of mildly elevated serum aminotransferase levels is NAFLD.

Very high aminotransferase levels (>3000 U/L) are usually due to ischemic hepatitis or acetaminophen toxicity.

An isolated alkaline phosphatase level may be of hepatic or nonhepatic (usually bone) origin. The former is associated with an elevated GGTP or 5'NT level.

Questions

The following question relates to the clinical vignette at the beginning of this chapter.

1. What is the next best step in the management of this patient's elevated liver biochemical test levels?

   A. Advise lifestyle modifications including weight loss and repeat the liver biochemical tests in 8 weeks

   B. Serologic tests for hepatitis B and C

   C. Serologic tests for autoimmune hepatitis

   D. Abdominal ultrasonography

   E. Liver biopsy

2. A 15-year-old boy is seen for evaluation of an upper respiratory tract infection. The history and physical examination are remarkable only for fatigue. Routine laboratory evaluation reveals a normal complete blood count and chemistry tests except for an elevated serum alkaline phosphatase level of 190 U/L. He is otherwise healthy and does not drink alcohol, smoke cigarettes, or use recreational drugs. He denies the use of prescription drugs, herbal remedies, or over-the-counter medications. There is no family history of liver disease or cirrhosis. Physical examination is unremarkable. The alkaline phosphatase level is repeated 2 weeks later and is 196 U/L. What is the next best step in evaluating this patient?

   A. Serum gamma-glutamyl transpeptidase (GGTP) level

   B. Antimitochondrial antibodies (AMA)

   C. Abdominal ultrasonography

   D. Liver biopsy

3. A 20-year-old African American college student is referred to the student health clinic for evaluation of a rash. The patient also complains of the new onset of dyspnea on exertion. He does not smoke cigarettes, drink alcohol, or use recreational drugs. His college performance has deteriorated since the fall term began, and he has become markedly fatigued. At night he occasionally feels warm and has night sweats that require him to change his bed clothes and his pillow case several times per week. He denies nausea, vomiting, diarrhea, or bloody stools. His past medical and surgical history is unremarkable. He has not been sexually active for over 6 months and was vaccinated for hepatitis B as an infant. His mother has a history of ulcerative colitis. His sister and maternal aunt have systemic lupus erythematosus. On physical examination the patient is an asthenic male in no acute distress. The vital signs are within normal limits. He has tender, erythematous nodular lesions on his lower extremities consistent with erythema nodosum. The remainder of the examination, including abdominal

(Continued)

and neurologic examinations, is normal. Laboratory tests show a normal complete blood count. The serum calcium level is 12 mg/dL, alkaline phosphatase 360 U/L, GGTP 418 U/L, ALT 80 U/L, AST 110 U/L, total bilirubin 2.0 mg/dL, and direct bilirubin 1.8 mg/dL. A parathyroid hormone level is normal. The titer of antinuclear antibodies titer is <1:20. Serologic tests for hepatitis B and C, cytomegalovirus, and Epstein Barr virus are negative. A chest X-ray reveals hilar adenopathy. Abdominal ultrasonography demonstrates hepatosplenomegaly but no intra- or extrahepatic bile duct dilatation. A lymph node biopsy reveals noncaseating granulomas. Which of the following is the most likely diagnosis?

A. Autoimmune hepatitis
B. Acute hepatitis B
C. Sarcoidosis
D. Celiac disease
E. Sickle cell disease

4. A 62-year-old woman is referred for evaluation of pruritus, which has been progressing over the past several months. She denies weight loss, fatigue, or a history of liver disease. She denies a history of illicit drug or alcohol use and does not take prescription or over-the-counter medications. Her family history is remarkable for thyroid disease in her mother and systemic lupus erythematosus in her sister. Physical examination is remarkable for xanthelasma on her eyelids. Routine laboratory tests including a complete blood count and comprehensive metabolic panel are normal except for an elevated serum alkaline phosphatase of 280 U/L and GGTP 330 U/L. Abdominal ultrasonography reveals a normal liver with no evidence of parenchymal abnormalities. Which of the following is the next best diagnostic step?

A. Fractionation of the alkaline phosphatase
B. Antimitochondrial antibodies (AMA)
C. Endoscopic retrograde cholangiopancreatography (ERCP)
D. Small bowel biopsy
E. Percutaneous liver biopsy

5. An 80-year-old woman is admitted to the hospital with a urinary tract infection (UTI). She has a history of heart failure, chronic obstructive lung disease, and diabetes mellitus. She takes multiple medications and has been placed on ampicillin–sulbactam for the UTI. Her routine laboratory tests including liver enzymes are normal. Urine and blood cultures grow *Escherichia coli*. Two days after admission her condition worsens, and she is transferred to the intensive care unit and intubated for acute respiratory failure. Following intubation she becomes hypotensive and requires medical therapy to support her blood pressure. Two days after that her serum liver enzymes reveal an aspartate aminotransferase (AST) level of 2570 U/L,

alanine aminotransferase (ALT) 1895 U/L, alkaline phosphatase (ALP) 160 U/L, and total bilirubin 2.9 mg/dL. The most likely cause of the abnormal liver biochemical test levels is which of the following:

A. Acute viral hepatitis

B. Drug-induced hepatotoxicity

C. Congestive hepatopathy

D. Ischemic hepatitis

E. Transfusion reaction

6. A 45-year-old man seeking life insurance presents for a physical examination. He is asymptomatic except for fatigue. The physical examination is unremarkable. The body mass index is 25.5. He admits to having used "recreational" drugs as well as binge drinking on the weekends when he was in college. He is sexually active with several partners. He has been vaccinated against hepatitis A and B. A urine drug screen is negative. Laboratory tests are normal except for ALT 65 U/L, AST 58 U/L. What is the next best step in the evaluation of this patient?

A. Recommend weight loss and repeat liver biochemical testing in 3 months

B. Reassure the patient and repeat liver biochemical testing in 3 months

C. Serologic testing for hepatitis C

D. Serum ceruloplasmin level

E. Serologic testing for celiac disease

Answers

1. A

The patient has asymptomatic elevations of the ALT and AST levels with normal bilirubin and ALP levels. The most common cause of mildly elevated serum aminotransferase levels in the US is nonalcoholic fatty liver disease (NAFLD). This patient is overweight, making the diagnosis of NAFLD likely. Therefore, lifestyle modifications emphasizing weight loss and repeating the tests in 8 weeks is a reasonable option. If the elevated ALT and AST levels persist, a work-up for chronic liver disease is warranted, including serologic tests for hepatitis B and C and autoimmune hepatitis as well as abdominal ultrasonography. Liver biopsy is not indicated at this time.

2. A

Benign elevation of the serum ALP level can be seen in adolescents due to rapid bone turnover associated with bone growth. This is the most probable cause of an elevated ALP level in this young man. Concurrent elevation of the GGTP level would prompt a work-up for cholestasis with abdominal

(Continued)

imaging; if the GGTP were normal, no further work-up would be necessary. AMA, a marker of primary biliary cirrhosis (PBC), is not likely to be useful in a male adolescent in whom PBC would be unlikely. Liver biopsy is not indicated at this time.

3. C

The patient's presentation with dyspnea, hilar adenopathy, erythema nodosum, and hypercalcemia is consistent with a diagnosis of sarcoidosis. This is further confirmed by lymph node biopsy findings of noncaseating granulomas. Hepatic involvement is common in patients with sarcoidosis and is characterized by an elevated serum ALP level that typically is out of proportion to elevation in serum aminotransferase or bilirubin levels.

4. B

This presentation is typical of primary biliary cirrhosis (PBC). AMA are detected in 95% of patients with PBC. Ultrasonography does not show evidence of biliary disease, and ERCP is therefore unnecessary. A liver biopsy may be contemplated in order to determine the stage of the patient's disease, but it would not be the appropriate next step in this clinical scenario. A small bowel biopsy may be considered to diagnose celiac disease, but the clinical presentation and pattern of liver biochemical test abnormalities are not typical of those associated with celiac disease.

5. D

The patient had normal liver enzymes on presentation with a UTI and developed markedly elevated aminotransferase levels after a hypotensive episode. This sequence of events suggests ischemic hepatitis. Congestive hepatopathy typically causes a cholestatic pattern of enzyme elevations and would not cause such a dramatic elevation in the aminotransferase levels. Drug-induced hepatotoxicity could potentially cause marked elevations in liver enzymes, but the more likely diagnosis in this clinical scenario is ischemic hepatitis.

6. C

Chronic hepatitis C is prevalent among former intravenous drug users who often are asymptomatic and are found incidentally to have mildly elevated aminotransferase levels on routine laboratory testing. If the patient had no risk factors for hepatitis C, it would be reasonable to stop potentially offending drugs and follow the liver biochemical tests. A serum ceruloplasmin level is helpful in the evaluation of patients with Wilson disease, an uncommon diagnosis after age 40. Celiac disease is often associated with mildly elevated serum aminotransferase levels, but in the setting of prior intravenous drug use, chronic hepatitis C is more likely.

Further Reading

Aragon, G. and Younossi, Z.M. (2010) When and how to evaluate mildly elevated liver enzymes in apparently healthy patients. *Cleveland Clinic Journal of Medicine*, 77, 195–204.

Pratt, D.S. (2010) Liver chemistry and function tests, in *Sleisenger and Fordtran's Gastrointestinal and Liver Disease: Pathophysiology/Diagnosis/Management*, 9th edn (eds M. Feldman, L.S. Friedman and L.J. Brandt), Saunders Elsevier, Philadelphia, pp. 1227–1238.

Pratt, D.S. and Kaplan, M.M. (2000) Evaluation of abnormal liver enzyme results in asymptomatic patients. *New England Journal of Medicine*, 342, 1266–1271.

Weblinks

http://www.clevelandclinicmeded.com/medicalpubs/diseasemanagement/hepatology/guide-to-common-liver-tests/

http://www.med.upenn.edu/gastro/documents/ClinLiverDisoutpatientliverfunctiontestsLFTs2009.pdf

Viral Hepatitis

Shanthi V. Sitaraman and Lawrence S. Friedman

CHAPTER 13

Clinical Vignette

A 21-year-old man presents with the insidious onset of anorexia, nausea, and upper abdominal discomfort. His symptoms developed approximately 2 weeks earlier when he returned from a cruise in the Caribbean. For the past 2 days he has noticed that his urine is darker than usual. He denies illicit drug use, medication (prescription or over-the-counter) use, or travel outside the US. He received a blood transfusion 6 years ago following a car accident in which he sustained a femoral fracture. His past medical history is otherwise unremarkable. Family history is noncontributory. He smokes 20 cigarettes a day and drinks two to three beers a day but has not smoked or had a beer for several days. He is a senior in college, is heterosexual, and has a single partner. He denies high-risk sexual practices. Physical examination reveals a blood pressure of 118/68 mmHg, pulse rate 76/min, and body mass index 20. He is afebrile. There are no cutaneous stigmata of chronic liver disease, tattoos, or needletracks. Conjuctival icterus is present. Chest and cardiovascular examinations are unremarkable. The abdominal examination is notable for a tender liver edge that is palpable just below the right costal margin. Rectal examination reveals brown stool that is negative for occult blood. Laboratory tests reveal a white blood cell count of 7200/mm^3, hemoglobin 13.1 g/dL, platelet count 260 000/mm^3. A comprehensive metabolic panel is normal. The serum alanine aminotransferase (ALT) level is 980 U/L, aspartate aminotransferase (AST) 960 U/L, alkaline phosphatase 200 U/L, total bilirubin 14.5 mg/dL, direct bilirubin 11.2 mg/dL, prothrombin time (PT) 12.4 seconds, and international normalized ratio (INR) 1.1. Additional testing shows the presence of immunoglobulin M antibody to hepatitis A virus (IgM anti-HAV). He is hepatitis B surface antigen (HBsAg) negative, antibody to HBsAg (anti-HBs) positive, IgG antibody to hepatitis B core antigen (IgG anti-HBc) positive, and antibody to hepatitis C virus (anti-HCV) negative.

Essentials of Gastroenterology, First Edition. Edited by Shanthi V. Sitaraman, Lawrence S. Friedman.
© 2012 John Wiley & Sons, Ltd. Published 2012 by John Wiley & Sons, Ltd.

Etiology

- There are five major hepatotropic viruses (viruses that have affinity for hepatocytes): hepatitis A virus (HAV), hepatitis B virus (HBV), hepatitis C virus (HCV), hepatitis D virus (HDV), and hepatitis E virus (HEV) (Table 13.1).
  - All hepatitis viruses are RNA viruses except for HBV, which is a partially double-stranded DNA virus.
  - HDV is a defective RNA virus that uses HBsAg as its envelope protein. Therefore, HBV coinfection is necessary for the propagation of HDV virions.
  - Ninety percent of cases of viral hepatitis in the US are caused by HAV, HBV, or HCV.
  - Damage to the liver is not due to cytopathic effects of the virus but to the immune response to the virus.
- Viruses that may affect the liver as a part of a systemic infection include Epstein-Barr virus, cytomegalovirus, herpes virus, parvovirus, and adenovirus.

Clinical Features

- Acute infection may result in subclinical (asymptomatic) disease, self-limited symptomatic disease, or fulminant hepatic failure (FHF).
- Infections caused by HAV, HBV, and HEV are usually symptomatic in adults but often asymptomatic in children. Acute infection caused by HCV is usually asymptomatic in both children and adults.
- Following an incubation period that varies with the virus, symptomatic acute hepatitis is characterized by a prodromal phase and an icteric phase. Typical symptoms in the prodromal phase include flu-like symptoms: fatigue, anorexia, nausea, vomiting, loss of taste for cigarettes, headache, arthralgias, and myalgias. The icteric phase typically occurs 1–2 weeks after the prodromal phase; symptoms include jaundice, tea-colored urine, pruritus, and right upper quadrant abdominal discomfort.
- Acute hepatitis may progress rapidly to acute liver failure, marked by poor hepatic synthetic function (prolonged PT >16 seconds or INR >1.5) and encephalopathy in the absence of chronic liver disease.
- FHF, defined as acute liver failure that occurs within 8 weeks of the onset of hepatitis, occurs in <2% of patients with acute HAV, HBV, or HEV infection.
- Typical laboratory test abnormalities in acute hepatitis include elevated serum aminotransferase levels (>500 U/L) and hyperbilirubinemia, primarily the direct (conjugated) fraction.

Table 13.1 Characteristics of hepatotropic viruses.

	HAV	HBV	HCV	HDV	HEV
Viral type	RNA	DNA	RNA	RNA	RNA
Modes of transmission	Fecal–oral	Parenteral, perinatal, sexual	Parenteral; infrequent: perinatal or sexual	Parenteral	Fecal-oral
Diagnostic test	IgM anti-HAV	See Table 2	Anti-HCV; confirmatory: HCV RNA	Anti-HDV	IgM anti-HEV
Chronic liver disease	No	Yes	Yes	Yes	No
Natural immunity	Yes	Yes	No	No	Yes
Vaccine	Yes	Yes	No	No	Yes (experimental)
Treatment options	Supportive care only	PEG-IFN-alpha or oral nucleoside or nucleotide analogs	PEG-IFN-alpha plus ribavarin plus protease inhibitor	PEG-IFN-alpha	Supportive care only

HAV, hepatitis A virus; HBV, hepatitis B virus; HCV, hepatitis C virus; HDV, hepatitis D virus; HEV, hepatitis E virus; IgM, immunoglobulin M; PEG-IFN, pegylated interferon.

- Patients with chronic hepatitis B or C are often asymptomatic. When present, fatigue is the most common symptom.
- Extrahepatic complications associated with HBV infection include:
  - Polyarteritis nodosa is a rare complication of HBV infection. Small- and medium-sized vessels are affected. It is seen in North American and European patients and rarely in Asian patients.
  - Glomerulonephritis is seen in patients from endemic areas. Essential mixed cryoglobulinemia (see below) may occasionally be associated with HBV infection. Palpable purpura and acrodermatitis may also be associated with HBV infection.
- Extrahepatic complications associated with chronic hepatitis C include:
  - Essential mixed cryoglobulinemia: HCV may form immune complexes with anti-HCV, often in association with the appearance of rheumatoid factor in the serum. The deposition of immune complexes in small blood vessels leads to organ damage. Features of cryoglobulinemia include rash, vasculitis, peripheral neuropathy, and glomerulonephritis.
  - Other extrahepatic complications of HCV infection: focal lymphocytic sialadenitis, autoimmune thyroiditis, porphyria cutanea tarda, lichen planus, and Mooren corneal ulcer.

> HAV or HBV infection as well as HEV infection in pregnant women can cause FHF. Encephalopathy in FHF is due to cerebral edema and is potentially fatal. Emergent intervention to decrease intracranial pressure is required, and FHF is generally a clear indication for liver transplantation.

Natural History

Hepatitis A Virus and Hepatitis E Virus

- Symptoms related to acute HAV or HEV infection resolve over several days to weeks.
- Acute hepatitis A and acute hepatitis E never progress to chronic liver disease. Relapsing hepatitis A is an uncommon sequela of acute hepatitis A, more common in elderly than younger persons, and characterized by a protracted course of symptoms and a relapse of symptoms and signs following apparent resolution. Occasional cases of acute hepatitis A are characterized by marked cholestasis (high serum bilirubin and alkaline phosphatase levels).
- HEV, which is endemic to South, Southeast, and East Asia, can be fatal in pregnant women.

Hepatitis B Virus and Hepatitis C Virus
- In approximately 90–95% of neonates, 25–30% of children, and less than 5% of immunocompetant adults, acute hepatitis B progresses to chronic HBV infection.
- Up to 85% of persons with acute HCV infection progress to chronic HCV infection; the remainder are considered to have resolved HCV infection and remain positive for anti-HCV in serum without evidence of viral replication (i.e., HCV RNA is undetectable in serum).
- Cirrhosis ultimately develops in 20% or more of patients with chronic hepatitis B or C.
- Patients with chronic hepatitis B and superimposed HDV infection tend to progress more rapidly to cirrhosis than those with chronic hepatitis B alone.

> Hepatocellular carcinoma is a serious complication of chronic hepatitis B (with or without cirrhosis), chronic hepatitis D, and HCV-related cirrhosis.

Diagnosis

Hepatitis A and E
- IgM anti-HAV and IgM anti-HEV are diagnostic of acute hepatitis A and hepatitis E, respectively.

Hepatitis B
- Acute hepatitis B:
  - HBsAg is the first serologic marker seen in persons with acute HBV infection. It signifies the presence of HBV virions in serum. The first antibody that appears is IgM anti-HBc.
  - The hallmark of acute hepatitis B is elevation of ALT levels and both HBsAg and IgM anti-HBc in serum. Figure 13.1 shows the time course of viral antigens and antibodies in acute self-limiting HBV infection.
  - After acute hepatitis B resolves, >95% of adult patients clear HBsAg, develop antibody to HBsAg (anti-HBs), and recover fully. See Table 13.2.
- Chronic hepatitis B:
  - Chronic hepatitis B is defined as persistence of HBsAg for at least 6 months. Persons with chronic hepatitis B are classified based on the presence or absence of active viral replication (HBV DNA > 2×10^3 IU / mL, HBeAg, elevated serum ALT levels, and active inflammation or fibrosis on a liver biopsy specimen, as outlined below and in Figure 13.2.

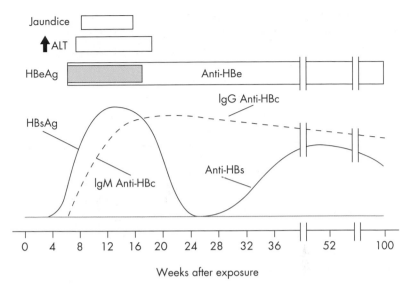

Figure 13.1 Time course of the expression of hepatitis B virus (HBV) antigens and antibodies in acute self-limited HBV infection. (ALT, alanine aminotransferase; anti-HBc, antibody to hepatitis B core antigen; anti-HBe, antibody to hepatitis B e antigen; anti-HBs, antibody to hepatitis B surface Ag; HBeAg, hepatitis B e antigen; HBsAg, hepatitis B surface antigen; Ig, immunoglobulin). (Redrawn with permission from original figure in Fauci, A.S., Kasper, D.L., Braunwald, E., et al. (2008) *Harrison's Principles of Internal Medicine,* 17th edn, McGraw-Hill, New York.)

- Immune-tolerant phase. Persons who are infected as neonates or as young children may have elevated levels of HBV DNA and detectable HBeAg in serum, but normal serum ALT levels, with minimal histologic evidence of liver damage.
- Immune-active phase. Some persons who are immune-tolerant may enter the immune-active phase of disease. Unresolved acute hepatitis B in an adult may progress to the immune-active phase of chronic hepatitis B. The HBV DNA and ALT levels remain elevated in serum, and there is histologic evidence of active inflammation and fibrosis.
- Inactive carrier. Typically, the immune-active phase ends with loss of HBeAg and the appearance of anti-HBe (HBeAg "seroconversion"). In these patients, the serum HBV DNA level is usually less than $2 \times 10^3 \, \text{IU/mL}$, the serum ALT level is normal, and there is minimal inflammation and fibrosis on liver biopsy specimens.

Table 13.2 Interpretation of hepatitis B serologic tests.

	HBsAg	IgG anti-HBs	IgG anti-HBc	IgM anti-HBc	HBeAg	Anti-HBe	HBV DNA (IU/mL)	ALT
Acute hepatitis B	+	−	−	+	+	−	$>2 \times 10^3$	Elevated
Natural immunity	−	+	+	−	−	−	Undetectable	Normal
Vaccination	−	+	−	−	−	−	Undetectable	Normal
Chronic hepatitis B (persistence of HBsAg for >6 months)								
Immune-tolerant phase	+	−	+	−	+	−	$>2 \times 10^3$	Normal
Immune-active phase	+	−	+	−	+	−	$>2 \times 10^3$	Elevated
Inactive carrier	+	−	+	−	−	+	$<2 \times 10^3$	Normal
Reactivation phase	+	−	+	−	−	+	$>2 \times 10^3$	Elevated

Anti-HBc, antibody to hepatitis B core antigen; anti-HBe, antibody to hepatitis B e antigen; anti-HBs, antibody to hepatitis B surface antigen; HBeAg, hepatitis B e antigen; HBsAg, hepatitis B surface antigen; Ig, immunoglobulin; IU, international units.

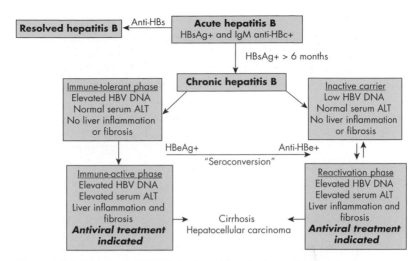

Figure 13.2 Outcomes of HBV infection. (ALT, alanine aminotransferase; anti-HBc, antibody to hepatitis B core antigen; anti-HBe, antibody to hepatitis B e antigen; elevated HBV DNA, $>2 \times 10^3$ IU/mL; HBeAg, hepatitis B e antigen; HBsAg, hepatitis B surface antigen; Ig, immunoglobulin.)

- Reactivation phase. Some persons who have undergone HBeAg seroconversion may later enter the "reactivation phase." These persons remain HBeAg negative (and anti-HBeAg positive) but have serum HBV DNA levels greater than 2×10^3 IU/mL, elevated serum ALT levels and histologic evidence of active inflammation and fibrosis. These persons presumably were infected with wild-type virus at some point, and, over time, they acquired mutations in either the pre-core or the core promoter region of the HBV genome, or both. In such patients with pre-core/core mutations, HBV continues to replicate, but HBeAg is not produced. The pre-core/core mutation state is seen in 20% of patients with chronic hepatitis B in the US and 30–50% of patients in Africa and Asia.
- Immunity to hepatitis B. The detection of anti-HBs in serum indicates immunity to HBV. When present as the only serologic marker, anti-HBs generally signifies immunity as a result of prior vaccination against HBV. The presence in serum of both IgG anti-HBc and anti-HBs indicates immunity as a result of past infection.

Hepatitis C

- Anti-HCV in serum, as measured by enzyme-linked immunosorbent assay (ELISA), may indicate active or prior HCV infection. Confirmation

of the result with a recombinant immunoblot assay (RIBA) indicates a true-positive ELISA result, although a RIBA test is not usually necessary.
- HCV RNA in serum indicates active infection. All positive anti-HCV test results should be followed by measurement of the HCV RNA level in the serum.
- Six major HCV genotypes have been described (1 through 6). Three HCV genotypes are prevalent in the US (1 (a and b), 2, and 3). Determination of the HCV genotype is recommended after diagnosis of HCV infection because the treatment and response to treatment vary with the genotype (see later). There is no correlation between genotype and rate of progression of fibrosis.

Hepatitis D
- IgM antibody to HDV (IgM anti-HDV) indicates acute infection, and total anti-HDV indicates chronic co-infection. If available, HDAg and HDV RNA in serum indicate active infection (acute or chronic).

Treatment and Prevention

Hepatitis A
- Acute hepatitis A is managed with supportive care (e.g., bed rest, fluids, fever-reducing medications), usually guided by symptoms.
- HAV vaccine is recommended for all infants as well as for adults who are at high risk of infection (e.g., travelers to developing countries, persons with human immunodeficiency virus (HIV) infection, patients with chronic liver disease, men who have sex with men, workers at daycare centers). The dose of HAV vaccine (inactivated HAV) is 1 mL and 0.5 mL intramuscularly in adults and children, respectively. A booster dose is recommended 6 months after the initial dose.
- Postexposure prophylaxis with immune globulin (0.02 mL/kg intramuscularly) is recommended for household and intimate contacts of patients with HAV infection. In healthy persons aged 1 to 40, the HAV vaccine can be administered instead of immune globulin.

Hepatitis B
- Acute HBV infection is managed with supportive care. Nucleoside or nucleotide analogs (see below) are sometimes administered in severe cases of acute HBV infection.
- Chronic HBV infection:
  - The agents currently used for the treatment of chronic hepatitis B include subcutaneous pegylated interferon alpha and the oral

nucleoside or nucleotide analogs: telbivudine, entecavir, tenofovir, adefovir, and lamivudine. The preferred first-line agents are entecavir and tenofovir.

○ Candidates for antiviral therapy include patients with chronic hepatitis B who have evidence of active viral replication (HBV DNA >2 × 10^4 IU/mL (HBeAg positive) or >2 × 10^3 IU/mL (HBeAg negative), elevated serum ALT levels, and inflammation or fibrosis on a liver biopsy specimen).

○ The primary goal of antiviral treatment of HBV infection is suppression of viral replication. Secondary goals of therapy are to reduce symptoms and delay the progression of chronic hepatitis to cirrhosis or hepatocellular carcinoma.

• Vaccination and prevention:
○ HBV vaccine: vaccines derived from recombinant HBsAg are used to stimulate the production of anti-HBs in uninfected persons. The available vaccines are highly effective, with serconversion rates of greater than 95%. Vaccine administration is recommended for all infants and for adults who are at increased risk of infection (e.g., those receiving dialysis, healthcare workers, persons with high-risk sexual practices). The recommended vaccination schedule for infants is at the time of birth (before hospital discharge), at 1–2 months, and at 6–18 months. The recommended vaccination schedule for adults is 0, 1, and 6 months.

○ Post-exposure prophylaxis: hepatitis B immune globulin (HBIG, 0.5 mL intramuscularly) provides passive immunization for persons who are exposed to persons with acute hepatitis B or for contacts of persons who are positive for HBsAg in serum. Recommendations are as follows:

■ perinatal exposure: HBIG plus initiation of the vaccine series at time of birth;

■ anticipated sexual contact with an acutely infected patient: HBIG plus vaccine series;

■ sexual contact with a chronic carrier: vaccine series;

■ household contact with an acutely infected person resulting in exposure: HBIG plus vaccine series;

■ household contact with a chronically infected person: vaccine series;

■ infants (<12 months) cared for primarily by an acutely infected patient: HBIG plus vaccine series;

■ inadvertent percutaneous or permucosal exposure: HBIG plus vaccine series.

Reactivation of quiescent HBV infection leading to potentially life-threatening hepatitis is common in inactive HBV (HBsAg positive) carriers who undergo treatment with chemotherapy or immunosuppressant therapy. All candidates for chemotherapy or immunosuppressant therapy should be tested for HBV, and if positive, should be treated with antiviral agents prior to initiation of chemotherapy or immunosuppressant therapy.

Patients with chronic hepatitis B (or with chronic hepatitis C and cirrhosis) should undergo biannual screening with abdominal ultrasonography; often the serum alpha fetoprotein (AFP) level is also measured biannually.

Hepatitis C

- Acute hepatitis C is detected infrequently. When diagnosed at an acute stage, early treatment with pegylated interferon alpha should be considered.
- Chronic hepatitis:
  - Current treatment includes peginterferon alpha-2a or peginterferon alpha-2b in combination with ribavirin and, in persons infected with HCV genotype 1, a protease inhibitor (see below).
  - The goal of treatment is to achieve a sustained viral response (SVR), defined as the absence of detectable HCV RNA in serum 6 months after the completion of antiviral treatment. It is generally accepted that the achievement of SVR indicates viral eradication, or cure, of HCV infection.
  - In patients infected with HCV genotype 1 or prior nonresponse to or relapse following treatment with pegylated interferon alpha and ribavirin, the addition of a protease inhibitor, telaprevir or boceprevir, to pegylated interferon and ribavirin increases SVR.
  - Recently, genome-wide association studies have identified single nucleotide polymorphisms in the *IL28B* gene (that encodes interferon lambda-3) as important determinants of treatment response to peginterferon.
    - Response to peginterferon is strongly associated with the CC genotype of the *IL28B* gene, with a SVR as high as 80% compared with 40% for the CT genotype and 30% for the TT genotype, in patients with treated peginterferon and ribavirin. (The CC genotype is also associated with a higher rate of spontaneous recovery following acute hepatitis C.)

The dose, duration, and attainment of SVR depend on the HCV genotype. With treatment with peginterferon and ribavirin, SVR is achieved in 75–80% of patients infected with HCV genotypes 2 and 3 treated for 24 weeks, and 40–45% of patients HCV genotype 1a or 1b treated for 48 weeks, but approximately 70% when a protease inhibitor is included in the regimen (with many patients requiring only 24 weeks of therapy).

Knowledge of a patient's *IL28B* genotype potentially will aid in treatment decisions. The role of *IL28B* genotype testing before treatment with three-drug combinations, including a a protease inhibitor, is under study.

Hepatitis D

- The treatment of patients co-infected with HBV and HDV is not well studied. HBV-HDV-co-infected patients are less responsive to peginterferon therapy than patients infected with HBV alone. Nucleoside and nucleotide analogs do not suppress HDV.

Pearls

Hepatitis B and C can lead to chronic liver disease, whereas hepatitis A and E do not lead to chronic liver disease.

Acute hepatitis B progresses to chronic infection in less than 5% of immunocompetant adults, whereas acute hepatitis B infection progresses to chronic liver disease in 90–95% of neonates and 25–30% of children.

Acute HCV infection progresses to chronic infection in up to 85% of persons.

Hepatitis A, B, and E can be prevented with the administration of vaccine. A vaccine has not been developed for hepatitis C.

Chronic hepatitis B and C can be treated with antiviral agents that prevent progression of disease.

Questions

Questions 1 to 3 relate to the clinical vignette at the beginning of this chapter.

1. Which of the following is the most likely diagnosis?
   A. Acute hepatitis A
   B. Acute hepatitis B
   C. Acute hepatitis A and previous hepatitis B infection
   D. Previous hepatitis A and acute hepatitis B
   E. Acute hepatitis A and previous hepatitis B vaccination

2. Which one of the following statements is TRUE regarding the patient's acute illness?

(Continued)

A. It is a result of an infection with a DNA virus.

B. He could have avoided the infection if he had been vaccinated prior to travel.

C. Measuring viral DNA levels in serum at the time of infection would have confirmed the diagnosis.

D. He is at risk of cirrhosis.

E. He has an increased risk of developing hepatocellular carcinoma.

3. Appropriate management of the patient includes:

A. Supportive care

B. Lamuvidine

C. Peginterferon alfa-2a

D. Supportive care plus immunoglobulin

E. Supportive care followed by HAV vaccine.

4. The following hepatitis B serologic profile is found in an asymptomatic 40-year-old man:

HBsAg	Positive
Anti-HBs	Negative
IgG anti-HBc	Positive
IgM anti-HBc	Negative
HBeAg	Positive
Anti-HBe	Negative

Which of the following is the best interpretation of this profile?

A. Past hepatitis B infection

B. Acute hepatitis B

C. Inactive HBV carrier

D. Chronic hepatitis B

E. Hepatitis B vaccination

5. Which of the following is a DNA virus?

A. Hepatitis A

B. Hepatitis B

C. Hepatitis C

D. Hepatitis D

E. Hepatitis E

6. Which one of the following antibodies signifies immunity to reinfection?

A. Anti-HBs

B. Anti-HBe

C. Anti-HBc

D. Anti-HCV

E. None of the above

7. A 57-year-old-man is seen in your office for increasing fatigue, anorexia, and jaundice. He was seen in the office 3 months ago for the same

symptoms, and you diagnosed acute hepatitis A based on the results of serologic tests. He says that his symptoms improved gradually during the next month, but he has noticed recurrence of symptoms over the past 3 weeks. The patient also has essential hypertension and has taken hydrochlorothiazide, 50 mg daily, for the past 3 years. On examination he appears jaundiced. The liver edge is palpable below the costal margin, and the liver span is 10 cm. There is no splenomegaly or ascites. Laboratory test results are listed below.

AST	872 U/L
ALT	780 U/L
Alkaline phosphatase	128 U/L
Bilirubin:	
Total	11.4 mg/dL
Direct	10.1 mg/dL
IgM anti-HAV	Positive
HBsAg	Negative
Anti-HBs	Positive
IgG anti-HBc	Negative
Anti-HCV	Negative

What is the most likely diagnosis of this patient's condition?
A. Relapsing hepatitis A
B. Acute hepatitis B
C. Chronic hepatitis B
D. Acute hepatitis C
E. Drug-induced hepatitis

8. A 35-year-old Asian woman who immigrated to the US 3 years ago undergoes an annual health examination. She feels well and is asymptomatic. Her fiancé is known to be negative for HBsAg. Physical examination is normal, and her serum aminotransferase levels are normal. Because she is Asian, you screen her for hepatitis B and find that she is positive for HBsAg. Additional testing shows that HBV DNA is undetectable, HBeAg negative, anti-HBe positive. Which of the following should you recommend for the patient's fiancé at this time?
A. Administer hepatitis B vaccine now
B. Administer hepatitis B serum immunoglobulin (HBIG) now
C. Prescribe lamivudine now
D. No prophylaxis or treatment for hepatitis B is required

9. A former intravenous drug user acquired chronic viral hepatitis from sharing needles. He has evidence of chronic hepatitis C and resolved

(Continued)

hepatitis B. Which of the following statements is TRUE of his HBV and HCV infections?
A. It is more common for hepatitis C than hepatitis B to become chronic in drug users
B. He is at risk for hepatocellular carcinoma because of his past history of hepatitis B infection
C. The risk of transmitting HCV to his wife is >20% if he does not use condoms
D. He is more likely to respond to antiviral treatment for chronic hepatitis C if he is infected with HCV genotype 1 than genotype 2 or 3

Answers

1. C
   The patient is positive for IgM anti-HAV, indicating acute hepatitis A. This diagnosis is consistent with the elevated serum aminotransferase and bilirubin levels. Although the patient reports a history of alcohol use, the serum aminotransferases are not consistent with alcoholic hepatitis. The serum aminotransferase levels in persons with alcoholic hepatitis are typically less than 500 U/L, and the AST/ALT ratio is <1 (see Chapter 14). The patient also has anti-HBs and IgG anti-HBc indicating past infection with HBV (natural immunity).
2. B
   HAV is an RNA virus. HAV vaccine is readily available, and the patient could have avoided HAV infection if he had received the vaccine prior to travel. Hepatitis A does not progress to chronic liver disease, and patients are not at risk of cirrhosis or hepatocellular carcinoma.
3. A
   Acute hepatitis A is managed with supportive care (bed rest, fluids, and fever-reducing medicines), usually guided by the severity of symptoms. Following recovery, patients develop natural immunity (appearance of IgG anti-HAV in serum) and hence do not need HAV vaccination. Antiviral medications have no role in the management of acute hepatitis A.
4. D
5. B
6. A
7. A
   Relapse of acute HAV infection can occur in 3–20% of patients with acute hepatitis A. Following a typical acute course of HAV infection, a remission phase occurs, with partial or complete resolution of clinical and biochemical manifestations. Relapse can occur shortly after symptom resolution and mimics the initial presentation, although it usually is clinically milder.

Recrudescence of symptoms and biochemical abnormalities, along with reappearance of IgM anti-HAV in serum, is diagnostic of relapsing hepatitis A. Recovery eventually occurs.

8. A

The patient is an inactive carrier of HBV and has a low chance of transmitting HBV to her partner. However, her fiancé should be given the hepatitis B vaccine series to protect against transmission in case the patient's hepatitis B reactivates.

9. A

At least 95% of immunocompetent adults with acute HBV infection recover and do not progress to chronic hepatitis B. However, a majority of patients acutely infected with HCV progress to chronic hepatitis C. In this patient, there is no risk of sequelae from HBV infection, which has resolved. The risk of sexual transmission of HCV is low (<2.5%). HCV genotypes 2 and 3 are more responsive than genotype 1 to antiviral therapy.

Further Reading

Balagopal, A., Thomas, D.L. and Thio, C.L. (2010) IL28B and the control of hepatitis C virus infection. *Gastroenterology*, 139, 1865–1876.

Ghany, M.G., Strader, D.B., Thomas, D.L., et al. (2009) Diagnosis, management, and treatment of hepatitis C: an update. American Association for the Study of Liver Diseases. *Hepatology*, 49, 1335–1374.

Servoss, J.C. and Friedman, L.S. (2006) Serologic and molecular diagnosis of hepatitis B virus. *Infectious Disease Clinics of North America*, 20, 47–61.

Sjogren, M.H. and Cheatham, J.G. (2010) Hepatitis A, in *Sleisenger and Fordtran's Gastrointestinal and Liver Disease: Pathophysiology/Diagnosis/Management*, 9th edn (eds M. Feldman, L.S. Friedman and L.J. Brandt), Saunders Elsevier, Philadelphia, pp. 1279-86.

Weblinks

http://www.cdc.gov/hepatitis/
http://digestive.niddk.nih.gov/ddiseases/pubs/viralhepatitis/
http://emedicine.medscape.com/article/185463-overview
http://gastro.ucsd.edu/fellowship/Documents/AASLD.HBV.guidelines.pdf

Alcoholic Liver Disease and Nonalcoholic Fatty Liver Disease

Andrew J. Simpson and Ryan M. Ford

CHAPTER 14

Clinical Vignette 1

A 52-year-old man is found unconscious and brought to the emergency department by an ambulance. The patient is unable to provide a history, but his breath smells of alcohol. Physical examination reveals a blood pressure of 160/104 mmHg, pulse rate 120/min, respiratory rate 24/min, and temperature 101 °F (38.3 °C). The patient is arousable only to painful stimuli, the conjunctivae are icteric, and the mucous membranes are dry. The pupils are reactive to light, and reflexes are 2+ and symmetrical; plantar reflex is flexor bilaterally. Chest and cardiovascular examinations are unremarkable. Abdominal examination reveals tender hepatosplenomegaly. There is no extremity or sacral edema. Skin examination is unremarkable. Laboratory tests are significant for a white blood cell (WBC) count of 19800/mm^3 with 80% neutrophils, 10% band forms, and 8% lymphocytes. The hemoglobin level is 10.0 g/dL, platelet count 100000/mm^3, aspartate aminotransferase (AST) 181 U/L, alanine aminotransferase (ALT) 85 U/L, total bilirubin 10.8 mg/dL, direct bilirubin 7.9 mg/dL, and international standardized ratio (INR) 1.8. Computed tomography (CT) of the head without contrast reveals no intracranial hemorrhage. Urinalysis reveals trace protein, 0 WBCs, 10 RBCs per high-power field, 1+ bilirubin, 2+ urobilinogen, and negative leukocyte esterase. A urine drug screen is negative.

Definition

- Alcoholic liver disease and nonalcoholic fatty liver disease (NAFLD) represent a spectrum of liver diseases characterized initially by the accumulation of triglycerides in hepatocytes.

Essentials of Gastroenterology, First Edition. Edited by Shanthi V. Sitaraman, Lawrence S. Friedman.

- The spectrum of alcoholic liver disease and NAFLD include:
  - steatosis (also called fatty liver): a reversible accumulation of triglycerides without inflammation;
  - steatohepatitis: steatotic hepatocytes with pericellular inflammation;
  - cirrhosis: advanced steatohepatitis with fibrosis and regenerating nodules;
  - cirrhosis can lead to end-stage liver disease (ESLD) and its complications, including portal hypertension and hepatocellular carcinoma (HCC) (see Chapters 15 and 16).
- Histologically, steatosis may be **macrovesicular**, in which lipid accumulation compresses and displaces the hepatocyte nucleus to the periphery of the cell, or **microvesicular**, in which lipid accumulates in small droplets.
  - Alcohol-induced fatty liver and NAFLD cause predominantly macrovesicular steatosis.
  - Microvesicular steatosis occurs as a result of impaired mitochondrial beta-oxidation of free fatty acids. Liver disease associated with microvesicular steatosis is more severe with multiple systemic effects and can be fatal. Causes of microvesicular steatosis include:
    - drugs: ethanol, valproic acid, high-dose intravenous tetracycline, amiodarone, aspirin, nevirapine, stavudine, didanosine, and piroxicam;
    - acute fatty liver of pregnancy;
    - inborn errors of metabolism affecting beta-oxidation of free fatty acids;
    - Reye's syndrome: a potentially fatal disease that is characterized by encephalopathy and multiorgan failure. It is associated with aspirin use in children with a viral illness but may also occur in the absence of aspirin use.

Alcoholic Liver Disease

General

- Steatosis typically develops after consumption of 80 g of alcohol (e.g., six beers or 8 ounces (240 mL) of 80-proof liquor) daily over one to several days.
- The development of cirrhosis is associated with the consumption of 40–80 g of alcohol daily in men and 20–40 g daily in women for a minimum of 10 years.
- Cirrhosis develops in 10–15% of alcoholics (see definition below).

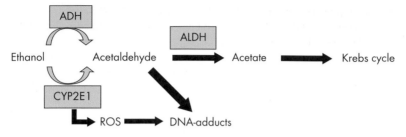

Figure 14.1 Alcohol metabolism. (ADH, alcohol dehydrogenase; ALDH, acetaldehyde dehydrogenase; CYP2E1, cytochrome P450 2E1; ROS, reactive oxygen species.)

Steatosis is completely reversible if alcohol consumption is stopped.

- Approximately 20% of ingested alcohol is absorbed into the systemic circulation through the stomach and metabolized by hepatocytes through oxidation of alcohol to acetaldehyde by the enzyme alcohol dehydrogenase (ADH) (Figure 14.1).
  - ADH is the rate-limiting enzyme in alcohol metabolism, and its activity varies with race, gender, and genetic polymorphisms.
  - Women, Native Americans, Asians, and the elderly have lower levels of gastric ADH. This may account in part for the observation that women are more susceptible than men to liver injury for a given dose of alcohol consumed.
- Gastric ADH may account for up to 10% of "first-pass" metabolism through oxidation of ethanol before intestinal absorption occurs. The dose of ethanol, concomitant food ingestion, and gastric emptying rate may affect first-pass gastric metabolism of ethanol.
- Acetaldehyde is an unstable metabolite of ethanol that forms adducts with macromolecules through the Schiff-base reaction. Acetaldehyde can impair mitochondrial function, destroy hepatocyte membranes, and interfere with normal transcriptional activity of the cell. It is more injurious to hepatocytes than ethanol.
- Acetaldehyde is rapidly converted to acetate, an inert and inactive metabolite, by aldehyde dehydrogenase (ALDH). Acetate is eventually converted to CO_2 and H_2O by the Krebs cycle.
- An alternative pathway for hepatic alcohol metabolism involves the microsomal ethanol-oxidizing system and cytochrome P450 (CYP) 2E1. This pathway also produces acetaldehyde and reactive oxygen species that contribute to fatty liver and depletion of glutathione.

○ This pathway is induced in chronic alcoholism and increases susceptibility to drug-induced liver injury from agents such as isoniazid, acetaminophen, or cocaine.

> Acetaldehyde is responsible for many of the systemic toxic effects of alcohol, such as nausea, headaches, palpitations, and flushing. The "Oriental flush syndrome" is due to mutations in the ALDH gene that result in deficiency of the enzyme, thereby leading to toxic effect of acetaldehyde in persons who consume alcohol.

Alcoholic Steatosis

* In most persons, ingesting alcohol leads to triglyceride accumulation within the cytoplasm of the hepatocyte. This process is reversible, but persons with chronic alcoholism may develop progressive liver injury (inflammation, fibrosis) over time.
* Patients with steatosis are asymptomatic. Physical examination may reveal hepatomegaly. Laboratory tests are frequently normal in persons with fatty liver. If serum aminotransferase levels are elevated, the AST:ALT ratio is typically ≥ 2.
* The diagnosis of fatty liver is based on clinical suspicion. The diagnosis of alcohol abuse is based on history and standardized screening tools such as the Alcohol Use Disorders Identification Test-Consumption (AUDIT-C) questions, and the CAGE (need to cut down, annoyed by criticism, guilty about drinking, need an eye-opener in the morning) questionnaire. Mean corpuscular volume (MCV) and the serum gamma-glutamyl transpeptidase (GGTP) level may be elevated in chronic alcoholism.
* Treatment is abstinence from alcohol, which quickly reverses fatty liver. To help maintain abstinence, intensive counseling with or without concominant medications (acamprosate, baclofen, naltrexone, disulfiram) is recommended.

Alcoholic Hepatitis

General
* Alcoholic hepatitis may occur with or without fatty liver. It may occur acutely in a subset of patients with chronic alcohol-induced liver disease, and it ranges in severity from mild to life-threatening.
* Alcoholic hepatitis is potentially fatal. The 5-year survival rate in patients with alcoholic hepatitis is estimated to be 50–75%. Even patients who recover are at increased risk for developing cirrhosis.

Clinical and Laboratory Features
- Patients may present with fever, anorexia, nausea, vomiting, jaundice, abdominal pain, or diarrhea.
- The most common finding on examination is tender hepatomegaly. Some patients may have prolonged fever, typically >102.2 °F (39 °C). On physical examination, patients with severe alcoholic hepatitis may have spider angiomas, splenomegaly, jaundice, ascites, hepatic encephalopathy, and peripheral edema.
- Laboratory tests may reveal an elevated WBC count with neutrophil predominance. Patients may have megaloblastic anemia. Serum AST and ALT levels are elevated in a ratio of at least 2:1 and are typically <500 U/L even with severe disease. The ALT may be normal, in part because of concomitant pyridoxine deficiency. The total bilirubin level can be as high as 40 mg/dL. The serum albumin level is typically low, often <2 g/dL. The prothrombin time is markedly prolonged in severe disease.

Diagnosis
- The diagnosis of alcoholic hepatitis is made by history, physical examination, and laboratory tests. Liver biopsy is seldom needed to make the diagnosis.
  - Classic histologic features in the liver include a polymorphonuclear leukocyte (PMN) infiltrate, Mallory bodies (or Mallory hyaline), steatosis, pericentral collagen deposition, hepatocyte ballooning degeneration, and varying degrees of fibrosis (see Chapter 26).

Prognosis
- Estimating the prognosis is important in determining the need for specific drug treatment. The 28-day mortality rate may be as high as 75% in patients with severe disease.
- Four clinical indices have been shown to predict mortality:
  - The Maddrey Discrimination Function (DF) is calculated as 4.6 × (the patient's prothrombin time – control prothrombin time in seconds) + total bilirubin (mg/dL). A DF >32 indicates severe disease and is associated with a mortality rate of up to 50% at 4 weeks.
  - The Model for End-Stage Liver Disease (MELD) score utilizes the serum bilirubin, INR, and serum creatinine (see Chapter 16).
  - The Glasgow alcoholic hepatitis score utilizes the patient's age, WBC count, blood urea nitrogen level, prothrombin time ratio (ratio of the patient's prothrombin time to the control value), and serum bilirubin level.
  - The Lille Model score incorporates age, serum bilirubin level on presentation, bilirubin level at day 7, serum creatinine, serum

albumin, and prothrombin time. Failure of the serum bilirubin to decline by day 7 is an adverse prognostic sign.

Treatment
- The most important therapy is abstinence from alcohol.
- Nutritional support improves long-term survival. It is no longer considered necessary to restrict the patient's protein calories, and enteral feedings are preferred, even if a nasogastric feeding tube is required. A high-calorie diet with multivitamins, thiamine, and folic acid supplementation is recommended.
- Medical treatments include:
  - Glucocorticoids:
    - used in patients with severe disease (encephalopathy, DF ≥32, MELD score ≥18, or Glasgow score ≥9);
    - the recommended regimen is prednisone 40 mg daily for 28 days, followed by 20 mg daily for 7 days and 10 mg daily for 7 days;
    - contraindications include gastrointestinal bleeding requiring blood transfusion and systemic infection;
    - prednisone is not effective in patients with hepatorenal syndrome.
  - Pentoxifylline:
    - used as an alternative agent to glucocorticoids in patients with a contraindication to the use of glucocorticoids or in patients with renal failure. The recommended dose is 400 mg orally three times daily for 4 weeks.

Alcoholic Cirrhosis

General
- Cirrhosis is an irreversible complication of alcoholic liver disease and other forms of chronic liver disease (see Chapter 15).
- Histopathologic findings indicating alcoholic cirrhosis do not reliably correlate with clinical findings.

Clinical and Laboratory Features
- Patients with compensated cirrhosis are often asymptomatic or may have nonspecific constitutional symptoms such as fatigue, anorexia, or weight loss.
- Patients with decompensated cirrhosis may present with jaundice, weakness, abdominal pain, or symptoms of portal hypertension, such as ascites, encephalopathy, or variceal bleeding (see Chapter 16).

- The physical examination may reveal hepatosplenomegaly; however, the examination is often normal in patients with well compensated cirrhosis.
- Patients with decompensated cirrhosis may show muscle wasting, jaundice, spider angiomas, palmar erythema, gynecomastia, a small liver, ascites, caput medusae, asterixis, and fetor hepaticus (a distinct odor to the breath that is caused by volatile aromatic substances that accumulate in the setting of cirrhosis).
- Findings on laboratory tests may include elevated serum aminotransferase and bilirubin levels, an increased INR, a low serum albumin level, anemia, an increased mean corpuscular volume, a low platelet count, and evidence of renal insufficiency.

Diagnosis

- The diagnosis of alcoholic cirrhosis is based on history, physical examination, and laboratory tests.
- Abdominal imaging by ultrasonography, CT, or magnetic resonance imaging (MRI) may show a nodular and shrunken liver, in addition to signs of portal hypertension (ascites, varices, and/or splenomegaly).

Patients with alcoholic cirrhosis are susceptibile to sudden decompensation. Factors that contribute to decompensation in an otherwise stable person with cirrhosis include acetaminophen toxicity, viral illness (e.g., influenza), portal vein thrombosis, and hepatocellular carcinoma (HCC). Once the diagnosis of cirrhosis is established, a patient is at risk of developing decompensated liver disease and HCC, even if the person abstains from alcohol or has no symptoms of chronic liver disease.

Prognosis

- The overall 5-year survival rate for patients with alcoholic cirrhosis is 50–75%. The survival rate decreases dramatically with the development of ascites, spontaneous bacterial peritonitis, hepatorenal syndrome, or hepatic encephalopathy (see Chapter 16).
- The clinical tools used most widely to determine prognosis in patients with alcoholic cirrhosis are the Child–Turcotte–Pugh (CTP) score (Child–Pugh classification) and the MELD score (see above). The CTP score is based on the serum bilirubin, ascites, serum albumin, INR, and encephalopathy.

Chronic hepatitis C virus (HCV) infection, obesity, and smoking are independent risk factors for the progression of alcoholic liver disease to cirrhosis.

Treatment

- The treatment of patients with alcoholic cirrhosis involves abstinence from alcohol, which is beneficial even in patients with decompensated cirrhosis.
- Nutritional supplementation with thiamine, folic acid, vitamin B12, and magnesium is often necessary.
- The management of portal hypertension is outlined in Chapter 16.
- Liver transplantation is definitive treatment for patients with decompensated cirrhosis; the MELD score is an important determinant for the eligibility for transplantation (see Chapter 16). Given the dramatic benefits of abstinence from alcohol, a period of abstinence is recommended prior to transplantation.

Nonalcoholic Fatty Liver Disease

Clinical Vignette 2

A 55-year-old woman was found to have elevated serum aminotransferase levels when she applied for life insurance. She presents to her primary care physician for evaluation. She is asymptomatic. Her past medical history is significant for type 2 diabetes mellitus, hypertension, hypercholesterolemia, obesity, and osteoarthritis. She has never used alcohol or tobacco and denies use of illicit drugs. She works as a bank teller. Her mother died from cirrhosis of unknown cause. There is a strong family history of obesity and type 2 diabetes mellitus; an older brother died of a myocardial infarction at age 58; her sister has chronic kidney disease and is dialysis dependent. She notes that weight loss programs and diet pills have not worked for her; chronic back and knee pain prohibit her from participating in vigorous exercise. Medications include pioglitazone, glyburide, metformin, enalapril, simvastatin, and a generic over-the-counter nonsteroidal anti-inflammatory drug (NSAID). Physical examination reveals an obese woman in no distress. The blood pressure is 150/94 mmHg, pulse rate 88/min, respiratory rate 18/min, and temperature 99.3 °F (37.4 °C). Her body mass index (BMI) is 44. An S_4 is heard on auscultation of the heart. The abdomen is obese precluding palpation of the liver or the spleen. Neurologic examination reveals decreased sensation in her toes, and her extremities demonstrate 2+ pitting edema. The remainder of the examination is unremarkable. Laboratory tests reveal a fasting total cholesterol of 312 mg/dL, low-density lipoprotein (LDL) cholesterol 172 mg/dL, high-density lipoprotein (HDL) 28 mg/dL, triglycerides 230 mg/dL, glucose 298 mg/dL, AST 100 U/L, ALT 150 U/L, and hemoglobin A1c 9.8%. Tests for viral hepatitis, human immunodeficiency virus, hereditary hemochromatosis, Wilson disease, autoimmune hepatitis, and alpha-1 antitrypsin deficiency are all unremarkable. Ultrasonography of the right upper quadrant reveals a few gallstones in the gallbladder; the liver is echogenic and heterogeneous.

General

- The estimated prevalence of NAFLD in the U.S. is 10–24%.
- NAFLD is typically diagnosed in the fifth and sixth decades of life; however, the frequency of NAFLD is increasing among obese children and adolescents.
- NAFLD affects men and women equally. Hispanics have the highest frequency of NAFLD (45%) compared with whites (33%) and African Americans (24%). Familial clustering of NAFLD has been reported.
- Many drugs and conditions are associated with NAFLD (Table 14.1), but NAFLD occurs most commonly with the metabolic syndrome, a constellation of clinical disorders that include type 2 diabetes mellitus, essential hypertension, low serum levels of HDL, elevated fasting serum triglycerides, obesity, hypothyroidism, and rarely polycystic ovary syndrome in women.
- The spectrum of NAFLD includes fatty infiltration of the liver without inflammatory changes (nonalcoholic fatty liver, or NAFL) and

Table 14.1 Causes of nonalcoholic fatty liver disease.

Metabolic syndrome:
    Obesity
    Diabetes mellitus
    Hypertension
    Hypertriglyceridemia
    Low high-density lipoprotein levels

Other disorders of lipid metabolism (e.g., abetalipoproteinemia)

Surgical procedures:
    Jejuno-ileal bypass
    Extensive small bowel resection
    Gastric bypass

Drugs:
    Amiodarone
    Methotrexate
    Glucocorticosteroids
    Hormonal therapy (e.g., tamoxifen, high-dose estrogen)

Others:
    Hepatitis C
    Inflammatory bowel disease
    Total parenteral nutrition
    Wilson disease

fatty infiltration of the liver with inflammatory changes (nonalcoholic steatohepatitis, or NASH). NASH may lead to hepatocyte cell death and fibrosis and ultimately cirrhosis.

NAFLD is the most prevalent liver disease in the US and the most common reason a patient is evaluated for elevated serum aminotransferase levels. NAFLD-related cirrhosis has become the second leading indication for liver transplantation in the US (after hepatitis C).

Pathophysiology

- Insulin resistance, particularly hepatic insulin resistance, is the hallmark of NAFLD. Hepatocytes of affected persons escape the normal response to insulin (e.g., glycogen synthesis and storage) and paradoxically synthesize excess glucose and free fatty acids. Skeletal muscle and adipose tissue also have maladaptive responses to hyperglycemia, resulting in increased hepatic concentrations of free fatty acids. The mechanism underlying insulin resistance is not clearly understood and is currently an intense area of investigation.

Clinical and Laboratory Features

- Most patients with NAFLD are asymptomatic. Some patients may have vague right upper quandrant pain or fatigue. Patients with NAFLD-associated cirrhosis may have stigmata of chronic liver disease (see Chapter 15).
- The past medical history is important and may reveal risk factors for NAFLD including diabetes mellitus, hyperlipidemia, and hypertension. Physical examination is nonspecific; hepatomegaly may be present in up to 75% of patients but may be difficult to appreciate due to obesity.
- Results of laboratory studies are nonspecific and most commonly show elevated serum ALT and AST levels (ALT usually greater than AST) and occasionally elevated alkaline phosphatase levels.
- Antinuclear antibodies and smooth muscle antibodies, which typically are associated with autoimmune hepatitis, may be present in low titers.
- NAFLD is often found incidentally on imaging studies and can be seen on ultrasonography (increased echogenicity, seen as "bright liver"), CT (lower density than spleen), or MRI (bright on T1-weighted imaging, see Figure 14.2).
- Histologic features of NAFL and NASH are indistinguishable from those of alcoholic fatty liver and alcoholic hepatitis, respectively.

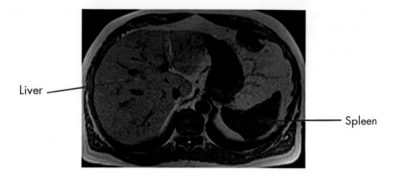

Liver

Spleen

Figure 14.2 Magnetic resonance imaging (MRI) showing hepatic steatosis. On this T1-weighted image, the liver is brighter than the spleen because of fat in the liver.

Diagnosis

- Alcoholic liver disease must be excluded before a diagnosis of NAFLD can be made.
- NAFLD is often a diagnosis of exclusion. Laboratory testing, including antibody to hepatitis C virus, hepatitis B surface antigen, iron indices, ceruloplasmin, alpha-1 antitrypsin level, antinuclear antibodies, smooth muscle antibodies, antimitochondrial antibodies, and trans-glutaminase antibodies, should be conducted to rule out other causes of liver disease.

Prognosis

- The long-term prognosis of patients with NAFLD is unknown. It is estimated that only 3% of patients with NAFL progress to cirrhosis over 7–8 years. Although NASH and alcoholic hepatitis are similar histologically, the prognosis of NASH appears to be substantially better.
- NASH is more concerning than NAFL in terms of overall prognosis; however, it is difficult to predict which patients with NAFLD will progress to NASH or NAFLD-related cirrhosis.

Treatment

- The mainstay of treatment for NAFLD is lifestyle modification:
  - diet, exercise, weight loss, and controlling other metabolic risk factors such as diabetes mellitus, hyperlipidemia, and hypertension;

○ the patient's diet should be balanced but limited in carbohydrate content, saturated fat, and calories.

- Pharmacotherapy for obesity is limited, although tight control of blood sugar in persons with diabetes mellitus is important.

- In patients with obesity, bariatric surgery (laparoscopic banding or gastric bypass) can help reverse steatosis and treat other health problems related to obesity and insulin resistance.

- Metformin and lipid-lowering agents are used to treat insulin resistance and hyperlipidemia, respectively. Statin drugs (3-hydroxy-3-methylglutaryl [HMG]-coenzyme A reductase inhibitors) should not be withheld because of mild aminotransferase elevations.

- Liver transplantation may be considered in persons who develop cirrhosis or hepatocellular carcinoma.

Pearls

The metabolic syndrome is a group of risk factors (obesity, elevated triglycerides, low HDL, hypertension, insulin resistance/diabetes mellitus) that portends a higher risk of NAFLD.

Weight loss can reverse NAFL and NASH and can prevent the development of cirrhosis.

Insulin resistance, particularly hepatic insulin resistance, is the hallmark of NAFLD. Hepatocytes of affected persons escape the normal response to insulin (e.g., glycogen synthesis and storage) and paradoxically synthesize excess glucose and free fatty acids.

Prompt recognition and institution of treatment for severe alcoholic hepatitis reduce mortality.

Questions

Question 1 relates to clinical vignette 1 at the beginning of this chapter.

1. What is the most likely diagnosis?
   A. Acetaminophen-induced fulminant hepatic failure
   B. Acute viral hepatitis
   C. Budd–Chiari syndrome
   D. Acute alcoholic hepatitis
   E. Wilson disease

(Continued)

Questions 2 and 3 relate to clinical vignette 2 earlier in this chapter.

2. Which of the following is the likely cause of the patient's elevated serum aminotransferase levels?
   A. Primary biliary cirrhosis
   B. NAFLD
   C. Alcoholic hepatitis
   D. Acute cholecystitis
   E. Drug-induced hepatotoxicity

3. Which of the following would you recommend to this patient?
   A. Lifestyle modification including a weight-loss program
   B. Cholecystectomy
   C. Discontinue simvastatin
   D. Oral cholestyramine
   E. Liver biopsy

4. A patient has acute alcoholic hepatitis. You are asked to comment on whether glucocorticoids would benefit this patient's hospital outcome. If the Maddrey Discriminant Function is determined to be greater than 32, which of the following is true?
   A. Pentoxifylline and glucocorticoids reduce the mortality rate
   B. Glucocorticoids are beneficial in patients with alcoholic hepatitis who have gastrointestinal bleeding
   C. Colchicine is an effective treatment for acute alcoholic hepatitis
   D. The patient should be placed on parenteral nutrition

5. Which of the following causes macrosteatosis?
   A. Acute fatty liver of pregnancy
   B. Alcohol
   C. High-dose intravenous tetracycline
   D. Reye's syndrome
   E. Valproic acid

6. Which of the following is a likely clinical feature in a patient with NASH?
   A. Low titers of antinuclear antibodies
   B. A family history of autoimmune thyroid disease
   C. Elevated ratio of serum AST to ALT
   D. Low serum ceruloplasmin level
   E. Increased high-density lipoprotein (HDL) cholesterol level

Answers

1. D

   This case has many of the classic features of acute alcoholic hepatitis. The patient has an odor of alcohol on the breath, hypertension, tachycardia, a moderate elevation of serum aminotransferase levels (with an AST:ALT ratio of over 2:1), a neutrophil-predominant leukocytosis, low-grade fever, hepatomegaly, decreased platelet count (that may be due to alcohol-induced bone marrow suppression), a mildly increased INR, and jaundice. Acetaminophen overdose and severe acute viral hepatitis usually present with serum aminotransferase levels above 1000 U/L and do not generally present with deep jaundice until later in the course of disease. Acute viral hepatitis is associated with a lymphocytic leukocytosis. Wilson disease is a chronic liver disease that may present as acute liver failure in younger patients and is usually associated with a low ceruloplasmin level. Budd–Chiari syndrome may present as acute abdominal pain with hepatomegaly, ascites, and even liver failure. Imaging studies generally show hepatic vein thrombosis, and there is often a history of or risk factor for a hypercoagulable state.

2. B

This patient has metabolic syndrome and many of the classic features of NAFLD, and more specifically nonalcoholic steatohepatitis (NASH). The serum ALT level is greater than the AST level, and abdominal ultrasonography shows bright echoes of fat within the liver. Primary biliary cirrhosis tends to cause a cholestatic elevation of liver tests and is typically associated with antimitochondrial antibodies. Although alcoholic liver disease and drug-induced liver injury cannot be entirely ruled out, the history, physical examination, and laboratory findings are more consistent with NAFLD. Gallstones are an incidental finding and commonly found in obese women. The patient has no clinical (e.g., right upper quadrant pain, fever) or radiographic (thickened gallbladder wall with pericholecystic fluid) features of acute cholecystitis.

3. B

The mainstay of treatment for NAFLD is lifestyle modification (diet, exercise, weight loss) and control of risk factors such as hypertension, diabetes mellitus, and hyperlipidemia. Simvastatin should be continued to treat hypercholesterolemia. Cholecystectomy is not indicated for asymptomatic gallstones in this patient. Cholestyramine is a bile-acid binding agent and has no role in the management of NAFLD. Liver biopsy may be considered but is not the next step in the management of this patient.

4. A

In patients with alcoholic hepatitis who have a high mortality rate as predicted by a Maddrey Discriminant Function of greater than 32, glucocorticoids and pentoxifylline have been shown to improve survival. Glucocorticoids are contraindicated if the patient has a severe infection, such as sepsis, or active gastrointestinal bleeding. Colchicine has not been

(Continued)

shown to be beneficial in alcoholic hepatitis. Nutritional support has been shown to improve long-term survival, but enteral, not parenteral, nutrition is the preferred method of feeding.

5. B

Alcohol is associated with predominantly macrovesicular steatosis. The other choices are associated with microvesicular steatosis in which smaller fat droplets are seen on liver biopsy specimens. Microvesicular steatosis is more toxic to hepatocytes than macrovesicular steatosis.

6. A

Antinuclear antibodies and smooth muscle antibodies are normally associated with autoimmune hepatitis but can be seen in low titers in patients with NASH. A personal or family history of autoimmune disease is not typically associated with the metabolic syndrome. Patients with autoimmune causes of liver disease, such as autoimmune hepatitis or primary biliary cirrhosis, may have a family history of other autoimmune diseases, such as Hashimoto's thyroiditis. Low serum ceruloplasmin levels are associated with Wilson disease. Decreased levels of HDL cholesterol are typically seen in the metabolic syndrome.

Further Reading

Akriviadis, E., Botla, R., Briggs, W., et al. (2000) Pentoxifylline improves short-term survival in severe acute alcoholic hepatitis: a double-blind, placebo-controlled trial. *Gastroenterology*, 119, 1637–1648.

Dunn, W., Jamil, L.H., Brown, L.S., et al. (2005) MELD accurately predicts mortality in patients with alcoholic hepatitis. *Hepatology*, 41, 353–358.

Maddrey, W.C., Boitnott, J.K., Bedine, M.S., et al. (1978) Corticosteroid therapy of alcoholic hepatitis. *Gastroenterology*, 75, 193–199.

O'Shea, R.S., Dasarathy, S., McCullough, A.J., et al. (2010) Alcoholic liver disease. Practice Guideline Committee of the American Association for the Study of Liver Diseases and the Practice Parameters Committee of the American College of Gastroenterology. *Hepatology*, 51, 307–328.

Sanyal, A.J., Chalasani, N., Kowdley, K.V., et al. (2010) Pioglitazone, vitamin E, or placebo for nonalcoholic steatohepatitis. *New England Journal of Medicine*, 362, 1675–1685.

Weblinks

http://pubs.niaaa.nih.gov/publications/aa64/aa64.htm
http://www.acg.gi.org/physicians/guidelines/AlcoholicLiverDisease.pdf
http://www.aasld.org/practiceguidelines/Documents/Practice%20 Guidelines/position_nonfattypg.pdf
http://www.digestive.niddk.nih.gov/ddiseases/pubs/nash/

Chronic Liver Disease

Preeti A. Reshamwala

CHAPTER 15

Clinical Vignette

A 59-year-old woman is seen in the office for complaints of fatigue, increasing abdominal girth, pruritus, and diarrhea for the past 4 months. The pruritus is diffuse and is most bothersome at nighttime. She has four to five watery stools each day that usually occur after a meal. She denies blood in the stool, rectal urgency, or tenesmus. She denies recent travel, sick contacts, antibiotic use, or a recent hospitalization. Her husband notes that she is often forgetful and repetitive. She has a history of diabetes mellitus and hypertension but currently takes no medications. She has no history of alcohol, tobacco, or illicit drug use. The family history is unremarkable. Physical examination reveals a blood pressure of 90/60 mmHg, pulse rate 98/min, and respiratory rate 16/min. She is afebrile, alert, and oriented, but with a slow response time. She has mild conjunctival icterus, bitemporal wasting, and multiple spider angiomas on the face and torso. A fluid wave, shifting dullness, and bulging flanks are noted on abdominal examination. She has 2+ lower extremity pitting edema. Rectal examination shows scant brown stool that is negative for occult blood. Laboratory tests show a serum alkaline phosphatase level of 345 U/L, total bilirubin 3 mg/dL, alanine aminotransferase (ALT) 48 U/L, aspartate aminotransferase (AST) 65 U/L, and international normalized ratio (INR) 2.8. Abdominal ultrasonography shows a cirrhotic-appearing liver with normal intra- and extrahepatic bile ducts. Serologic tests are negative except for antimitochondrial antibodies (AMA).

Essentials of Gastroenterology, First Edition. Edited by Shanthi V. Sitaraman, Lawrence S. Friedman.
© 2012 John Wiley & Sons, Ltd. Published 2012 by John Wiley & Sons, Ltd.

General

- Chronic liver disease is a process of progressive destruction and regeneration of the liver parenchyma. Although multiple pathophysiologic mechanisms of injury exist (see later), the final common pathway is hepatic fibrosis that replaces damaged hepatocytes. Although the process may be reversible, continued deposition of dense extracellular matrix can lead to cirrhosis, an irreversible condition that can lead to end-stage liver disease and portal hypertension (see Chapter 16).
- Chronic liver disease may be caused by a number of conditions (Table 15.1). The most common causes of chronic liver disease worldwide are excessive alcohol intake (see Chapter 14), chronic hepatitis B and C (see Chapter 13), and nonalcoholic fatty liver disease (see Chapter 14).

> Cirrhosis is an often irreversible and potentially fatal consequence of untreated chronic liver disease.

Clinical Features

- Most patients with chronic liver disease are asymptomatic. When present, symptoms and signs depend on the etiology, degree of parenchymal damage, and presence of cirrhosis, which may be compensated or decompensated.
- Patients with well compensated cirrhosis may present with anorexia, weight loss, weakness, and fatigue. From 80 to 90% of the liver parenchyma must be destroyed before decompensated cirrhosis is manifested clinically. Persons with decompensated disease may present with ascites, spontaneous bacterial peritonitis, hepatic encephalopathy, and variceal bleeding from portal hypertension (see Chapter 16).
- A thorough history is the first step in identifying the etiology of chronic liver disease. Risk factors that predispose patients to liver disease should be elicited; these include alcohol consumption, risk factors for hepatitis B and C transmission (e.g., birth in endemic areas, high-risk sexual behaviors, intravenous drug use, body piercing, tattooing, prior blood transfusions), and a personal or family history of liver, autoimmune, or metabolic diseases.

Diagnosis

- If liver disease is suspected, a complete blood count and comprehensive metabolic panel should be obtained. Further diagnostic work-up

Table 15.1 Causes of chronic liver disease.

Viral	Autoimmune	Metabolic	Other pediatric	Miscellaneous
Hepatitis B	Autoimmune hepatitis	Alpha-1 antitrypsin deficiency	Biliary atresia	Alcoholic liver disease
Hepatitis C	Primary biliary cirrhosis	Wilson disease	Alagille syndrome	Nonalcoholic fatty liver
Hepatitis D	Primary sclerosing	Hemochromatosis	Congenital biliary cysts	disease
	cholangitis	Disorders of amino acid	Cystic fibrosis	Medications and toxins
		metabolism (e.g., tyrosinemia)		Granulomatous liver disease
		Disorders of carbohydrate		(e.g., sarcoidosis)
		metabolism (e.g., fructose		Cryptogenic chronic liver
		intolerance, galactosemia,		disease/cirrhosis
		glycogen storage diseases)		
		Disorders of lipid metabolism		
		(e.g., abetalipoproteinemia)		
		Porphyria		
		Urea cycle enzyme defects (e.g.,		
		ornithine decarboxylase		
		deficiency)		

should be dictated by the pattern of elevated serum aminotransferase, alkaline phosphatase, and bilirubin levels, as outlined in Chapters 12 and 24.
- Characteristic diagnostic test abnormalities for common chronic liver disease are summarized in Table 15.2.

Autoimmune Hepatitis

- Autoimmune hepatitis (AIH) is a chronic inflammatory condition of the liver characterized by elevated serum autoantibodies, interface hepatitis on histologic examination, and hypergammaglobulinemia.
- Women are more likely to be affected with AIH than men and often are diagnosed in the fifth to sixth decade of life.
- The pathogenesis of AIH is unknown. It is believed to involve a robust immune response to foreign or self antigen resulting in destruction of hepatocytes by a combination of cell- and antibody-mediated cytotoxicity.
- AIH can present as a chronic smoldering disease, cirrhosis without prior documentation of AIH, or acute hepatitis including acute liver failure.
- The elements of diagnosis of AIH include the following:
  - elevated serum aminotransferase levels: serum aminotransferases may be as high as ten or more times the upper limit of normal depending on the clinical presentation;
  - hypergammaglobulinemia with a significantly elevated immunoglobulin G;
  - serum autoantibodies, which include antinuclear antibodies (ANA), smooth muscle antibodies (SMA), and/or anti-liver-kidney-microsomal antibodies (anti-LKM) type 1, may be detected;
  - interface hepatitis (inflammation of the portal tracts extending into the hepatic lobules) on histologic examination of the liver (Figure 15.1): the infiltrate is often predominantly plasmacytic. The bile ducts are generally spared from inflammatory destruction. There may be varying degrees of fibrosis depending on the chronicity of the condition;
  - exclusion of other causes of chronic liver disease, such as chronic hepatitis B, chronic hepatitis C, alcoholic liver disease, Wilson disease, and hemochromatosis.
- Prednisone, usually in combination with azathioprine, is the mainstay of treatment. Budesonide is a potential alternative glucocorticoid to prednisone. Patients who present with acute liver failure may be treated with intravenous glucocorticoids.

Table 15.2 Laboratory test abnormalities in common chronic liver diseases.

Disease	Laboratory test abnormalities
Alcoholic liver disease	AST:ALT ratio ≥2; elevated serum GGTP level
Alpha-1 antitrypsin deficiency	Decreased serum alpha-1 antitrypsin level; genetic screening available but not routinely performed
Autoimmune hepatitis	ANA and/or SMA
Chronic hepatitis B	HBsAg and HBeAg
Chronic hepatitis C	HCV antibody; HCV RNA
Hereditary hemochromatosis	Transferrin saturation ≥45% or unsaturated iron-binding capacity ≥155 μg/dL; *HFE* gene mutation
Nonalcoholic fatty liver disease	Elevated serum AST and/or ALT level; ultrasonography suggestive
Primary biliary cirrhosis	Elevated serum ALP level; AMA
Primary sclerosing cholangitis	MRCP or ERCP
Wilson disease	Serum ceruloplasmin <20 mg/dL (normal: 20–60 mg/dL) or low serum copper level (normal: 80–160 μg/dL); basal 24-hour urinary copper excretion >100 μg (normal: 10-80 μg); genetic screening available but not commonly performed

ALP, alkaline phosphatase; ALT, alanine aminotransferase; AMA, antimitochondrial antibodies; ANA, antinuclear antibody; AST, aspartate aminotransferase; ERCP, endoscopic retrograde cholangiopancreatography; GGTP, gamma-glutamyl transpeptidase; HBeAg, hepatitis B e antigen; HBsAg, hepatitis B surface antigen; HCV, hepatitis C virus; MRCP, magnetic resonance cholangiopancratography; SMA, smooth muscle antibodies.

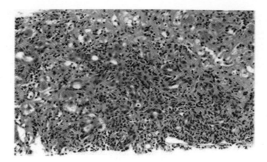

Figure 15.1 Photomicrograph of the liver in autoimmune hepatitis. Note severe interface hepatitis and an intense plasma cell infiltrate. Hematoxylin and eosin, ×10. (Courtesy of Dr. S. Sharma, Emory University, Atlanta, GA, USA.)

- Alternative treatment options for patients with severe side effects or intolerance to standard therapy include immunosuppressants such as mycophenolate mofetil, tacrolimus, and cyclosporine; these drugs often require more frequent monitoring of serum levels and are associated with side effects as well.
- Liver transplantation is an effective treatment and may be considered in patients with decompensated cirrhosis or acute liver failure due to AIH.

Characteristic features of AIH include elevated serum aminotransferases levels, elevated serum immunoglobulin levels, serum autoantibodies, and interface hepatitis with plasma cells on histologic examination of the liver.

Primary Biliary Cirrhosis (PBC)

- Primary biliary cirrhosis (PBC) is an autoimmune disorder characterized by granulomatous destruction of small intrahepatic bile ducts. The result is chronic cholestasis and, in up to one third of patients, cirrhosis.
- The disease affects females and males in a ratio of 9:1.
- The pathogenesis of PBC is unknown. Over 95% of patients with PBC have detectable antimitochondrial antibodies (AMA). AMA target a family of enzymes, including the pyruvate dehydrogenase complex, that are found on the inner membrane of mitochondria.
- A majority of persons with PBC are asymptomatic. Typical symptoms of PBC include fatigue and pruritus. Other symptoms include jaundice, right upper quadrant pain, and anorexia.

- Patients are at increased risk for fat-soluble vitamin deficiency (vitamins A, D, E, K), bone disease (hepatic osteodystrophy), and hypercholesterolemia. Steatorrhea can occur in the late stages of PBC. These clinical problems develop as a result of impaired entero-hepatic circulation of bile salts, which are deficient because of chronic cholestasis (see Chapter 20).
- Other physical findings may include xanthomas, xanthelasma, spider angiomas, and jaundice.
- Laboratory tests typically show a cholestatic picture (see Chapter 20). The serum alkaline phosphatase level is elevated in almost all patients with PBC. The bilirubin level is normal in early stages of the disease and increases as the disease progresses. Serum aminotransferase levels are mildly elevated; levels more than five times the upper limit of normal should raise suspicion of other diseases or of a PBC–AIH "overlap" syndrome.
- Other serologic markers, including ANA, SMA, rheumatoid factor, and antithyroid antibodies, may be detected in up to 50% of patients with PBC.
- An important characteristic histopathologic finding is granulomatous biliary injury, also called the florid duct lesion (see Chapter 26). Florid duct lesions are seen in only a small number of patients. "Ductopenia," defined as a reduced number of bile ducts in >50% of portal tracts visualized under high-power microscopy, is seen in more advanced stages of PBC.
- Treatment generally includes ursodeoxycholic acid, a fat-soluble bile acid (see Chapter 20), which has been shown to delay both histologic progression of the disease and the time to liver transplantation.

Due to impaired enterohepatic circulation, patients with advanced PBC are at increased risk of fat-soluble vitamin deficiency (vitamins A, D, E, K), bone disease (hepatic osteodystrophy), and hypercholesterolemia with a predominant elevation of plasma high density lipoprotein (HDL) levels. Patients are generally not at increased risk of cardiovascular disease; therefore, treatment of hypercholesterolemia in patients with PBC is usually not necessary. Patients with PBC should be screened regularly for osteoporosis by dual-energy X-ray absorptiometry (DEXA) scan.

Primary Sclerosing Cholangitis

- Primary sclerosing cholangitis (PSC) is a chronic inflammatory condition of the intra- and extrahepatic bile ducts resulting in strictures (or narrowing) of the biliary tract and consequent cholestasis.

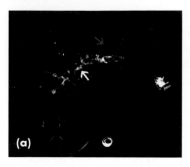 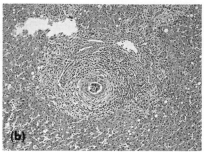

Figure 15.2 Primary sclerosing cholangitis. (a) Magnetic resonance cholangiopancreatography showing irregular appearance of the intrahepatic ducts with areas of dilatation (white arrow) and small strictured ducts (red arrow). (Courtesy of Dr. D. Martin, Emory University, Atlanta, GA, USA). (b) Liver biopsy specimen showing the typical "onion skin" appearance of periductular fibrosis. Hematoxylin and eosin, ×20. (Courtesy of Dr. S. Sharma, Emory University, Atlanta, GA, USA.)

- PSC is primarily a disease of large ducts, in contrast to PBC, which is primarily a disease of the bile ductules in the portal tracts.
- Symptoms can be vague and may include right upper quadrant pain, pruritus, and weight loss.
- Patients with PSC are at risk of bacterial cholangitis due to biliary stasis and bacterial overgrowth. Acute cholangitis, a suppurative infection of the bile duct, is a medical emergency and should be treated in consultation with a gastrointestinal endoscopist (see Chapter 21).
- Approximately 70% of patients with PSC also have concomitant inflammatory bowel disease, usually ulcerative colitis.
- No specific autoantibody is diagnostic of PSC. The diagnosis of PSC is made when patients have a cholestatic pattern of liver biochemical test abnormalities (elevated serum alkaline phosphatase and bilirubin levels disproportionate to the serum aminotransferase levels) in the setting of a cholangiogram that shows biliary strictures alternating with areas of dilatation. Typically, the bile ducts appear "beaded" and the radicles are pruned or truncated on a cholangiogram (Figure 15.2).
- Magnetic resonance cholangiopancreatography (MRCP) is the preferred diagnostic test (Figure 15.2), with a high sensitivity and specificity. Endoscopic retrograde cholangiopancreatography (ERCP) is often deferred due to the risk of procedure-related complications such as pancreatitis but can be used as a therapeutic procedure to dilate and place a stent across a significant (dominant) bile-duct stricture to permit drainage of bile, decrease the risk of acute cholangitis, and reduce morbidity.

- A liver biopsy is not required to make a diagnosis of PSC. The typical finding on histologic examination of the liver is onion-skin fibrosis surrounding a bile duct. About 10% of patients have onion-skin fibrosis of only small intrahepatic bile ductules with no abnormalities on cholangiography, a condition often referred to as small-duct PSC, which appears to have a better prognosis than PSC associated with strictures involving the extrahepatic bile duct.
- No effective medical therapy exists for PSC; management is aimed at treating the symptoms and monitoring the patient for acute cholangitis. Like PBC, PSC is also a cholestatic liver disease and can result in fat-soluble vitamin deficiency and osteodystrophy. Ursodeoxycholic acid does not appear to affect the course of PSC.
- Liver transplantation is an effective treatment and should be considered in patients with advanced PSC.
- A dominant stricture in the bile duct or the major hepatic ducts should raise concern for cholangiocarcinoma, which can occur in up to 10% of patients with PSC.

Hemochromatosis

- Hereditary hemochromatosis (HH) comprises several inherited disorders of iron homeostasis characterized by increased intestinal absorption of iron that results in deposition of iron in the liver, pancreas, heart, and other organs.
- HH is the most common genetic abnormality in Caucasians, with a gene carrier frequency of approximately 1 in 200 persons. HFE-related HH is an autosomal recessive disorder most common in persons of northern European ancestry. Most patients with HH are homozygous for the C282Y mutation of the HFE gene. Some patients are compound heterozygotes (C282Y/H63D).
- Causes of secondary iron overload include iron overload anemias (e.g., aplastic anemia, thalassemia major, sideroblastic anemia), parenteral iron overload (e.g., red cell transfusions, hemodialysis), and chronic liver diseases (e.g., alcoholic liver disease, chronic hepatitis B and C, nonalcoholic steatohepatitis).
- The pathophysiologic mechanisms leading to iron overload in HH are not fully understood. Increased intestinal absorption of dietary iron, decreased expression of the iron-regulatory hormone hepcidin, altered function of the HFE protein, and iron-induced tissue injury and fibrogenesis have been implicated. The predominant mechanism is thought to be related to dysregulated expression of hepcidin by the mutated HFE protein. Hepcidin is a hormone synthesized by the liver that regulates iron absorption from enterocytes.

- Most persons with HH remain asymptomatic. When present, symptoms include weakness and lethargy, arthralgias, abdominal pain, and loss of libido or potency in men. In symptomatic patients, hepatomegaly is a common finding on examination. Although rare now, a pathognomonic finding on physical examination includes bronzed or slate-gray skin pigmentation. Other signs of chronic liver disease such as splenomegaly, ascites, jaundice, and peripheral edema may be present. Diabetes mellitus usually occurs in patients who have developed cirrhosis.
- Other clinical manifestations include cardiomyopathy, arrhythmias, heart failure, and a characteristic arthropathy that involves the second and third metacarpophalangeal joints.
- The diagnosis of HH should be considered in any patient with typical symptoms, a positive family history, or (most commonly) abnormal screening iron test results. Measurements of the serum iron level and total iron binding capacity or transferrin, with calculation of the transferrin saturation (TS), and a serum ferritin level should be obtained.
- The diagnosis of HH is based on identification of increased iron stores with elevated serum ferritin levels and TS. If the TS is >45% in women and >50% in men, the serum ferritin level is elevated, or an unsaturated iron-binding capacity $\geq 155\,\mu g/dL$, genetic testing should be considered.
- Siblings of persons who are homozygous for the *C282Y* mutation or a compound heterozygote (*C282Y/H63D*) should undergo genetic screening for the HFE mutation.
- A liver biopsy is indicated for histopathologic evaluation (see Chapter 26) and quantification of hepatic iron content in affected patients with a serum ferritin >1000 ng/mL or elevated serum aminotransferase levels.
- Imaging of the liver can reveal hepatomegaly or evidence of cirrhosis, and magnetic resonance imaging may detect hepatic iron overload (but is not yet sensitive enough to be used as a screening test).
- Patients with HH are treated with phlebotomy, initially one unit and occasionally two units weekly, to deplete iron stores in the body. The goal is to achieve a serum ferritin level of <50 ng/mL and a TS <50%. Then, maintenance phlebotomies, one unit three or four times a year, are continued. Iron desaturation in a patient who does not have cirrhosis will prevent progression to cirrhosis. Each unit of blood removed contains 250 mg of iron; many patients with genetic HH have a hepatic iron burden of 50 g.
- Intravenous chelation therapy with desferoxamine may be offered to patients who do not tolerate phlebotomy.

- For patients who develop cirrhosis as a consequence of HH, liver transplantation can be considered.

> Up to 30% of patients with cirrhosis due to HH develop hepatocellular carcinoma (HCC). Screening for HCC with imaging of the liver every 6 months is recommended in these patients.

Wilson disease (WD)

- WD is a chronic hepatic and neurologic condition resulting from excessive copper deposition.
- WD is an autosomal recessive disorder. The genetic defect is a mutation in the *ATP7B* (also called Wilson adenosine triphosphatase, [ATPase]) gene. *ATP7B* is expressed predominantly in hepatocytes, the placenta, and the kidney. The gene encodes a P-type (cation transport enzyme) ATPase that transports copper into bile. Mutations lead to accumulation of copper within hepatocytes, thereby causing oxidative damage.
- WD commonly presents in younger persons. Patients may present with chronic or fulminant liver disease, a progressive neurologic disorder without clinically prominent hepatic dysfunction, or acute hemolysis. A neurologic presentation occurs in the second or third decade of life, and symptoms may include depression, tremor, movement disorders, dystonia, and even psychosis. The classic Kayser–Fleischer ring is caused by copper deposition in Descemet's membrane of the cornea. A careful slit-lamp examination is mandatory in patients with suspected WD. Sunflower cataracts may be seen in some patients with WD.
- Genetic testing is expensive and often unavailable; therefore, patients with unexplained liver disease and a low or low–normal ceruloplasmin level should have a 24-hour urine collection to detect elevated copper concentrations and a slit-lamp examination for Kayser–Fleischer rings.
- Liver biopsy for histology (see Chapter 26) and copper quantification is generally performed. A hepatic copper concentration >250 µg/g liver is typical of Wilson disease; a concentration ≤40 µg/g excludes the diagnosis.
- Copper chelation with D-penicillamine or trientine is an effective treatment for WD. Oral zinc may be considered in asymptomatic or pregnant patients or as maintenance therapy. If treatment is initiated early, most patients live a normal healthy life.
- Liver transplantation, when indicated, is curative.

Alpha-1 Antitrypsin Deficiency (A1ATD)

- A1ATD is the second most common metabolic disease affecting the liver. It is an autosomal recessive disorder that predominantly affects the liver and the lung.
- Alpha-1 antitrypsin (A1AT) is a protease inhibitor that promotes the degradation of serine proteases in the serum and tissues. Neutrophil elastase is one of the most important serine proteases that is inhibited by A1AT. A1ATD is a consequence of a mutation in SERPINA1 that results in deficiency of this protein, thereby leading to uninhibited neutrophil elastase activity and the development of pulmonary emphysema in affected patients.
- Emphysema occurs due to destruction of normal lung tissue. Precocious emphysema is often a clue to the diagnosis. With the most common phenotype (ZZ), liver disease occurs as a result of the inability of the abnormal protein to be secreted from the endoplasmic reticulum and Golgi, because the protein is misfolded and has an abnormal tertiary structure; it accumulates in the hepatocytes and results in hepatocyte destruction, which may lead to cirrhosis.
- A biopsy specimen of the liver in a patient with A1ATD can be stained with a periodic acid-Schiff (PAS) stain to demonstrate the excess abnormal proteins (see Chapter 26).
- A1ATD can be diagnosed in the neonatal period or can manifest later in life with jaundice, liver dysfunction, or cirrhosis.
- The diagnosis is based on a decreased serum level of A1AT and phenotype testing for the genetic defect; the A1AT level alone is not sufficient to confirm the diagnosis.
- Treatment of A1ATD liver disease is aimed at supportive care of portal hypertension and complications associated with end-stage liver disease. A1AT replacement therapy does not improve the liver disease.
- Liver transplantation is curative because the donor liver will synthesize normal A1AT protein.

Vascular Disorders of the Liver

Portal Vein Thrombosis (PVT)

- The most common vascular disorder of the liver is PVT, which occurs most commonly in patients with cirrhosis and results from sluggish portal blood flow and a possible prothrombotic state associated with cirrhosis.
- PVT can also occur in noncirrhotic patients with malignancy, infection, trauma, or a hereditary prothrombotic state (e.g., factor V Leiden mutation, prothrombin 20210A mutation, deficiencies of protein C, protein S, or antithrombin, sickle cell disease, and hyperhomocysteinemia).

- Acute PVT can present with severe abdominal pain and fever, and occasionally with possibly bloody diarrhea. With extensive thrombosis, bowel ischemia and infarction can ensue.
- Chronic PVT may result in cavernous transformation of the portal vein (portal cavernoma).
- Doppler ultrasonography, computed tomography, or magnetic resonance imaging (MRI) may reveal PVT.
- Most patients with acute PVT can be treated with anticoagulation with restoration of blood flow.
- Anticoagulation for chronic PVT is generally not recommended.

Budd–Chiari Syndrome (BCS)

- BCS refers to hepatic venous outflow tract obstruction. BCS can result from thrombosis or other secondary causes of outflow obstruction.
- BCS can present with acute abdominal pain, ascites, and hepatomegaly; often it is associated with a prothrombotic state.
- Investigation for underlying malignancy or a prothrombotic state (e.g., a myeloproliferative disorder associated with the *V617F* mutation of the *JAK2* gene, factor V Leiden mutation, prothrombin 20210A mutation, deficiencies of protein C, protein S, or antithrombin, sickle cell disease, and hyperhomocysteinemia) should be performed.
- MRI or venography is generally diagnostic (Figure 15.3).
- The clinical features are similar to those for sinusoidal obstruction syndrome (veno-occlusive disease).

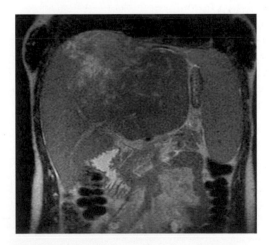

Figure 15.3 Magnetic resonance imaging in a patient with Budd–Chiari syndrome. A characteristic spider-web pattern of venous collaterals is seen at the dome of the liver. (Courtesy of Dr. B. Kalb, Emory University, Atlanta, GA, USA.)

- Anticoagulation therapy should be considered, especially in patients who present acutely.
- A transjugular intrahepatic portosystemic shunt (TIPS) is indicated in patients with portal hypertension, and liver transplantation can be considered for those patients with progressive symptoms and evidence of liver failure or when TIPS is ineffective.

Pearls

Chronic liver disease may be caused by a number of conditions. Multiple pathophysiologic mechanisms of injury exist, but the final common pathway is hepatic parenchymal fibrosis and cirrhosis.

A variety of biochemical and serologic tests can aid in the determination of the cause of chronic liver disease.

Abdominal ultrasonography is a noninvasive, fast, and cost-effective test that should be used as a first-line radiographic study for imaging the liver; however, it is insensitive for detecting cirrhosis.

Questions

Questions 1 and 2 relate to the clinical vignette at the beginning of this chapter.
1. Which of the following is the most likely diagnosis?
    A. Autoimmune hepatitis
    B. Primary biliary cirrhosis (PBC)
    C. Heart failure
    D. Chronic hepatitis C
    E. Drug-induced liver injury
2. The patient asks you about potential implications of her diagnosis on her overall health. You inform her that she is at risk for which of the following?
    A. Fat-soluble vitamin deficiencies
    B. Osteoporosis
    C. Hypercholesterolemia
    D. Hepatocellular carcinoma
    E. All of the above
3. A 21-year-old man presents for evaluation of jaundice and pruritus that has been worsening over the past 8 weeks. He has ulcerative colitis that is being treated with mesalamine and is in remission. He denies abdominal pain, fever, chills, or weight loss. He does not drink alcohol, smoke cigarettes, or use illicit drugs. Physical examination shows jaundice. Laboratory tests show a serum alkaline phosphatase level of 693 U/L, total bilirubin 7 mg/dL, ALT 65 U/L, and AST 83 U/L. Serologic tests for viral hepatitis,

antimitochondrial antibodies, smooth muscle antibodies, and antinuclear antibodies are negative. Serum ceruloplasmin and alpha-1 antitrypsin levels are normal. Ultrasonography of the abdomen shows mildly dilated intra- and extrahepatic bile ducts. Magnetic resonance cholangiopancreatography (MRCP) shows a beaded pattern with multiple biliary strictures and focal areas of ductal dilatation proximal to the strictures. A long "dominant" stricture is noted in the mid bile duct. The most likely diagnosis is which of the following?

A. Autoimmune hepatitis
B. Primary biliary cirrhosis
C. Viral hepatitis
D. Nonalcoholic fatty liver disease
E. Primary sclerosing cholangitis (PSC)

4. A 16-year-old girl presents to the emergency department with obtundation. There is no history of drug or alcohol use. Her parents note that she has become increasingly withdrawn at home and school; there is no report of suicide attempts. Physical examination reveals an unresponsive young woman with conjuctival icterus. Laboratory evaluation is remarkable for a hemoglobin level of 9 g/dL (normal 20–50 mg/dL), international normalized ratio 3.8, total bilirubin 11.6 mg/dL with an indirect fraction at 9 mg/dL, and ceruloplasmin 8 mg/dL. A toxicology screen is negative. Which of the following should be the next step in management this patient?

A. 24-hour urine copper measurement
B. Administer intravenous glucocorticoids
C. Immediate transfer to a liver transplant center
D. Urgent phlebotomy
E. Begin copper chelation therapy

5. A 55-year-old woman with Graves' disease is evaluated in the office for a persistently elevated serum alkaline phosphatase level. Physical examination is unremarkable except for shiny deposits over her eyelids. Laboratory testing reveals a serum alkaline phosphatase level of 355 U/L, ALT 35 U/L, AST 25 U/L, and total cholesterol 500 mg/dL. Other tests including complete blood count, prothrombin time, platelet count, serum electrolytes, serum creatinine, and total bilirubin are within normal limits. Ultrasonography of the abdomen is unremarkable. Which of the following is the best test to identify the cause of the elevated serum alkaline phosphatase level?

A. Liver biopsy
B. Antineutrophil cytoplasmic antibodies (ANCA)
C. Magnetic resonance cholangiopancreatography (MRCP)
D. Antimitochondrial antibodies (AMA)
E. Serum immunoglobulins

(*Continued*)

Answers

1. B

The most likely diagnosis is PBC as evidenced by the patient's clinical presentation with fatigue and pruritus (and symptoms of advanced liver disease), cholestatic liver biochemical test pattern (elevated serum alkaline phosphatase and bilirubin levels disproportionate to the serum aminotransferases), and antimitochondrial antibodies.

2. E

Patients with PBC are at increased risk for fat-soluble vitamin deficiencies (vitamins A, D, E, K), bone disease (hepatic osteodystrophy), and hypercholesterolemia due to impaired enterohepatic circulation. In addition, they are at increased risk of developing hepatocellular carcinoma.

3. E

This is a classic presentation of PSC. PSC is a chronic inflammatory condition of the intra- and extrahepatic bile ducts resulting in strictures (or narrowings) of the biliary tract, with resulting cholestasis. The diagnosis of PSC is made when patients have a cholestatic pattern of liver biochemical test abnormalities and cholangiography reveals biliary strictures and intervening areas of dilatation. About 70% of patients with PSC also have concomitant inflammatory bowel disease. The clinical picture does not fit the other choices.

4. C

This patient has acute Wilson disease and should be referred immediately to a liver transplant center. This is a classic presentation in a young patient with altered mentation preceded by neurocognitive changes (depression and withdrawal) that is seen when copper is deposited in the central nervous system. She also has evidence of hemolytic anemia (elevated indirect hyperbilirubinemia) and a low serum ceruloplasmin level. Slit-lamp examination may reveal Kayser–Fleisher rings or rarely sunflower cataracts. Liver transplantation is curative.

5. D

The next step in the evaluation of this middle-aged woman with evidence of cholestatic liver disease should be a serum AMA. AMA are present in 95% of patients with PBC. Additionally, total cholesterol levels are often elevated in patients with cholestatic liver disease due to impaired enterohepatic circulation. The patient has thyroid disease, which is prevalent in patients with PBC. ANCA and serum immunoglobulins are not useful in the diagnosis of PBC. MRCP would be considered if there were evidence of extrahepatic biliary obstruction, but ultrasonography is normal.

Further Reading

Leonis, M.A. and Balistreri, W.F. (2010) Other inherited metabolic disorders of the liver, in *Sleisenger and Fordtran's Gastrointestinal and Liver Disease: Pathophysiology/ Diagnosis/Management*, 9th edn (eds M. Feldman, L.S. Friedman and L.J. Brandt), Saunders Elsevier, Philadelphia, pp. 1259–1278.

Lindor, K.D., Gershwin, M.E., Poupon, R., et al. (2009) Primary biliary cirrhosis. *Hepatology*, 50, 291–308.

Manns, M., Czaja, A.J., Gorham, J.D., et al. (2010) Diagnosis and management of autoimmune hepatitis. *Hepatology*, 51, 2193–2213.

Roberts, E.A. and Schilsky, M.L. (2008) Diagnosis and treatment of Wilson disease: an update. *Hepatology*, 47, 2089–2111.

van Bokhoven, M.A., van Deursen, C.T. and Swinkels, D.W. (2011) Diagnosis and management of hereditary haemochromatosis. *British Medical Journal*, 342, c7251.

Weblinks

http://digestive.niddk.nih.gov/ddiseases/pubs/cirrhosis/
http://www.cpmc.org/advanced/liver/patients/topics/
hep_autoimmune.html
http://www.aafp.org/afp/2006/0901/p756.html

Portal Hypertension

Sonali S. Sakaria and Ram Subramanian

CHAPTER 16

Clinical Vignette

A 55-year-old man presents to the emergency department with a 2-month history of increasing abdominal girth, fatigue, and lower extremity edema. He reports diffuse abdominal pain, fever, and chills for the past week. He denies confusion, diarrhea, melena, hematemesis, or rectal bleeding. His past medical and family history are unremarkable. He is married and has no children. He does not smoke cigarettes, drink significant amounts of alcohol, or use illicit drugs. Physical examination reveals a blood pressure of 90/50 mmHg, pulse rate 106/min, respiratory rate 18/min, and temperature of 101.5°F (38.5°C). Conjunctival icterus is present. Abdominal examination reveals a tense abdomen with a fluid wave and shifting dullness. The abdomen is diffusely tender to palpation. Normal bowel sounds are present. The liver edge is not palpable. Laboratory tests are significant for a serum sodium of 125 mmol/L, creatinine 1.8 mg/dL, aspartate aminotransferase 68 U/L, alanine aminotransferase 58 U/L, total bilirubin 6.8 mg/dL, platelet count 80000/mm^3, white blood cell (WBC) count 14000/mm^3, hemoglobin 10.2 g/dL, hematocrit 33%, and international normalized ratio (INR) 1.7.

Definition

- Portal hypertension is defined as an increase in the pressure gradient between the portal vein and the hepatic vein as measured by the hepatic venous pressure gradient (HVPG).
- Portal hypertension is a key consequence of decompensated cirrhosis and may result in life-threatening conditions including gastrointestinal hemorrhage from esophageal and gastric varices,

---

Essentials of Gastroenterology, First Edition. Edited by Shanthi V. Sitaraman, Lawrence S. Friedman.

portal hypertensive gastropathy, hepatorenal syndrome, pulmonary complications, spontaneous bacterial peritonitis, and hepatic encephalopathy.

Pathophysiology

Normal Portal Circulation

- The portal vein drains blood directly from the esophagus and stomach and from the mesenteric veins, which drain the small and large intestine, pancreas, gallbladder, and spleen. The portal vein is formed by the confluence of the splenic vein and the superior mesenteric vein (see also Chapter 11).
- The portal venous system is a high-compliance, low-resistance system that has the ability to accommodate high blood-flow volumes without increasing portal venous pressure.
- The hepatic artery, also a high compliance vessel, converges with the portal vein to flow into the hepatic sinusoids, thus providing a dual blood supply to the liver.

Hemodynamic Changes in Portal Hypertension

- Portal hypertension results from an increase in portal resistance (R) or portal blood flow (F) (or both), and can be represented by Ohm's law, $\Delta P = F \times R$, where ΔP represents the pressure gradient across the portal circulation, F is a function of blood flow, and R is resistance to portal blood flow.
- In North America and Europe the most common cause of portal hypertension is cirrhosis. Other common causes of portal hypertension worldwide include extrahepatic portal vein thrombosis, idiopathic portal hypertension, and schistosomiasis.
- In cirrhosis, portal hypertension and its complications are a key consequence of the synergistic effect of intrahepatic (sinusoidal) resistance to portal blood flow and increased portal blood flow from the splanchnic circulation.
  - ○ Intrahepatic resistance: the resistance to portal flow consists of both fixed and functional components.
    - The fixed component results from sinusoidal fibrosis and compression by regenerative nodules.
    - The functional component, vasoconstriction, is a key consequence of reduced intrahepatic nitric oxide (NO) levels. NO is normally a vasodilator, and in cirrhosis intrahepatic levels of NO are significantly reduced, resulting in enhanced intrahepatic vasoconstrictor activity. Other vasomotor constrictors, including endothelins, are overexpressed in decompensated cirrhosis and exacerbate

      intrahepatic sinusoidal resistance, thereby promoting collateral splanchnic circulation.

  ○ Increased portal blood flow: despite reduced intrahepatic NO levels, a paradoxical increase in NO production occurs in the splanchnic and systemic circulation and results in increased portal blood flow.

  ○ **The major pathophysiologic circulatory derangement in decompensated cirrhosis leading to complications results from systemic and splanchnic vasodilatation along with intrahepatic vasoconstriction and increased resistance in the hepatic sinusoids.** These changes activate the renin–angiotensin–aldosterone axis; in addition, there are increased circulating levels of norephinephrine and antidiuretic hormone (ADH). These hormones are activated to cause an increase in effective arterial blood volume due to avid renal reabsorption of sodium and increased afferent arteriolar resistance in the nephron.

Measurement of Portal Pressure

- The measurement of the HVPG is the method used most commonly to measure portal pressure.
- The HVPG is obtained by measuring the wedged hepatic venous pressure (WHVP). A balloon catheter is wedged into a branch of the hepatic vein, and the balloon is inflated, thereby occluding the vessel. The pressure reading obtained, WHVP, must be corrected for increases in abdominal pressure by subtracting the inferior vena caval pressure. This difference in pressures represents the HVPG.
- A normal HVPG is 3–5 mmHg.
- Elevated HVPG levels (>10–12 mmHg) are predictive of the development of complications of portal hypertension.

Complications
Variceal Hemorrhage

- Gastroesophageal varices are present in approximately 50% of patients with cirrhosis, and their presence corresponds directly with the severity of liver disease.
- Aggressive and early management of cirrhotic patients presenting with suspected variceal hemorrhage is critical in light of the high mortality associated with this complication of portal hypertension. The presentation of acute variceal hemorrhage carries a >20% mortality rate at 6 weeks.

Pathophysiology

- Splanchnic vasodilatation results in increased portal blood flow. Intrahepatic resistance to flow is also increased. The result is formation of portosystemic variceal collaterals. The collaterals most likely to result in bleeding are found around the esophagus and, less frequently, in the stomach.
- Variceal wall tension is the primary factor determining the risk of variceal hemorrhage and is determined by the vessel diameter and the pressure within the vessel. The formation of varices typically occurs when the HVPG is ≥12 mmHg.

Clinical and Laboratory Features

> Portal hypertension should be suspected in all patients with gastrointestinal bleeding and peripheral stigmata of liver disease (e.g., jaundice, ascites, splenomegaly, spider angiomas, and encephalopathy).

- Patients with variceal bleeding most commonly present with hematemesis, melena, or both.
- Variceal bleeding is commonly associated with hemodynamic compromise (hypotension, tachycardia, hypovolemic shock).
- Laboratory studies usually reveal a prolonged prothrombin time, low platelet count, hypoalbuminemia, and hyperbilirubinemia.

Diagnosis

- The diagnosis of esophageal and gastric varices is made by esophagogastroduodenoscopy (EGD). EGD will reveal esophageal or gastric varices with active bleeding and/or stigmata of recent hemorrhage. Such stigmata include pigmented spots (cherry red spots) and red wale signs (longitudinal red streaks) on a varix.

Treatment

- Patients with acute variceal bleeding should be admitted to an intensive care unit and should be stabilized hemodynamically (see Chapter 22).
  - Pharmacologic therapy:
    - In acute variceal bleeding, the goal of pharmacologic agents is to reduce portal blood flow and decrease intrahepatic resistance.
    - Octreotide (a somatostatin analog) causes splanchnic vasoconstriction and reduces portal flow. In acute variceal bleeding, octreotide, 50 μg administered intravenously as a bolus followed

by a continuous infusion of 50 µg/hr for 72 hours, has been shown to be a beneficial adjunct to endoscopic therapy in stopping bleeding.

- Empiric antibiotics must be administered to reduce the risk of bacterial infections including spontaneous bacterial peritonitis (SBP). Ceftriaxone administered intravenously or a fluoroquinolone (e.g., norfloxacin 400 mg twice daily) administered orally for 7 days is recommended.

○ Endoscopic therapy:
- Emergent EGD should be performed as soon as the patient is hemodynamically stable.
- The preferred endoscopic therapeutic modality is endoscopic variceal ligation (EVL), in which a varix is suctioned into a cap on the tip of the endoscope and a rubber band is applied around the varix to strangulate it, thereby causing thrombosis of the varix.

○ Balloon tamponade:
- Balloon tamponade may be necessary when control of variceal hemorrhage is not feasible with combined pharmacologic and endoscopic therapy.
- A tube (Sengstaken–Blakemore tube or Minnesota tube) with gastric and esophageal balloons is inserted through the mouth into the esophagus with subsequent inflation of the gastric balloon and esophageal balloon sequentially to tamponade varices.
- This procedure is associated with substantial morbidity and should be used only as a temporizing measure until definitive treatment such as transjugular intrahepatic portosystemic shunt (TIPS) is performed (see below).

○ Transjugular intrahepatic portosystemic shunt:
- A TIPS should be considered for uncontrolled esophageal variceal hemorrhage after failed pharmacologic and endoscopic therapy or for gastric variceal hemorrhage unresponsive to pharmacologic therapy.
- A TIPS reduces elevated portal pressure by creating a communication between the hepatic vein and an intrahepatic branch of the portal vein.
- A TIPS is placed by transjugular hepatic vein cannulation with subsequent cannulation of the portal vein. A stent is then placed over a guide wire to connect the hepatic vein and a branch of the portal vein with the goal of reducing portal pressure below 12 mmHg (or at least by 20%).
- Contraindications to a TIPS include severe right-sided heart failure, severe hepatic failure, polycystic liver disease, severe hepatic encephalopathy, and occlusive portal vein thrombus.

- Complications of TIPS include hepatic encephalopathy, pulmonary hypertension, and heart failure.

Endoscopic treatment of varices (EVL) is generally performed as first-line interventional therapy for acute bleeding esophageal varices. A TIPS is used as first-line interventional therapy for bleeding gastric varices that do not respond to pharmacologic treatment. (In some countries, injection of gastric varices with "glue" (cyanoacrylate) via endoscopy is another option for the treatment of bleeding gastric varices.)

Prevention of Variceal Bleeding
- Pharmacologic therapy:
  - Nonselective beta blockers (propranolol, nadolol, carvedilol) are used as primary (to prevent first variceal bleeding) or secondary (to prevent rebleeding of varices) prophylaxis. For secondary prophylaxis, treatment with a beta blocker should be initiated after the patient has stopped bleeding and is hemodynamically stable.
- Endoscopic therapy:
  - All patients with cirrhosis should be screened by EGD for varices. Those with large esophageal varices at high risk of bleeding should be started on a nonselective beta blocker. If a beta blocker is not tolerated or contraindicated, prophylactic EVL can be performed. Patients with gastric varices should be started on a nonselective beta blocker.
  - For patients with small varices, no prophlaxis is recommended.
  - Patients with esophageal variceal hemorrhage should undergo serial EVL.

Hepatic Encephalopathy (HE)

Definition
- HE refers to reversible neurologic and psychiatric symptoms usually seen in patients with chronic liver disease and portal hypertension.
- Up to 70% of patients with cirrhosis will develop HE.
- HE is a poor prognostic indicator with 3-year survival rates approximating 20% without liver transplantation.

Pathophysiology
- The pathophysiology of HE is poorly understood. The best described factor implicated in the development of HE is ammonia, a neurotoxin that leads to astrocyte swelling, alterations in neurotransmitters, and brain edema.

Table 16.1 Grading of hepatic encephalopathy based on the West Haven criteria.

Grade	Clinical features
I	Decreased attention span/concentration; abnormal sleep pattern; mildly slowed mentation; mild confusion; minimal changes in memory
II	Lethargy; inappropriate behavior; slurred speech; personality changes
III	Somnolence; disorientation; marked confusion; incomprehensible speech
IV	Unresponsive to verbal or noxious stimuli; coma

- Ammonia arises predominantly in the colon as a byproduct of the metabolism of proteins and nitrogen-containing compounds utilized by bacteria. Under normal conditions, ammonia enters the portal circulation and is metabolized by hepatocytes. Failure of hepatic clearance of ammonia in persons with cirrhosis and portal hypertension leads to increased arterial ammonia levels and encephalopathy.

> Although elevated ammonia levels are seen in 90% of patients with HE, serum levels of ammonia do not correlate with symptoms. Therefore, the measurement of venous ammonia in clinical practice is an expensive test with little clinical value in managing the patient with HE.

Clinical Features
- The presentation of HE may range from subtle symptoms and signs, such as changes in the sleep–wake cycle, lethargy, inability to perform activities of daily living, forgetfulness, and alterations in handwriting to frank coma.
- HE is usually precipitated by an inciting event such as gastrointestinal bleeding, infection, electrolyte abnormalities, and medications.
- The West Haven criteria grade HE from I to IV based on varying levels of consciousness, intellectual function, and behavior (Table 16.1).

Diagnosis

- The diagnosis of HE requires a high level of suspicion and careful attention to the cognitive and neurologic examination. A careful clinical history is essential to make a diagnosis of subclinical or minimal encephalopathy.
- Elevated serum ammonia levels in a patient with cirrhosis and altered mental status support the diagnosis of HE; however, the serum ammonia level is neither sensitive nor specific for the diagnosis.
- HE in chronic liver disease is clinically and pathophysiologically different from HE associated with acute liver failure. In acute failure encephalopathy is a consequence of cerebral edema and is a medical emergency.

Treatment

- The cornerstone of treatment of HE includes identifying and correcting precipitating factors such as:
  - gastrointestinal bleeding;
  - infection;
  - acid–base disturbances;
  - electrolyte disturbances;
  - dehydration;
  - constipation;
  - medications (e.g., sedatives, tranquilizers, narcotics);
  - medication nonadherence (e.g., lactulose).
- If a patient has high-grade encephalopathy (e.g., coma), he or she should be admitted to an intensive care unit where elective intubation for airway protection is prudent. In such patients computed tomography (CT) of the brain without iodinated contrast is important to rule out other etiologies of altered mental status including hemorrhage, prior infarcts, or a space-occupying lesion (e.g., tumor, abscess).
- Pharmacologic therapy:
  - Lactulose, a nonabsorbable disaccharide, has long been a first-line pharmacologic agent used in the treatment of HE.
    - Lactulose decreases colonic transit time and decreases ammonia production by acidifying colonic contents, thereby converting NH_3 to the less absorbable NH_4^+.
    - Lactulose is administered orally; however, in patients who are at risk for aspiration, lactulose may be given per rectum.
    - The dose of lactulose should be titrated so that patients have three soft bowel movements per day.
    - Side effects of lactulose include abdominal cramping, flatulence, diarrhea, and electrolyte imbalance.

- Overuse of lactulose may lead to dehydration and metabolic alkalosis, which paradoxically can worsen HE.
  ○ Antibiotics:
    - Antibiotics have been used as second-line agents after lactulose or in patients who are intolerant of lactulose. Increasingly, rifaximin is used as a first-line agent.
    - Antibiotics are thought to modify the intestinal flora and lower stool pH, thereby decreasing ammonia production and enhancing its excretion.
    - Rifaximin 550 mg orally twice daily is currently the antibiotic recommended to treat HE. The systemic bioavailability of rifaximin is much lower than that of other antibiotics used to treat HE; therefore, there are fewer side effects. Its efficacy and safety make rifaximin more conducive to long-term patient compliance compared with other antibiotics.
    - Neomycin (0.5–1 g orally every 12 hours) administered in conjunction with lactulose or alone has been used in the past for treatment of HE but has largely been replaced by rifaximin because of serious side effects including ototoxicity and renal toxicity.
    - Metronidazole and vancomycin have also been shown to be effective in some trials, but there are insufficient data to support their routine use.

Lactulose, a nonabsorbable disaccharide, is the mainstay of treatment for HE. The dose of lactulose should be titrated so that patients have three soft bowel movements per day. Overuse of lactulose may lead to dehydration and metabolic alkalosis and may worsen HE or precipitate hepatorenal syndrome. Rifaximin is an important addition to the armamentarium for the treatment of HE.

Hepatorenal Syndrome

Definition

- Hepatorenal syndrome (HRS) is defined as functional acute renal failure seen in the setting of cirrhosis and portal hypertension or acute liver injury in which intense renal arterial vasoconstriction and progressive renal failure occur in the face of dilated splanchnic arterial vasculature.
- Histologically the kidneys are normal in HRS, and indeed their function may be restored by transplantation into a noncirrhotic recipient.

- HRS occurs in 25% of patients hospitalized with cirrhosis and carries a high mortality rate.
- There are two types of HRS.
  - Type I:
    - defined as a doubling of initial serum creatinine level to >2.5 mg/dL or a 50% reduction in the initial 24-hour creatinine clearance to a level <20 mL/min in less than 2 weeks;
    - rapidly progressive and fatal if untreated.
  - Type II:
    - serum creatinine >1.5 mg/dL and <2.5 mg/dL;
    - sometimes associated with chronic use of diuretics and refractory ascites;
    - indolent course with increase in serum creatinine levels occurring over weeks to months.

Pathophysiology
- The kidneys perceive persistent ineffective arterial blood volume and adapt by activating sodium retention mechanisms including the renin–angiotensin–aldosterone system, resulting in enhanced renal vascular constriction and avid sodium reabsorption. The persistence of an ineffective arterial blood volume resulting from enhanced renal vasoconstriction further reduces the glomerular filtration rate (GFR), and renal failure ensues.

Diagnosis
- The diagnosis of HRS requires a high index of clinical suspicion.
- A "spot" urinary sodium concentration is less than 10 mEq/L.
- Diagnostic criteria for HRS include:
  - cirrhosis with ascites;
  - serum creatinine >1.5 mg/dL;
  - failure of the serum creatinine to improve to <1.5 mg/dL after 2 days of diuretic withdrawal and volume expansion with albumin;
  - absence of shock;
  - absence of exposure to nephrotoxic drugs;
  - absence of parenchymal kidney disease (indicated by proteinuria of more than 500 mg/day, microhematuria (>50 red blood cells/high power field), or abnormal renal ultrasonographic findings).

HRS is seen in up to 25% of patients with SBP. SBP may not be accompanied by overt symptoms or signs, and all patients with HRS should be evaluated for SBP.

Treatment

- Many medications such as diuretics, lactulose, angiotensin-converting enzyme inhibitors, angiotensin-receptor blockers, and nonsteroidal anti-inflammatory drugs may influence intravascular volume status and renal perfusion. These medications should be identified and discontinued in any patient with suspected HRS.
- A volume challenge with albumin should be administered to attempt to improve functional hypovolemia and improve renal perfusion. The dose of intravenous albumin is as follows: a bolus of 1 g/kg/day on presentation (maximum dose 100 g), then 20–60 g daily.
- Precipitants of hepatorenal syndrome, including gastrointestinal hemorrhage, volume depletion from excessive use of lactulose, and spontaneous bacterial peritonitis, should be identified and treated.
- Pharmacologic agents targeted at producing splanchnic vasoconstriction should be initiated:
  - octreotide 100 μg subcutaneously three times daily; increase to a maximum dose of 200 μg subcutaneously three times daily or begin a 25-μg intravenous bolus and continue at a rate of 25 μg/hr; **AND**
  - midodrine (an alpha adrenergic agonist) 2.5–5 mg orally three times daily; increase to a maximum dose of 15 mg three times daily. Titrate to a mean arterial pressure increase of at least 15 mmHg;
  - other options include intravenous terlipressin (not available in the US) or norepinephrine.
- Because HRS is associated with a high mortality rate, it is critical to prescribe prophylactic measures to prevent HRS:
  - albumin should be administered for all large-volume paracenteses (>5 L removed);
  - albumin administration on days 1 and 3 in the treatment of SBP has been shown to decrease the incidence of HRS.
- Renal replacement therapy (e.g., dialysis) can be used to bridge patients to liver transplantation.
- Liver transplantation is curative.

> HRS is associated with a high mortality rate and should be identified expeditiously and treated promptly. Precipitating factors should be identified and corrected.

Ascites

Definition

- Pathologic accumulation of fluid within the peritoneal cavity.

Pathophysiology
- Two main factors lead to ascites: sodium retention, as previously discussed, and increased hydrostatic pressure within the hepatic sinusoids, leading to transudation of fluid into the peritoneal space, exceeding the capacity of the lymphatic system to remove the fluid.

Clinical Features
- Patients usually present with increased abdominal girth and distention. They may have shortness of breath.
- Physical examination may reveal dullness to percussion, particularly in the flanks, shifting dullness, and a fluid wave.

Diagnosis
- All patients who present with the new onset of ascites in an outpatient or inpatient setting, as well as those with ascites admitted to the hospital, should undergo a diagnostic paracentesis.
- Ascitic fluid should be sent for cell count including a differential count of the white blood cells (WBCs), albumin concentration, and total protein concentration; a Gram stain and bacterial culture are optional.
- The WBC count in uncomplicated (uninfected) cirrhotic ascites is <500 cells/mm^3, and the polymorphonuclear (PMN) neutrophil count is <250/mm^3.
- The serum–ascites albumin gradient (SAAG) is used to categorize ascites. It is calculated by subtracting the ascitic fluid albumin concentration from the serum albumin concentration. A SAAG ≥1.1 g/dL is characteristic of cirrhotic ascites. Other causes of ascites with a SAAG ≥1.1 g/dL include alcoholic hepatitis, Budd–Chiari syndrome, portal vein thrombosis, passive congestion, and fatty liver of pregnancy. The most common condition associated with a low SAAG (<1.1 g/dL) is peritoneal carcinomatosis. Other causes of a low-SAAG ascites include biliary or pancreatic leaks, nephrotic syndrome, and tuberculous peritonitis.

Treatment
- Identify the precipitating cause such as dietary indiscretion or noncompliance with treatment.
- Sodium intake should initially be restricted to ≤2 g/day.
- Fluid restriction is indicated only for hyponatremia. In patients with severe hyponatremia (<125 mEq/L), a vaptan (e.g., tolvaptan) may be prescribed.
- Pharmacotherapy:
  - Spironolactone and furosemide in a ratio of 100:40 mg (e.g., 100 mg and 40 mg) once daily increased gradually (every 3–5 days) to a

maximum of 400 mg and 160 mg per day. Amiloride (10 mg daily) may be substituted for spironolactone and does not cause gynecomastia. The spironolactone and furosemide regimen maintains normokalemia and achieves diueresis in >90% of patients with cirrhotic ascites.

- ○ Serum electrolyte and creatinine levels should be monitored.
- ○ Diuretics should be discontinued in patients who develop encephalopathy, a serum sodium concentration <120 mEq/L despite fluid restriction, and a serum creatinine level >2.0 mg/dL.
- Large-volume paracentesis (LVP) may be performed in patients with tense ascites or ascites refractory to diuretics. LVP should be avoided in patients with diuretic-sensitive cirrhotic ascites. Intravenous albumin (10 g per liter of fluid removed) should be administered to prevent circulatory dysfunction if >5 L of ascitic fluid is removed. Terlipressin has been shown to be equivalent to albumin in preventing paracentesis-related circulatory dysfunction.
- Refractory ascites is defined as ascites not responsive to dietary sodium restriction, maximal diuretic therapy, or serial paracentesis. In such cases TIPS placement and liver transplantation should be considered.

Spontaneous Bacterial Peritonitis (SBP)

Definition
- Acute infection of ascitic fluid.
- SBP is associated with increased mortality and is a known precipitant of HRS and encephalopathy.

Clinical Features
- Approximately 90% of patients with SBP are asymptomatic. Therefore, all hospitalized patients with cirrhosis and known ascites or new-onset ascites should undergo a diagnostic paracentesis.

Diagnosis
- The diagnosis is made by the demonstration of an ascitic fluid absolute PMN count ≥250 cells/mm^3 in the absence of known peritonitis of other etiologies.
- The most common pathogens include:
  - ○ *Escherichia coli*;
  - ○ *Klebsiella pneumoniae*;
  - ○ *Streptococcus pneumoniae*.

Treatment

- Cefotaxime 2g every 8 hours intravenously or a similar third-generation cephalosporin for 5–7 days.
- Antibiotic coverage can be tailored once culture results are available.
- Intravenous administration of albumin on days 1 and 3 has been shown to decrease renal impairment and mortality rates.
- Prophylactic antibiotic therapy to prevent SBP is recommended in patients with an ascitic fluid protein concentration <1.0 g/dL or a previous episode of SBP. Norfloxacin 400 mg once daily is typically prescribed. Antibotic prophylaxis is also recommended in patients with acute variceal bleeding (see earlier).

Hepatopulmonary Syndrome (HPS)

Definition

- The triad of an increased alveolar–arterial (A–a) gradient, pulmonary vascular vasodilatations, and underlying liver disease (usually cirrhosis).

Pathophysiology

- Capillary vasodilatation results from increased circulating vasodilators (i.e., NO) primarily at the lung bases. Two subtypes of capillary vasodilatation exist:
  - type I: capillary vasodilatation is the predominant feature;
  - type II: arteriovenous malformations (AVMs), or abnormal connections between arteries and veins, are the predominant feature.
- Pulmonary vasodilatation causes intrapulmonary shunting leading to hyperperfusion of the lungs and reduced oxygenation of venous blood transported via the pulmonary arteries and returned to the heart. Consequently, there is rapid blood flow through the dilated pulmonary circulation that leads to inadequate oxygenation of erythrocytes and clinical hypoxia.

Clinical Features

- **Platypnea** is defined as dyspnea that worsens when the patient sits upright but improves when the patient is lying down. Platypnea, a clinical symptom, occurs because of **orthodeoxia**, a condition in which hypoxemia is exacerbated by sitting upright because more blood circulating at the lung bases is shunted away from alveoli. There are more arteriovenous shunts in the lower than upper lung fields in cirrhotic patients who have HPS.

- Other symptoms and signs include shortness of breath, cyanosis, digital clubbing, and hypoxia.

Diagnosis
- Hypoxia: PaO_2 <70 mmHg on room air blood gas measurement.
- Increased arterial–alveolar gradient without CO_2 retention.
- A "bubble" echocardiogram may reveal delayed appearance of air bubbles in the left heart within 3–6 beats after visualization in the right heart. Such a finding suggests trapped air bubbles in newly developed pulmonary shunts.
- A 99mTc macro-aggregated albumin lung perfusion scan can be used to confirm the diagnosis.

Treatment
- Supplemental oxygen for type I HPS.
- Embolization of AVMs by an interventional radiologist can be performed to reduce symptoms in type II HPS.
- Liver transplantation will reverse HPS.

Portopulmonary Hypertension

Definition
- Pulmonary arterial hypertension with elevated pulmonary resistance and a normal pulmonary artery wedge pressure in the setting of portal hypertension.

Pathophysiology
- The mechanisms underlying portopulmonary hypertension are incompletely understood. Theories include increased vascular flow causing shear stress that may trigger remodeling of the vascular endothelium and portosystemic shunting and a decrease in the phagocytic capacity of the cirrhotic liver, thereby allowing circulating bacteria and toxins to enter the pulmonary circulation and causing cytokine release and triggering vascular inflammatory changes.

Clinical Features
- Dyspnea on exertion (most common presenting symptom), chest pain, fatigue, hemoptysis, orthopnea, and signs of volume overload are typically present. Physical examination may reveal a loud second pulmonic heart sound (P2), murmurs of tricuspid and pulmonic regurgitation, and a right ventricular heave.

Diagnosis

- Right heart catheterization typically reveals a mean pulmonary artery pressure >25 mmHg, normal pulmonary wedge pressure, and elevated pulmonary vascular resistance >125 dynes.sec.cm^{-5}.
- Histopathology of the lung may show intimal fibrosis, smooth muscle hypertrophy, and characteristic plexiform lesions in small arteries and arterioles.

Patients with portopulmonary hypertension do not usually have hypoxemia, a key feature distinguishing it from HPS.

Treatment

- Liver transplantation for patients with mild portopulmonary hypertension (mean PA pressure <35 mmHg) is curative.
- Patients with moderate or severe (mean PA pressure ≥35 mmHg) portopulmonary hypertension have increased mortality associated with liver transplantation.
- Patients with moderate or severe portopulmonary hypertension are often placed on pharmacologic pulmonary vasodilator therapy with the primary goals of reducing mean pulmonary artery pressure to <35 mmHg and then considering liver transplantation.

Hepatic Hydrothorax

Definition

- The accumulation of fluid in the pleural space in a patient with portal hypertension and no underlying cardiopulmonary disease.

Pathophysiology

- The fluid is thought to originate in the abdominal cavity and flows into the pleural space through defects in the diaphragm.
  - On a microscopic level, these defects are breaks in the collagen bundles that constitute the tendinous portion of the diaphragm.
  - Increased intra-abdominal pressure causes the peritoneum to herniate through these breaks, thereby resulting in pleuroperitoneal blebs.
  - Eventually, the blebs rupture and allow free passage of intraperitoneal fluid preferentially into the pleural space given the negative intrathoracic pressure.
- Hepatic hydrothorax occurs when the rate of fluid accumulation exceeds the rate of reabsorption.

Clinical Features

- Dyspnea, cough, and pleuritic chest pain are typical symptoms. Patients usually present with ascites.
- If severe, hepatic hydrothorax can lead to severe respiratory distress.
- Hepatic hydrothorax typically occurs on the right side (80%), although it may occur on the left or bilaterally.

Diagnosis

- Thoracentesis should be performed to rule out infection and other causes of pleural effusion.
- Pleural fluid analysis in hepatic hydrothorax:
  - transudative with few cells and low protein concentrations;
  - spontaneous bacterial empyema (or pleuritis):
    - a total fluid PMN count $\geq 250/mm^3$ with a positive fluid culture; or
    - a fluid PMN count $\geq 500/mm^3$ with a negative fluid culture.

Treatment

- Medical management of hepatic hydrothorax should focus on treating ascites (see earlier).
- Therapeutic thoracentesis and paracentesis should be performed in dyspneic patients.
- Spontaneous bacterial empyema is treated with intravenous antibiotics as for SBP.
- Insertion of a large chest tube is generally not effective in the treatment of hepatic hydrothorax due to the risk of precipitating hypovolemic shock and re-expansion pulmonary edema.
- There have been studies assessing the utility of video-assisted thoracoscopy (VATS) with pleurodesis for the treatment of hepatic hydrothorax. Success rates are limited by a lack of apposition between the visceral and parietal pleura. Additionally, any surgical procedure in a patient with decompensated liver disease may increase mortality.
- Patients who are refractory to medical management and thoracentesis may also require more invasive approaches including a TIPS placement.
- Liver transplantation should be considered in patients with refractory hepatic hydrothorax.

Cirrhotic Cardiomyopathy

Definition

- Cirrhotic cardiomyopathy refers to a constellation of cardiac abnormalities that include electrophysiologic repolarization changes such as a prolonged QT interval, enlargement or hypertrophy of cardiac chambers, and blunted ventricular response to physiologic, pathologic, or pharmacologic stress in the face of a normal to increased cardiac output and contractility at rest.

Pathophysiology
- The pathophysiology of cirrhotic cardiomyopathy is unknown. Abnormal beta adrenergic receptor function, altered levels of cytokines, endogenous cannabinoids, and NO, and cardiomyocyte plasma membrane changes have been reported.

Clinical Features
- Patients are usually asymptomatic or have mild symptoms such as shortness of breath or chest pain.
- Overt heart failure can be precipitated by a TIPS, liver transplantation, or major surgery.
- Cirrhotic cardiomyopathy may contribute to the worsening of the hepatorenal syndrome.

Treatment
- Liver transplantation reverses cirrhotic cardiomyopathy.

Prognostic Scoring Systems for Cirrhosis

Various scoring systems have been developed to determine prognosis and the need for transplantation.

Child–Turcotte–Pugh Score
- This uses five variables (bilirubin, INR, albumin, ascites, and encephalopathy), each allocated a score of 1–3, to compute an overall score and 3 Child-Pugh classes – A, B, and C (Table 16.2).
- A limitation of this scoring system is the subjective evaluation of the degree of ascites and encephalopathy.

The Model for End-Stage Liver Disease (MELD) Score
- This is another model to assess severity of end-stage liver disease; it is considered to overcome some of the limitations of the Child–Pugh classification by eliminating subjectivity.

Table 16.2 Child–Turcotte–Pugh score.

Parameter	1 point	2 points	3 points
Total bilirubin* (mg/dL)	<2	2–3	>3
Serum albumin (g/L)	>3.5	2.8–3.5	<2.8
International normalized ratio (INR)	<1.7	1.7–2.2	>2.2
Ascites	None	Mild	Severe
Hepatic encephalopathy	None	Grade I–II	Grade III–IV

Points	Class	1-year survival rate	2-year survival rate
5–6	A	100%	85%
7–9	B	81%	57%
10–15	C	45%	35%

*In cholestatic diseases (primary biliary cirrhosis and primary sclerosing cholangitis), the bilirubin references are changed; the upper limit for 1 point is 4mg/dL and the upper limit for 2 points is 10mg/dL.

- It was developed at the Mayo Clinic and modified by the United Network for Organ Sharing to facilitate objective allocation of donor organs for patients in need of liver transplantation, with the severity of liver disease guiding prioritization.
- The MELD score predicts 3-month mortality for patients with end-stage liver disease.
- The score ranges from 6 to 40 based on three variables – INR, creatinine, and bilirubin – plus the need for renal replacement therapy.

- Three-month mortality rates according to MELD score are as follows:
  - <9: 1.9%;
  - 10–19: 6.0%;
  - 20–29: 19.6%;
  - 30–39: 52.6%;
  - 40 or more: 71.3%.
- Patients with a MELD score >15 have been shown to have improved survival with liver transplantation.

Liver Transplantation

- Liver transplantation offers patients with acute or chronic liver disease improved survival and quality of life.
- Indications:
  - fulminant hepatic failure;
  - liver-based metabolic deficiency (e.g., ornithine transcarbamylase deficiency, hyperoxalurea);
  - cirrhosis with a MELD score of ≥15; or cirrhosis with one of the following complications:
    - recurrent or refractory ascites;
    - hepatocellular carcinoma (three tumors each ≤3 cm or one tumor ≤5 cm, with the tumor burden confined to liver);
    - hepatorenal syndrome;
    - recurrent portal hypertensive bleeding with or without a portosystemic shunt;
    - hepatopulmonary syndrome;
    - mild portopulmonary hypertension;
    - refractory hepatic hydrothorax.
  - biliary atresia;
  - hepatoblastoma;
  - Alagille syndrome;
  - hereditary tyrosinemia;
  - glycogen storage diseases;
  - metastatic neuroendocrine tumors.
- Contraindications to liver transplantation:
  - continued alcohol or substance abuse;
  - advanced cardiopulmonary disease;
  - morbid obesity;
  - extrahepatic malignancy;
  - severe systemic infection or sepsis;
  - inability to comply with pre- and post-transplant regimens.

Pearls

Approximately 50% of all patients with cirrhosis have gastroesophageal varices. It is recommended that all patients with cirrhosis be screened for the presence of varices by EGD. Those with large esophageal varices at risk for bleeding should be started on a nonselective beta blocker or undergo EVL for primary prevention.

A majority of patients with cirrhosis will develop HE. HE is a prognostic indicator of poor survival (3-year survival 20% without liver transplantation).

Patients with SBP are often asymptomatic. All hospitalized patients with cirrhosis and ascites should undergo a diagnostic paracentesis.

Questions

Questions 1 and 2 relate to the clinical vignette at the beginning of this chapter.

1. The next step in the management of the patient presented is which of the following?
   A. Diuretic therapy with furosemide and spironolactone
   B. Diagnostic paracentesis
   C. Large-volume paracentesis
   D. Echocardiogram
   E. Ultrasonography of the liver

2. The patient is admitted to the hospital, and a diagnostic paracentesis is performed. The peritoneal fluid analysis should include which of the following?
   A. Albumin
   B. Cell count
   C. Bacterial culture
   D. All of the above
   E. None of the above

3. The most common pathogen causing spontaneous bacterial peritonitis (SBP) is which of the following?
   A. *Clostridium perfringens*
   B. *Escherichia coli*
   C. Coagulase-negative *Staphyloccocus aureus*
   D. *Mycobacterium tuberculosis*
   E. *Helicobacter pylori*

4. A 45-year-old man has known cirrhosis resulting from chronic hepatitis C and alcoholism. He is brought by ambulance to the emergency department after a witnessed syncopal event preceded by two episodes of hematemesis. On arrival, the blood pressure is 68/40 mmHg and pulse rate 120/min. He is afebrile, alert, and oriented. What is the first step in the management of this patient?

A. Nasogastric tube placement
B. Placement of two large-bore intravenous lines
C. Noncontrast computed tomography of the head
D. Electrocardiogram
E. Placement of an oral airway

5. Which of the following statements regarding portal hypertension is true?
   A. It results from increased intrahepatic resistance and an increase in portal blood flow.
   B. It is measured by calculating the difference between the central venous pressure and the hepatic vein pressure.
   C. It is mediated by carbon dioxide released from endothelial cells.
   D. It is associated with increased peripheral vasomotor tone.
   E. It results in an increase in effective arterial blood volume to the nephron.

Answers

1. B
   The suspicion for SBP in this patient is high. Given increased mortality rates associated with SBP, initiation of early antibiotic therapy is essential. A paracentesis should be performed as soon as possible. A large-volume paracentesis is unnecessary.

2. D
   A patient with newly diagnosed ascites must undergo paracentesis to evaluate the etiology of ascites and to rule out infection. Fluid albumin and total protein concentrations, cell and differential counts, and bacterial culture should be obtained.

3. B
   Gram-negative rods, particularly *Escherichia coli*, are the most common pathogens implicated in SBP.

4. B
   In a patient with hemodynamic instability, obtaining intravenous access and aggressive volume resuscitation must be performed expeditiously. If the patient were not breathing, placement of an airway would be needed immediately, before placement of peripheral intravenous lines.

5. A
   Portal hypertension results from intrahepatic resistance to blood flow and increased portal venous blood inflow. The increased intrahepatic resistance is mediated by sinusoidal fibrosis and compression by regenerative nodules. Increased portal venous blood flow is caused by decreased release of nitric oxide in the intrahepatic sinusoids coupled with increased release of nitric oxide and vasodilatation in both the splanchnic and systemic circulation.

Further Reading

Garcia-Tsao, G. (2006) Portal hypertension. *Current Opinion in Gastroenterology*, 22, 254–262.

Runyon, B.A., AASLD Practice Guidelines Committee. (2009) Management of adult patients with ascites due to cirrhosis: an update. *Hepatology*, 49, 2087–2107.

Shah, V.H. and Kamath, P.S. (2010) Portal hypertension and gastrointestinal bleeding, in *Sleisenger and Fordtran's Gastrointestinal and Liver Disease: Pathophysiology/Diagnosis/Management*, 9th edn (eds M. Feldman, L.S. Friedman and L.J. Brandt), Saunders Elsevier, Philadelphia, pp. 1489–1516.

Sharma, P. and Rakela, J. (2005) Management of pre-liver transplantation patient-part 2. *Liver Transplantation*, 11, 249–260.

Weblinks

http://www.turner-white.com/pdf/brm_Gast_pre10_1.pdf
http://www.med.upenn.edu/gastro/documents/
   Gastroenterologyportalhypertensionandcomplications.pdf
http://www.aafp.org/afp/2006/0901/p767.html
http://www.jefferson.edu/gi/education/documents/
   ComplicationsChronicLiverDiseaseHerrine-06.pdf

Pancreas and Biliary System

Field F. Willingham

Pancreatic Anatomy and Function

Field F. Willingham

CHAPTER 17

Clinical Vignette

A 36-year-old woman presents to the emergency department with a one-day history of epigastric pain radiating to the back. She has had several similar episodes, but the current episode is the most severe. She complains of nausea and has had three episodes of nonbloody emesis. She denies diarrhea, constipation, melena, hematemesis, fatigue, or weight loss. Her past medical and surgical history is unremarkable. Her only medication is an oral contraceptive pill. She drinks one to two glasses of wine per month. She does not smoke. Physical examination reveals a blood pressure of 144/85 mmHg, pulse rate 89/min, and temperature 100.2 °F (37.9 °C). She has mild tenderness to palpation in the epigastrium and right upper quadrant. There is no rebound tenderness or guarding. Bowel sounds are normal. The remainder of the examination is unremarkable. Abdominal ultrasonography reveals a normal gallbladder with no wall thickening, pericholecystic fluid, or gallstones. There is fluid noted around the pancreas. Laboratory tests including liver enzymes are normal. The serum lipase level is 269 U/L and the amylase level is 223 U/L.

Anatomy

- The pancreas is a retroperitoneal organ that lies posterior to the stomach.
- The head of the pancreas lies in the curvature of the duodenum and to the right of the portal vein confluence (formed by the union of the superior mesenteric vein and splenic vein) (Figure 17.1).

Essentials of Gastroenterology, First Edition. Edited by Shanthi V. Sitaraman, Lawrence S. Friedman.
© 2012 John Wiley & Sons, Ltd. Published 2012 by John Wiley & Sons, Ltd.

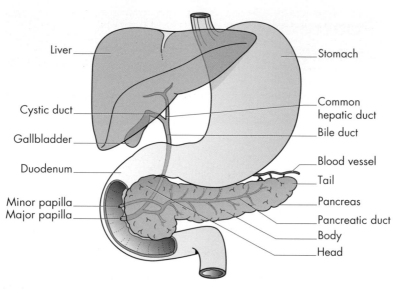

Figure 17.1 The anatomy of the pancreas, pancreatic ducts, and the bile duct.

Tumors in the head of the pancreas may cause compression of the duodenum leading to gastric outlet obstruction.

- The neck of the pancreas lies anterior to the portal vein.
- The body of the pancreas lies between the portal confluence and the abdominal aorta.

Due to its proximity to the local vasculature, pancreatic adenocarcinoma frequently invades the portal vein, celiac axis, and/or superior mesenteric artery early in the course. Therefore, pancreatic cancer is often advanced and unresectable at the time of presentation.

- The splenic vein and artery course along the length of the pancreas. Splenic vein thrombosis can occur in patients with pancreatitis and pancreatic tumors.
- The tail of the pancreas terminates in the superior portion of the splenic hilum.
- The uncinate process of the pancreas tucks in posteriorly behind the superior mesenteric artery and vein.

Tumors in the head of the pancreas may cause dilatation of the bile duct and pancreatic duct, resulting in the "double-duct sign". The sensitivity of the double-duct sign for detecting pancreatic cancer is 77–85%.

- The midline portion of the pancreatic body lies anterior to the lumbar spine.

Blunt severe force in the anterior–posterior direction of the abdominal cavity is most likely to cause injury to the body of the pancreas as it crosses anterior to the lumbar spine.

- The distal portion of the bile duct runs through the pancreatic parenchyma in the head and joins with the pancreatic duct.

Mass lesions in the head of the pancreas may present with painless jaundice resulting from extrinsic compression of the distal bile duct.

- The common channel formed by the union of the bile duct and pancreatic duct terminates at and drains through the major papilla.

Gallstones passing from the gallbladder may obstruct biliary and pancreatic outflow, thereby resulting in elevated liver biochemical test levels and gallstone pancreatitis.

- The accessory pancreatic duct, called the duct of Santorini, drains through the minor papilla and usually communicates with the main pancreatic duct, the duct of Wirsung.
- The pancreatic duct has its greatest diameter in the head of the pancreas. The diameter of the pancreatic duct typically follows the "3-2-1 rule": the diameter measures approximately 3 mm in the head, 2 mm in the body, and 1 mm in the tail.
- The exocrine pancreas constitutes approximately 90% of the pancreas.
- The functional unit of the exocrine pancreas consists of the acinus and a corresponding ductule (Figure 17.2).
- Between the acinus and the ductule are the centroacinar cells.
- The ductules drain into larger interlobular ducts, which drain into the main pancreatic duct.

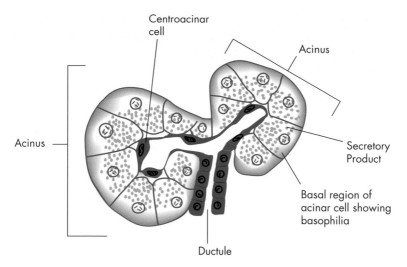

Figure 17.2 Diagram of a pancreatic acinus and ductule. Zymogen granules are stored at the apical aspect of the acinar cells. Enzymatic secretion is stimulated by small peptides, fat, and carbohydrate in the duodenum and is upregulated by cholecystokinin and acetylcholine. (Adapted from Dr. Thomas Caceci and Dr. Samir El-Shafey; Virginia Tech, Blacksburg, VA, USA.)

Embryology

- Pancreatic development begins around the fourth week of gestation.
- The pancreas develops from the endoderm and begins as dorsal and ventral buds.
- The dorsal bud grows more rapidly than the ventral bud and forms the majority of the pancreas (the superior portion of the head, the body, and the tail).
- The ventral pancreas initially arises in the duodenum on the opposite side from the dorsal bud.
- The ventral bud rotates and fuses with the dorsal bud to become the inferior portion of the head and the uncinate process.
- The ventral and dorsal ducts anastomose to form the main pancreatic duct. The proximal portion of the dorsal duct becomes the duct of Santorini in most adults.

Developmental Anomalies

- Pancreas divisum:
  - Pancreas divisum is the most common pancreatic congenital anomaly.

- In pancreas divisum, the dorsal and ventral ducts do not fuse during development. The main dorsal pancreatic duct drains through the minor papilla, and the ventral duct drains separately through the major papilla.
- It is estimated that pancreas divisum may be present in up to 7% of the population.
- There may be a higher risk of pancreatitis in patients with pancreas divisum. This is thought to be due to reduced outflow of pancreatic secretions through a diminutive or stenotic minor papilla.
- Pancreas divisum may be found in 19% of patients with idiopathic pancreatitis undergoing endoscopic retrograde cholangiopancreatography.
- Patients with recurrent pancreatitis due to pancreas divisum may be managed with sphincterotomy of the minor papilla and temporary placement of a pancreatic duct stent.

- Annular pancreas:
  - Annular pancreas describes a congenital anomaly in which a band of pancreatic tissue surrounds the second portion of the duodenum.
  - The condition results from abnormal fusion of the dorsal and ventral buds, which form a ring of pancreatic tissue around the duodenum.
  - There is a bimodal age distribution of the clinical presentation of annular pancreas, with a relatively increased frequency of presentation in the neonatal period and in adults in the fourth and fifth decades.

> In infants, annular pancreas may present on imaging with the "double-bubble sign." The double-bubble sign reflects the regions of dilatation in the proximal duodenum and the distal stomach.

  - Annular pancreas is treated by performing a surgical bypass (duodenoduodenostomy or gastrojejunostomy), because the pancreatic tissue may extend into the duodenal wall.
- Ectopic pancreas:
  - Ectopic pancreas refers to the presence of pancreatic tissue outside the pancreatic gland.
  - Ectopic pancreatic tissue may be found in many anatomic locations but is most frequently observed in the stomach, duodenum, and distal small intestine.
  - Ectopic pancreas is usually an incidental finding.

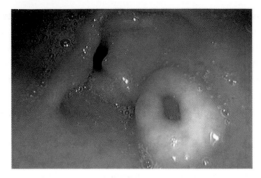

Figure 17.3 The classic appearance of a pancreatic rest in the gastric antrum adjacent to the pylorus on esophagogastroduodenoscopy. A pancreatic rest is a focus of ectopic pancreatic tissue with a characteristic central umbilication.

○ A **pancreatic rest** is a focus of ectopic pancreas that has a classic appearance of a small nodule with a central umbilication and is typically seen in the stomach as an incidental finding during esophagogastroduodenoscopy (Figure 17.3).

Physiology

Pancreatic Secretion

- Digestive enzymes are synthesized, stored, and secreted by the acinar cells. The enzymes are stored as inactive precursors (zymogens) in the zymogen granules located in the apical aspect of the acinar cells (see Figure 17.2).
- Activation of the zymogens is a multistage process that involves several proteolytic steps that occur sequentially during the transport of the nascent enzyme from its site of synthesis on ribosomes and endoplasmic reticulum to its final destination in the luminal space of the duodenum.
- The acinar cells are stimulated via basolateral membrane receptors, which trigger secretion of zymogen into the lumen of the acinus.
- In the last stage, trypsinogen is converted into an active form, trypsin, by enteropeptidase (also called enterokinase), an enzyme produced by the crypts of Lieberkühn in the duodenum. Trypsin, in turn, converts the other pancreatic proenzymes into their active forms in the duodenum.

Inappropriate activation of pancreatic proenzymes within the pancreas leads to pancreatitis.

- The pancreas secretes 1–2.5 L of fluid per day. As a consequence, dehydration can occur in patients with a pancreatic fistula when secretions are not delivered to the intestinal lumen for subsequent reabsorption.
- There are two major types of pancreatic secretion: the aqueous fraction and the enzymatic fraction:
  - The **aqueous fraction** is rich in bicarbonate and acts to neutralize the acidic chyme in the duodenum. The inorganic products of pancreatic secretion also include water, sodium, potassium, and chloride. The aqueous fraction is secreted by the centroacinar cells and ductal cells. Aqueous secretion is stimulated by the presence of H^+ ions in the duodenum and upregulated by secretin and acetylcholine.
  - The **enzymatic fraction** of pancreatic secretion acts on carbohydrates, proteins, and fat and plays a key role in digestion and absorption.
- Pancreatic enzymes are secreted by the acinar cells:
  - The pancreatic enzymes amylase and lipase are secreted in the active form.
  - As mentioned earlier, proteases, trypsinogen and chymotrypsinogen, are secreted in an inactive form and require further steps for activation.
  - Enzymatic secretion is stimulated by small peptides, fat, and carbohydrates in the duodenum. Enzymatic secretion is upregulated by cholecystokinin and acetylcholine.
- As pancreatic flow increases, often due to secretin stimulation, the relative concentration of bicarbonate increases.
- Table 17.1 compares pancreatic enzymes and several gastrointestinal hormones.

Chronic disease of the exocrine pancreas, such as cystic fibrosis and chronic pancreatitis, leads to loss of pancreatic mass and deficiency of pancreatic enzymes and may result in maldigestion. Maldigestion, in turn, leads to weight loss and nutritional deficiencies.

Endocrine Function
- The primary role of the endocrine pancreas is to secrete insulin and other hormones to control serum levels of glucose and triglycerides and amino acid balance.
- The endocrine portion of the pancreas constitutes approximately 10% of the gland and is made up of the islets of Langerhans.

Table 17.1 Enzymes and gastrointestinal hormones involved in digestion.

Enzyme or hormone	Source	Function	Regulation	Comment
Amylase	Pancreas and salivary glands	Digests dietary starch and glycogen	Stimulated by the vagus nerve, acetylcholine, CCK	Isolated hyperamylasemia may not be related to pancreatic disease
Lipase	Primarily pancreas	Hydrolyzes triglycerides and fatty acids	Stimulated by the vagus nerve, acetylcholine, CCK	More specific to the pancreas than amylase
Gastrin	G-cells (in the antrum and duodenum)	Stimulates secretion of gastric acid, intrinsic factor, and pepsinogen Increases gastric motility	Stimulated by gastric distension, amino acids, peptides, the vagus nerve Inhibited by secretin and very low gastric pH	Hypersecretion may be seen with gastrinoma (Zollinger–Ellison syndrome), leading to peptic ulceration and associated complications

Hormone	Cell source	Functions	Stimulus/inhibition	Clinical notes
CCK	I-cells (in the duodenum and jejunum)	Stimulates gallbladder contraction and pancreatic enzyme secretion; Inhibits gastric acid secretion	Stimulated by fat and acid	A HIDA scan uses a synthetic form of CCK to stimulate gallbladder contraction. Gallbladder dysfunction is defined as an ejection fraction less than 35%
Secretin	S-cells (in the duodenum)	Stimulates pancreatic secretion; Inhibits gastric acid secretion	Stimulated by acid and fat in the duodenum	Secretin is involved in alkalinizing the duodenum; pancreatic enzymes are inactivated by an acidic pH
Somatostatin	D-cells (in the pancreatic islets and gastric and intestinal mucosa)	Inhibits gastric acid and pepsinoger secretion; Decreases gallbladder contraction; Inhibits release of insulin and glucagon	Stimulated by acid; Inhibited by the vagus nerve	An inhibitory hormone. Synthetic somatostatin, octreotide, is used to treat carcinoid syndrome, acute variceal bleeding, and acromegaly

CCK, cholecystokinin; HIDA, hydroxy iminodiacetic acid

- The majority of the cells in the islets are beta cells, which produce insulin.
- Other cell types within each islet are the alpha, delta, and PP cells.
- The alpha cells secrete glucagon; the delta cells secrete somatostatin; and the PP cells secrete pancreatic polypeptide.
- Autonomic nerves, metabolites such as glucose, circulating hormones, and local paracrine hormones regulate the function of the islets.

Pearls

The splenic vein and artery course along the length of the pancreas. Splenic vein thrombosis may lead to gastric varices in the absence of esophageal varices. Unlike cirrhosis, this presentation is not related to portal hypertension.

It is estimated that symptoms of pancreatic insufficiency do not present until 85–90% of the pancreatic mass is compromised.

Questions

Questions 1 and 2 relate to the clinical vignette at the beginning of this chapter.

1. Which of the following is the most likely diagnosis?
   A. Primary sclerosing cholangitis
   B. Acute cholecystitis
   C. Ascending cholangitis
   D. Acute pancreatitis
   E. Peptic ulcer disease

2. Which of the following is the next best step in the evaluation of the patient's condition?
   A. Esophagogastroduodenoscopy
   B. Cholecystectomy
   C. Endoscopic retrograde cholangiopancreatography (ERCP)
   D. Magnetic resonance imaging (MRI)/ magnetic resonance cholangiopancreatography (MRCP)
   E. Serum amylase isoforms

3. A 26-year-old man is involved in a motor vehicle collision. He was the driver of the vehicle and was wearing his seat belt. The vehicle is "totaled," and the passengers are transported to the nearest trauma center. The

driver complains of marked abdominal pain. Computed tomography shows fluid surrounding the pancreas. A traumatic injury would most likely be localized to which of the following regions?

A. Stomach

B. Head of the pancreas

C. Body of the pancreas

D. Gallbladder

E. Spleen

4. An 84-year-old man is admitted to the hospital with lethargy and a change in mental status. Physical examination reveals a thin frail man. The blood pressure is 92/54 mmHg, pulse rate 115/min, and temperature 102 °F (38.9 °C). He is mildly jaundiced and oriented to person but not to place or time. Abdominal examination reveals mild tenderness to palpation in the epigastrium. There is no rebound tenderness or guarding. Bowel sounds are present. Abdominal ultrasonography reveals dilatation of the bile duct to 12 mm, multiple gallstones in the gallbladder, but no gallbladder wall thickening or pericholecystic fluid. Laboratory tests show a normal complete blood count, total bilirubin level of 5 mg/dL, aspartate aminotransferase 145 U/L, alanine aminotransferase 79 U/L, amylase 196 U/L, and lipase 246 U/L. The patient is started on intravenous fluids and broad-spectrum antibiotics. Which of the following is most appropriate at this time?

A. Laparoscopy

B. Cholecystectomy

C. Cholecystostomy tube placement

D. Endoscopic retrograde cholangiopancreatography (ERCP)

E. Magnetic resonance cholangiopancreatography (MRCP)

5. A 55-year-old man presents to his primary care doctor with a complaint of abdominal discomfort, bloating, and early satiety. The primary care physician obtains an abdominal X-ray, which reveals air–fluid levels in the stomach and first portion of the duodenum. Esophagogastroduodenoscopy is performed and reveals narrowing in the second portion of the duodenum with normal-appearing duodenal mucosa. The patient's findings are consistent with which of the following diagnosis?

A. Annular pancreas

B. Cystic fibrosis

C. Duodenal atresia

D. Pancreatic heterotopia

E. Pancreas divisum

(Continued)

Answers

1. D

2. D

This patient has mild acute pancreatitis as evidenced by epigastric pain and mildly elevated serum amylase and lipase levels. She likely has pancreatitis secondary to pancreatic divisum. Ultrasonography did not reveal features of cholecystitis such as gallbladder wall thickening, pericholecystic fluid, or gallstones. Ascending cholangitis is unlikely in the absence of fever, jaundice, or elevated liver enzyme levels. Peptic ulcer typically presents with epigastric pain and possibly with bleeding, but not with elevated serum amylase and lipase levels. Primary sclerosing cholangitis presents with elevated liver biochemical test levels in a cholestatic pattern (elevated serum bilirubin and alkaline phosphatase levels). ERCP would be considered if the bilirubin and alkaline phosphatase levels were elevated or there was other evidence of cholangitis or bile duct dilatation but would not be the next test in this case. Amylase isoforms can be obtained to determine if the salivary amylase level is elevated in serum and can be helpful in a patient with isolated hyperamylasemia. This patient has elevation of both amylase and lipase levels (lipase is more specific for the pancreas) associated with abdominal pain and fluid around the pancreas, and the elevated amylase level is not likely to be from a salivary source. MRI/MRCP would be helpful to evaluate the pancreatic parenchyma, which is not seen well on abdominal ultrasonography. MRI/MRCP will also help visualize the pancreatic and biliary ductal systems. If MRI/MRCP shows pancreas divisum, ERCP may be considered as a therapeutic intervention to perform sphincterotomy of the minor papilla.

3. C

This patient sustained a pancreatic injury following a motor vehicle collision; this is a common occurrence following a "seat-belt injury." The most frequently injured segment of the pancreas is the body, which passes anterior to the spine. Traumatic pancreatic injuries frequently can be missed on abdominal imaging. The spleen can be injured in motor vehicle collisions; however, in this case ultrasonography revealed fluid around the pancreas and no damage to the spleen.

4. D

This patient has ascending cholangitis and gallstone pancreatitis. After fluid resuscitation and administration of antibiotics, ERCP is indicated for biliary decompression. The bile duct is dilated, and the serum aminotransferase and pancreatic enzyme levels are elevated. Together with the presence of gallstones, this pattern is most suggestive of bile duct obstruction secondary to choledocholithiasis. The patient has Charcot's triad with fever, jaundice, and abdominal pain, as well as Reynold's pentad with the addition of hypotension and altered mental status. There is no evidence of cholecystitis on ultrasonography. Placement of a cholecystostomy tube may be considered for urgent decompression of the gallbladder in patients who are in the intensive care unit and in whom ERCP cannot be performed due to hemodynamic instability. MRCP would be unlikely to change the diagnosis, is not therapeutic, and could delay definitive management.

5. A

This patient has annular pancreas, a condition in which the pancreatic parenchyma encircles the second portion of the duodenum. A double-bubble sign on an abdominal X-ray is characteristic of annular pancreas. A double-bubble sign may also be seen with duodenal atresia. Duodenal atresia typically presents in neonates and is rarely diagnosed in childhood or adulthood. Cystic fibrosis typically presents in neonates, infants, and children. Gastrointestinal manifestations of cystic fibrosis include pancreatic insufficiency, steatorrhea, failure to thrive, and abdominal pain. Pancreas divisum does not present with duodenal narrowing and obstruction. Pancreatic heterotopia is often an incidental finding on endoscopy and does not cause obstructive symptoms.

Further Reading

Costanzo, L.S. (1998) *Physiology*, 1st edn, W.B. Saunders, Pennsylvania, pp. 289–333.

Owyang, C. and Williams, J.A. (2003) Pancreatic secretion, in *Textbook of Gastroenterology*, 4th edn (ed T. Yamada), Lippincott Williams & Wilkins, Pennsylvania, pp. 340–366.

Pandol SJ. Pancreatic secretion, in *Sleisenger and Fordtran's Gastrointestinal and Liver Disease: Pathophysiology/Diagnosis/Management*, 9th edn (eds M. Feldman, L.S. Friedman and L.J. Brandt), Saunders Elsevier, Philadelphia, pp. 921–929.

Acute Pancreatitis

Steven Keilin

CHAPTER 18

Clinical Vignette

A 48-year-old man presents with a 2-day history of nausea and upper abdominal pain. He describes the abdominal pain as gnawing, constant, radiating to the back, and associated with decreased appetite. The pain is not aggravated by movement, coughing, or breathing and improves with sitting or leaning forward. He reports that over the previous weekend he was on vacation with friends and consumed up to 10 beers each day. His past medical history is remarkable for hypertension and dyslipidemia. His medications include hydrochlorothiazide, simvastatin, and ibuprofen 1–2 tablets per week for joint pain. He has never had surgery. His family history is remarkable for hypertension and diabetes mellitus in his father. He is married and has three children, who are healthy. He used to smoke cigarettes but quit 10 years ago. He has consumed one to two beers daily for many years and admits to binge drinking on most weekends. On physical examination, the blood pressure is 136/88 mmHg, pulse rate 112/min, and respiratory rate 12/min. He is afebrile. There are no cutaneous stigmata of liver disease, tattoos, or needle tracts. There is no conjunctival icterus. The abdomen is tender to palpation in the epigastrium, but there is no guarding or rebound tenderness. There is no hepatosplenomegaly. Bowel sounds are present and normal. Rectal examination is normal. Laboratory tests show a white blood cell count of 13500/mm^3, serum aspartate aminotransferase (AST) 105 U/L, alanine aminotransferase (ALT) 48 U/L, alkaline phosphatase 92 U/L, and total bilirubin 0.8 mg/dL. The remainder of the blood work is normal.

Essentials of Gastroenterology, First Edition. Edited by Shanthi V. Sitaraman, Lawrence S. Friedman.
© 2012 John Wiley & Sons, Ltd. Published 2012 by John Wiley & Sons, Ltd.

General

- Acute pancreatitis is an acute inflammatory condition of the pancreas that may extend to local and distant extrapancreatic tissues.
- The clinical diagnosis of acute pancreatitis is based on the presence of two of the following three features: (1) serum amylase and lipase levels elevated three times the upper limit of normal; (2) epigastric abdominal pain (often radiating to the back); and (3) typical imaging features on computed tomography (CT) or magnetic resonance imaging (MRI).
- Acute pancreatitis accounts for more than 200 000 hospital admissions each year in the US.

Etiology

The majority (80%) of cases of acute pancreatitis are caused by gallstones or alcohol.

Gallstones

- Gallstones account for 45% of cases of acute pancreatitis.
- In addition to gallstones, microlithiasis (small [<3 mm] stones) and sludge (biliary debris) cause acute pancreatitis.
- Gallstones cause acute pancreatitis by obstructing the pancreatic duct or through reflux of bile or debris from the bile duct into the pancreatic duct.

Alcohol

- Alcohol accounts for 35% of cases of acute pancreatitis.
- Acute pancreatitis typically occurs after binge drinking. About 10% of heavy drinkers will develop acute pancreatitis.
- Persons with acute pancreatitis due to alcohol may have underlying chronic pancreatitis.

Other Causes

These account for 10% of cases of acute pancreatitis:

- Hypertriglyceridemia (serum triglyceride level >1000 mg/dL).
- Hyperparathyroidism/hypercalcemia.
- Medications (asparaginase, azathioprine, 6-mercaptopurine, dapsone, didanosine, enalapril, estrogen and tamoxifen (by raising serum triglycerides), isoniazid, mesalamine, methyldopa, metronidazole, nonsteroidal anti-inflammatory drugs, pentamidine, procainamide,

simvastatin, sulfonamides, sulindac, tetracyclines, thiazides, valproic acid).
- Infections (tuberculosis, *Mycobacterium avium* complex infection, cytomegalovirus infection, Coxsackie virus infection, ascariasis).
- Vascular diseases (polyarteritis nodosa, systemic lupus erythematosus, ischemic damage to the pancreas).
- Anatomic causes:
  ○ pancreas divisum: affects up to 7% of the population, but pancreatitis occurs in 15% of persons with pancreas divisum;
  ○ sphincter of Oddi dysfunction.
- Genetic causes (associated with chronic pancreatitis that may present acutely):
  ○ cystic fibrosis;
  ○ hereditary pancreatitis:
    ▪ protease serine 1 (PRSS1), (also called cationic trypsinogen) – a mutation in the *PRSS1* gene renders trypsinogen resistant to autolysis, thereby leading to the activation of trypsinogen within the pancreas;
    ▪ serine protease inhibitor Kazal type 1 (SPINK1) – a mutation in the *SPINK1* gene, which codes for trypsin inhibitor, leads to trypsin activation within the pancreas.
- Post-endoscopic retrograde cholangiopancreatography (post-ERCP). Acute pancreatitis occurs in an estimated 5% of diagnostic ERCPs and in 25% of persons with sphincter of Oddi dysfunction who undergo ERCP.
- Autoimmune pancreatitis: often associated with concomitant autoimmune disorders like Sjögren's syndrome, autoimmune thyroiditis, sclerosing cholangitis (see Chapter 19).
- Pancreatic cancer.

Idiopathic Acute Pancreatitis
- The cause of pancreatitis is unknown in 10% of cases.

Differential Diagnosis

- Peptic ulcer disease
- Gastritis/gastropathy
- Intestinal perforation
- Acute cholecystitis
- Mesenteric ischemia
- Small intestinal obstruction
- Ruptured abdominal aortic aneurysm
- Acute hepatitis.

Pathophysiology

- Normal mechanisms that protect the pancreas (see also Chapter 17) include:
  - ○ the activation of pancreatic proenzymes occurs outside of the pancreas within the duodenal lumen;
  - ○ enterokinase, the enzyme responsible for activating pancreatic proenzymes, is located only in the duodenum;
  - ○ trypsin inhibitor (SPINK1) partially blocks the activity of trypsin.
- Mechanisms of injury in acute pancreatitis (Figure 18.1) include:
  - ○ activation of pancreatic proenzymes into active forms occurs within the pancreatic acinar cells, thereby leading to autodigestion of pancreatic tissue;
  - ○ failure of normal protective mechanisms to inactivate trypsin such as SPINK1 dysfunction;
  - ○ microcirculatory injury and damage to the vascular endothelium in the pancreas lead to the activation of the complement system, release of proinflammatory mediators, and translocation of bacteria into the systemic circulation.

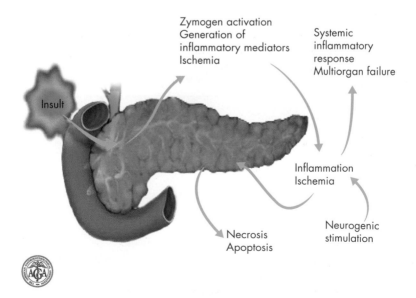

Figure 18.1 Mechanisms of injury in acute pancreatitis.

Clinical Features

- Typical symptoms:
  - pain – 90–95% of patients with acute pancreatitis present with abdominal pain that is usually localized to the epigastrium or right upper quadrant and often radiates to the back. The pain may be worse after eating;
  - nausea and vomiting – in 90% of patients;
  - fever and chills may occur but do not necessarily indicate infection;
  - anorexia and decreased appetite may also be seen.
- Physical examination:
  - common findings include tachycardia, fever, epigastric or right upper quadrant tenderness, localized guarding and rebound tenderness in the epigastrium, and decreased bowel sounds;
  - findings associated with severe pancreatitis include hypotension, jaundice, tachypnea, and a palpable mass (which may indicate a pseudocyst); pancreatic necrosis may track along the falciform ligament and into the retroperitoneum and can be seen as ecchymoses in the periumbilical region (Cullen's sign) and flanks (Grey-Turner's sign).

Complications

- Local:
  - pancreatic: pseudocyst, ascites, fistula, fluid collection, abscess, necrosis (sterile and infected);

> Organisms most frequently seen in infected pancreatic necrosis include *Escherichia coli*, *Klebsiella* spp., *Pseudomonas* spp., *Enterococcus* spp., and rarely *Candida albicans*.

  - nonpancreatic: ileus, bile duct obstruction, gastric outlet obstruction, duodenal ulcer, splenic vein thrombosis.
- Systemic:
  - cardiovascular: hypotension, tachycardia, shock;
  - pulmonary: pleural effusion, pulmonary edema, acute respiratory distress syndrome (ARDS);
  - renal: decreased urine output, acute renal failure;
  - hematologic: vascular thrombosis, disseminated intravascular coagulation;

○ metabolic: metabolic acidosis, hyperglycemia, hypocalcemia;
○ infectious: sepsis, bacteremia, fungemia.

Prognosis

• The majority (75–80%) of cases of acute pancreatitis are mild and self-limiting.
• 20–25% of cases are severe, and despite aggressive efforts at initial resuscitation, up to 50% of these patients will develop multiorgan failure or pancreatic necrosis.
  ○ The mortality rate in patients with severe, acute pancreatitis is 10–30%:
    ▪ approximately 75% of deaths are associated with the presence of pancreatic necrosis;
    ▪ early mortality (<7 days) is usually due to multiorgan failure;
    ▪ late mortality (>7 days) is usually due to sepsis or other infectious complications.

Assessment of Severity

• Several scoring systems have been developed to predict severity, in order to identify severe, acute pancreatitis and predict pancreatic necrosis, mortality, and the need for prompt aggressive fluid resuscitation and intensive patient monitoring.
• Ranson's criteria: measured at admission and at 48 hours (Tables 18.1 and 18.2).
• Acute Physiology And Chronic Health Evaluation (APACHE) III:
  ○ used to predict mortality in critically ill patients admitted to the intensive care unit;

Table 18.1 Ranson's criteria.

Admission	At 48 hours
Age >55	Hematocrit value decrease >10%
WBC >16 000 mm^3	BUN increase >5 mg/dL
Serum glucose >200 mg/dL	Calcium <8 mg/dL
Serum LDH >350 U/L	Base deficit ≥4 mEq/L
Serum AST >250 U/L	Fluid sequestration >6 L
	PaO$_2$ <60 mmHg

AST, aspartate aminotransferase; BUN, blood urea nitrogen; LDH, lactate dehydrogenase; WBC, white blood cell count.

Table 18.2 Ranson's criteria: the presence of three or more criteria predicts a severe course and increased mortality.

Number of criteria*	Mortality (%)
3–4	15
5–6	40
7–8	100

*See Table 18.1.

- ○ can be measured at any time during the hospital admission;
- ○ cumbersome method; some parameters may not be relevant to prognosis in acute pancreatitis.
- • CT severity index (Balthazar score):
  - ○ CT severity index utilizes the presence and degree of pancreatic necrosis and the presence or absence of peripancreatic fluid collections on CT to predict morbidity and mortality;
  - ○ the limitations of the CT severity index include variability in radiologists' interpretation of CT findings and lack of correlation of the score with the presence of organ failure, extrapancreatic complications, or peripancreatic vascular complications.
- • Atlanta classification:
  - ○ developed to allow comparison among all aforementioned scoring systems (Ranson's, APACHE, and CT severity index); however, it only defines mild and severe acute pancreatitis.
- • BISAP scoring system:
  - ○ simple five-point scoring system that includes: **B**lood urea nitrogen (>25 mg/dL), **I**mpaired mental status, **S**ystemic inflammatory response (SIRS), **A**ge (>65), **P**resence of pleural effusion (also called the **B**edside **I**ndex of the **S**everity of **A**cute **P**ancreatitis);
  - ○ BISAP is used to identify patients within the first 24 hours of admission at increased risk of in-hospital mortality.
- • Other indicators of severity or pancreatic necrosis: blood urea nitrogen, hematocrit value, C-reactive protein (CRP), serum interleukin-6, urinary trypsinogen activation peptide level.
- • HAPS score:
  - ○ **H**armless **A**cute **P**ancreatitis **S**core;
  - ○ absence of rebound abdominal tenderness, a normal hematocrit value, and a normal serum creatinine level predict a nonsevere course with 98% accuracy.

Diagnosis

Laboratory Tests

- Pancreas specific: the diagnosis of acute pancreatitis relies on elevations of serum amylase and lipase levels greater than three times the upper limit of normal. See Tables 18.3 and 18.4.
  - Amylase tends to rise earlier, within hours, and can remain elevated for 3–5 days.
  - Lipase is more specific for pancreatic disease and may remain elevated for longer periods than amylase.
  - The degree of pancreatic enzyme elevation or trend over time does not correlate with the patient's prognosis.
- Others:
  - Liver biochemical tests:
    - elevations of the serum bilirubin and alkaline phosphatase levels are often seen with gallstone pancreatitis (see Chapter 21);
    - greater than threefold elevation of the serum alanine aminotransferase (ALT) level is highly specific but not sensitive for gallstone pancreatitis;

Table 18.3 Other causes of hyperamylasemia.

Ectopic pregnancy
Intestinal perforation
Macroamylasemia
Medications
Mesenteric ischemia
Parotitis/salivary gland disease
Peptic ulcer disease
Renal failure

Table 18.4 Other causes of hyperlipasemia.

Gastritis/gastroenteritis
Intestinal obstruction
Intestinal perforation
Liver disease
Medications (e.g., chemotherapeutic agents)
Peptic ulcer disease

- elevation of the serum aspartate aminotransferase (AST) level greater than the serum ALT level may indicate acute pancreatitis due to alcohol consumption.
  - The white blood cell (WBC) count is commonly elevated; however, an elevated WBC count does not necessarily indicate infection.
  - Hyper- or hypoglycemia, hypocalcemia, and renal insufficiency are of prognostic significance.
  - Serum triglyceride levels should be checked and if elevated >1000 mg/dL may indicate hypertriglyceridemia as the cause of pancreatitis.

Imaging Modalities
- Abdominal X-ray:
  - plain films of the abdomen are often normal in acute pancreatitis; however, they are used to exclude other causes of abdominal pain;
  - may show ileus ("sentinel loop"), displacement or abnormal contour of other organs such as the stomach and colon ("colon cut-off sign"), gallstones, or pancreatic calcifications.
- Ultrasonography:
  - used to identify gallstones;
  - may also show bile duct dilatation, ascites, or decreased echogenicity of the pancreas;
  - because overlying bowel gas often obscures the pancreas, ultrasonography is a poor test to diagnose acute pancreatitis.
- Computed tomography (CT) with intravenous contrast (Figure 18.2)
  - CT is usually not necessary initially; however, it should be obtained if the patient is not improving clinically.
  - CT may be used to:
    - exclude other intra-abdominal disorders;
    - assess the severity of pancreatitis;
    - determine if complications are present.
  - CT is useful for detecting:
    - bile duct stones and bile duct dilatation;
    - pancreatic pseudocysts;
    - pancreatic necrosis and fluid collections (with administration of intravenous contrast).
  - CT can be used to guide needle aspiration or biopsy to assess for infected pancreatic necrosis.
  - Contraindications to performing CT include:
    - contrast allergy;
    - renal insufficiency.
- Magnetic resonance imaging (MRI) and magnetic resonance cholangiopancreatography (MRCP):

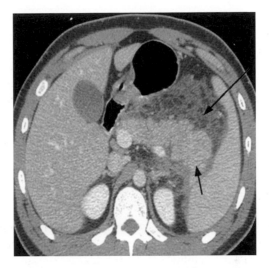

Figure 18.2 Computed tomography in a patient with acute pancreatitis. Findings include focal or diffuse enlargement (short arrow), heterogeneous enhancement of the pancreas, obliteration of fat planes around the pancreas, and peripancreatic fluid collections (long arrow).

- ○ MRI/MRCP uses gadolinium as a contrast agent; therefore, the test can be used in patients with an allergy to contrast dye.
- ○ MRI/MRCP is useful for detecting:
  - bile duct stones and bile duct dilatation;
  - pancreatic duct disruption;
  - pancreatic cysts and neoplasms;
  - pancreas divisum.
- ○ MRI/MRCP does not permit needle-guided biopsies and is more expensive than CT.
- Endoscopic retrograde cholangiopancreatography (ERCP):
  - ○ ERCP is preferable as a therapeutic rather than a purely diagnostic tool.
  - ○ ERCP should be used with caution in patients with severe acute pancreatitis, because acute pancreatitis may worsen with the procedure.
  - ○ ERCP is useful for detecting and treating:
    - bile duct stones (Figure 18.3) or microlithiasis;
    - bile duct stricture;
    - pancreas divisum;
    - pancreatic duct disruption;
    - sphincter of Oddi dysfunction.

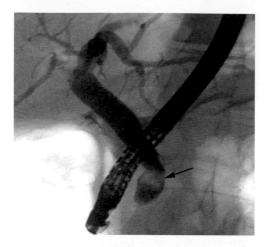

Figure 18.3 Endoscopic retrograde cholangiopancreatography showing a bile duct stone. A filling defect is seen in the distal bile duct (arrow) with dilatation of the bile duct proximal to the stone.

- ○ Commonly performed interventions include:
  - ▪ bile duct stone removal;
  - ▪ stent placement to relieve bile duct obstruction or treat pancreatic duct disruption.

Treatment

Prevention
- Preventive strategies include cessation of alcohol and smoking and discontinuation of potentially causative medications.

Conservative and Supportive Care
- The majority (80%) of cases will resolve with supportive measures.
- Aggressive fluid resuscitation with Ringer's lactate or normal saline 250–300 mL/hr intravenously for the first 48 hours is the mainstay of management of acute pancreatitis.
- Patients should be given nothing by mouth.
- Nasogastric suction should be considered in patients who have protracted vomiting.
- Electrolyte abnormalities should be corrected.
- Analgesics and anti-emetics should be given as needed.

Nutrition
- Oral diet should be initiated by day 3 if the patient's pain is improved and the patient's appetite returns.
  - Start with clear liquids and advance to a low-fat diet.
- If the patient's symptoms do not improve within 72 hours, parenteral or enteral feeding should be initiated.
- Total parenteral nutrition (TPN):
  - has been used traditionally;
  - does not stimulate pancreatic secretion;
  - has been shown to decrease mortality;
  - however, TPN is expensive and is associated with complications such as line infections, thrombophlebitis, electrolyte disturbances, and liver dysfunction (including cholestasis).
- Enteral nutrition through a nasogastric or nasojejunal feeding tube:
  - may stimulate pancreatic secretion;
  - is less expensive than TPN;
  - maintains intestinal integrity and prevents intestinal atrophy;
  - reduces the rate of infections and shortens length of hospitalization.

Enteral nutrition is preferred to TPN. There appears to be no difference in efficacy between nasojejunal and nasogastric feeding.

Antibiotics

The routine use of prophylactic antibiotics is not recommended for mild acute pancreatitis, and its use is controversial in severe acute pancreatitis. Routine use of antibiotics does not affect the rate of infection or mortality. Use of antibiotics also increases the risk of fungal infections and infections with resistant organisms.

- Antibiotics are recommended in the following situations:
  - persistent fever or leukocytosis while the source is being identified;
  - pancreatic necrosis, both sterile ($\geq30\%$ of pancreas) and infected (Figure 18.4), although the use of antibiotics in sterile necrosis is controversial;
  - bacteremia;
  - infected pancreatic pseudocyst;
  - an abscess or infected peripancreatic fluid collection.

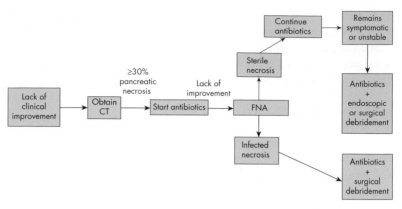

Figure 18.4 Algorithm for the approach to the management of pancreatic necrosis in a patient with acute pancreatitis. (CT, computed tomography; FNA, fine-needle aspiration.)

- Antibiotics that have good pancreatic penetration include imipenem, meropenem, cefepime, and moxifloxacin.

Gallstones and Bile Duct Stones
- Indications for ERCP:
  - severe acute gallstone pancreatitis in a hemodynamically stable patient;
  - cholangitis;
  - recurrent idiopathic pancreatitis to rule out microlithiasis, sphincter of Oddi dysfunction, or pancreas divisum;
  - if required during pregnancy, it is safest to do ERCP during the second trimester.
- Indication for cholecystectomy:
  - Gallstones: recurrent pancreatitis occurs in about 30% of patients with gallstone pancreatitis; therefore, cholecystectomy is recommended.
  - Cholecystectomy should be performed during the hospitalization for acute pancreatitis, if possible, or within 2–4 weeks of discharge.

Pancreatic Pseudocyst
- Observation: it usually takes 4–6 weeks for a pseudocyst to mature. Therefore, immediate intervention is usually not necessary.

- Indications for drainage of a pseudocyst include worsening abdominal pain, infected pseudocyst, gastric outlet or bile duct obstruction, associated leak, and ascites.
- Drainage of the pseudocyst may be performed percutaneously, endoscopically, or surgically.

Pancreatic Ascites
- Patients should be placed on TPN.
- Octreotide administered intravenously has been shown to be beneficial.
- Antibiotics may be used, but the benefit is unclear.
- Diuretics are not helpful.
- Drainage options include:
  ○ endscopic stent placement into the pancreatic duct to bridge the leak or relieve duct obstruction;
  ○ percutaneous drainage;
  ○ surgical drainage.

Pancreatic Necrosis
- All patients with sterile pancreatic necrosis (>30%) and infected pancreatic necrosis should be placed on antibiotics (see earlier).
- Further treatment with endoscopic or surgical debridement depends on whether the pancreatic necrosis is sterile or infected (see Figure 18.4).

Pearls

Acute pancreatitis is a potentially fatal disease with a mortality rate of 5–10%.

Eighty percent of all cases are caused by gallstones or alcohol.

The diagnosis of acute pancreatitis relies on elevations of serum amylase and lipase levels greater than three times the upper limit of normal

Patients with acute pancreatitis need hospitalization with close monitoring and frequent assessment.

There is no specific treatment for acute pancreatitis. Supportive care includes intravenous fluids, parenteral analgesia, anti-emetics, and attention to the patient's nutritional status.

Antibiotics should be reserved for patients with documented infection or pancreatic necrosis.

Questions

Questions 1 and 2 relate to the clinical vignette at the beginning of the chapter.

1. The differential diagnosis includes all of the following except:
   A. Gastric ulcer
   B. Alcoholic hepatitis
   C. Acute pancreatitis
   D. Gastroesophageal reflux disease
   E. Acute cholecystitis

2. The next best test to perform to make a diagnosis is:
   A. Endoscopic retrograde cholangiopancreatography
   B. Abdominal ultrasonography
   C. Serum amylase and lipase levels
   D. Esophagogastroduodenoscopy
   E. Magnetic resonance imaging

3. A 38-year-old obese woman with a history of hypertension, dyslipidemia, and cholecystectomy presents with her third episode of acute pancreatitis. Which of the following is the LEAST likely cause of acute pancreatitis in this patient?
   A. Hydrochlorothiazide
   B. Hypertriglyceridemia
   C. Hypercholesterolemia
   D. Idiopathic
   E. Pancreas divisum

4. A 67-year-old man has been hospitalized for 4 days with acute alcoholic pancreatitis. He is febrile (101.8 °F [38.7 °C]). The white blood cell count is 18 500/mm^3 and serum creatinine level 2.1 mg/dL. Abdominal pain persists. What is the next step in management of his condition?
   A. Start a clear liquid diet
   B. Start antibiotics
   C. Perform computed tomography scan of the abdomen
   D. Perform endoscopic ultrasonography
   E. Perform magnetic resonance imaging of the abdomen

5. Enteral nutrition has been shown to be more beneficial than parenteral nutrition in acute pancreatitis. The benefits of enteral nutrition compared with parenteral nutrition include all of the following EXCEPT:
   A. Does not stimulate pancreatic secretion
   B. Shortens the length of hospitalization
   C. Maintains intestinal integrity
   D. Lowers the rate of infection
   E. Is less expensive

6. In which of the following patients with acute pancreatitis should antibiotics be started?

A. A patient with a fever of 100.4 °F (38 °C) on admission
B. A patient with a white blood cell count of 12 300/mm^3 on admission
C. A patient with persistent abdominal pain on day 3 of hospitalization
D. A patient with a large asymptomatic pseudocyst on computed tomography
E. A patient with >30% necrosis on computed tomography

Answers

1. D
The patient's symptoms, history of ibuprofen and alcohol use, along with abnormal laboratory test results can be associated with all of the listed diagnoses except gastroesophageal reflux disease, which typically is associated with heartburn, but not associated with laboratory abnormalities.

2. C
Elevated serum amylase or lipase levels in a patient with abdominal pain typical of acute pancreatitis will confirm the diagnosis of acute pancreatitis. Amylase and lipase are not included in a comprehensive metabolic panel and have to be ordered separately. Abdominal imaging is not necessary initially but should be obtained if the patient does not improve or requires evaluation for other causes of abdominal pain if the serum amylase and lipase are normal. Once a diagnosis of acute pancreatitis is made, abdominal ultrasonography is indicated to look for gallstones, and computed tomography may be indicated in patients with severe acute pancreatitis.

3. C
All of the choices are associated with acute pancreatitis except hypercholesterolemia.

4. E
The patient's elevated white blood cell count and persistent abdominal pain are concerning for complications of acute pancreatitis such as pancreatic necrosis, a fluid collection, or an abscess. Abdominal imaging should be performed. Intravenous contrast is contraindicated because of renal failure. Magnetic resonance imaging (without gadolinium) is an alternative approach.

5. A
Enteral nutrition, in contrast to parenteral nutrition, has the potential to stimulate pancreatic secretion. Nevertheless, enteral feeding has several advantages over parenteral nutrition and is the preferred method of nutrition in acute pancreatitis.

6. E
Antibiotics are recommended for persistent fever or leukocytosis, while the source is being identified; pancreatic necrosis, both sterile (>30%) and infected; bacteremia; an infected pancreatic pseudocyst; an abscess; or an infected peripancreatic fluid collection.

Further Reading

Banks, P.A. and Freeman, M.L. Practice Parameters Committee of the American College of Gastroenterology. (2006) Practice guidelines in acute pancreatitis. *American Journal of Gastroenterology*, 101, 2379–2400.

Gupta, K. and Wu, B. (2010) Acute pancreatitis. *Annals of Internal Medicine*, 153, ITC51–55.

Loveday, B.P., Srinivasa, S., Vather, R., et al. (2010) High quantity and variable quality of guidelines for acute pancreatitis: a systematic review. *American Journal of Gastroenterology*, 105, 1466–1476.

Tenner, S. and Steinberg, W.M. (2010) Acute pancreatitis, in *Sleisenger and Fordtran's Gastrointestinal and Liver Disease: Pathophysiology/Diagnosis/Management*, 9th edn (eds M. Feldman, L.S. Friedman and L.J. Brandt), Saunders Elsevier, Philadelphia, pp. 959–982.

Weblinks

http://www.nlm.nih.gov/medlineplus/ency/article/000287.htm

http://www.clevelandclinicmeded.com/medicalpubs/diseasemanagement/gastroenterology/acute-pancreatitis/

http://www.aafp.org/afp/2007/0515/p1513.html

Chronic Pancreatitis

Anthony Gamboa, Xuan Zhu, and Qiang Cai

CHAPTER 19

Clinical Vignette

A 47-year-old man is seen in the office for a 10-month history of abdominal pain. The pain is localized to the epigastrium and radiates to the back, worse with eating, and associated with nausea. Over the past 8 months, he has had an unintentional weight loss of 15 lb (6.8 kg) and six episodes of oily-appearing diarrhea per day. He takes ibuprofen for his abdominal pain with minimal relief. The past medical history includes hypertension, type 2 diabetes mellitus, and depression. For the past 25 years, he has consumed approximately six beers daily and has smoked one pack of cigarettes per day. On physical examination, the vital signs are within normal limits. The patient is leaning forward in his chair. There is mild abdominal tenderness in the epigastric area with no rebound tenderness or guarding. Bowel sounds are present and normal. There is no organomegaly. Laboratory tests reveal a normal complete blood count, glucose 206 mg/dL, aspartate aminotransferase 180 U/L, alanine aminotransferase 101 U/L, amylase 105 U/L, and lipase 210 U/L. A plain abdominal film reveals calcifications in the mid-upper abdomen. Computed tomography is remarkable for coarse calcifications of the pancreas and a dilated pancreatic duct with a diameter of 5 mm. A 2×2 cm fluid collection is noted adjacent to the pancreas.

General

- Chronic pancreatitis (CP) is defined as irreversible injury to the pancreas caused by chronic inflammation and fibrosis leading to impairment of the exocrine and endocrine functions of the pancreas (Figure 19.1).

Essentials of Gastroenterology, First Edition. Edited by Shanthi V. Sitaraman, Lawrence S. Friedman.
© 2012 John Wiley & Sons, Ltd. Published 2012 by John Wiley & Sons, Ltd.

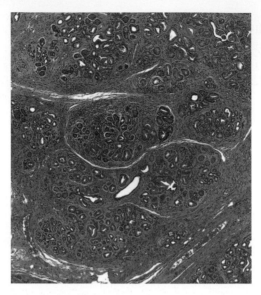

Figure 19.1 Histopathology of chronic pancreatitis demonstrating atrophy and interstitial fibrosis. Hematoxylin and eosin, 40×.

- The incidence of CP in the US is 3–10 cases per 100 000 persons, with a prevalence of 27–35 per 100 000.

Etiology and Pathogenesis

- **Alcohol:**
  - The majority of cases of CP in western countries are caused by chronic alcoholism. The median age of onset of CP is 36 years.
  - Most patients have a history of drinking 150 g/day for at least 5–10 years (a standard 12-ounce [350 mL] beer contains approximately 18 g of alcohol).
  - Only 5–10% of heavy drinkers develop CP. Proposed cofactors that contribute to the development of CP include genetic variations, including polymorphisms of proteins involved in cellular antioxidant defense or alcohol metabolism, consumption of high-protein and high-fat diets, hyperlipidemia, exposure to bacterial endotoxins, and smoking.
  - The strongest cofactor seems to be smoking. Ninety percent of patients with alcoholic CP are smokers. Smoking is also an independent risk factor for the development of CP. Smoking leads to the rapid development of pancreatic calcifications.

- The pathogenesis may follow a necrosis–fibrosis pathway, in which repeated episodes of acute pancreatitis lead to irreversible fibrosis and atrophy. This is also referred to as the SAPE (sentinel acute pancreatitis event) hypothesis. Alcohol also causes zymogens to be prematurely activated, leading to autodigestion of the pancreas. Finally, alcohol use causes increased secretion of proteins and ionized calcium from acinar cells with a relative decrease in bicarbonate secretion. This leads to precipitation of proteins and obstruction of ductules.
- **Idiopathic:**
  - 10–30% of cases of CP are idiopathic. Contributing factors include genetic abnormalities, modest alcohol consumption in susceptible patients, surreptitious alcohol use, trauma, and smoking.
- **Obstruction:**
  - Chronic obstruction of the pancreatic duct can cause CP proximal to the obstruction, and relief of the obstruction occasionally reverses damage to the pancreas.
  - Causes of obstruction include pancreatic, ductal, or ampullary tumors, benign ductal strictures, and pancreatic divisum with stenosis of the minor papilla.
  - In eastern countries, bile duct disorders, such as gallstone disease, are thought to be a major cause of CP.
- **Tropical pancreatitis:**
  - Tropical pancreatitis is the most common form of CP in southwest India and other tropical areas including Africa, southeast Asia, and Brazil.
  - The etiology is unknown, but there is an association with mutations in the serine protease inhibitor Kazal type 1 (*SPINK1*) gene, which encodes a trypsin inhibitor (see Chapter 18) and thereby leads to trypsin activation within the pancreas. Environmental triggers may include malnutrition, including deficiencies in calories or micronutrients, and infections.
  - A striking feature of tropical pancreatitis is that diabetes mellitus is an inevitable consequence, and >90% of patients develop pancreatic calcifications.
- **Hereditary pancreatitis:**
  - Hereditary CP is associated with mutation of the protease serine 1 (*PRSS1*) gene and is transmitted in an autosomal dominant manner with a penetrance of 80%.
  - The *PRSS1* gene encodes trypsinogen, and mutations lead to increased autoactivation of trypsin within the pancreas. This allows increased activation of various zymogens to their active proteolytic forms, leading in turn to autodigestion of the pancreas.

- **Other genetic factors:**
  - Other mutations may act as cofactors or increase susceptibility to or the severity of CP. These include mutations in *SPINK1* and the cystic fibrosis transmembrane conductance regulator (*CFTR*) gene.
  - Mutations of the *CFTR* gene that are not severe enough to cause cystic fibrosis may predispose to CP.
- **Autoimmune pancreatitis:**
  - Autoimmune pancreatitis is a chronic inflammatory and fibrosing disease of the pancreas.
  - The characteristic feature of autoimmune pancreatitis is a dense infiltration of the pancreas and other organs by plasma cells and lymphocytes. The plasma cells secrete immunoglobulin G (IgG) or IgG4.
- **Metabolic disorders:**
  - Hypertriglyceridemia and hypercalcemia are associated with CP.

Up to 70% of cases of CP in Western countries are caused by alcohol; however, only 5–10% of alcoholics develop chronic pancreatitis. A convenient mnemonic for the causes of CP is TIGAR-O: toxic–metabolic, idiopathic, genetic, autoimmune, recurrent and severe acute pancreatitis, or obstructive.

Clinical Features

- Abdominal pain:
  - Abdominal pain is the most common symptom of CP and contributes significantly to the quality of life in patients with CP. The pain is typically epigastric and may radiate to the back and sometimes around to the flank in a band-like manner. The pain is worse with eating and may be associated with nausea and vomiting. Leaning forward relieves the pain in some patients.
  - Pain may be absent in some patients who present with pancreatic insufficiency.
- Fat maldigestion:
  - Exocrine dysfunction typically occurs after acinar cell reserve is reduced by 90%. With an inadequate lipase, fat maldigestion and steatorrhea occur. Patients may have loose, oily stools with a foul odor.
  - Osteopenia and osteoporosis are common due to malabsorption of vitamin D. Deficiencies in other fat-soluble vitamins – A, E, and K – and vitamin B12 may also occur.

○ Protein and carbohydrate deficiencies may occur at later stages and to a lesser degree than fat maldigestion.
• Impaired glucose tolerance and diabetes mellitus:
○ Impaired glucose tolerance resulting in diabetes mellitus results from destruction of the islet cells and is similar to type I diabetes mellitus; however, alpha cells are also destroyed, so patients lose the ability to secrete glucagon, thereby making hypoglycemia more common and more severe.
○ Patients with CP who have a family history of diabetes mellitus are more likely to develop diabetes mellitus.
• Physical examination:
○ The only consistent finding on physical examination is epigastric tenderness.

The differential diagnosis of CP includes peptic ulcer disease, symptomatic gallstones, bile duct stricture, recurrent acute pancreatitis, and pancreatic cancer.

Diagnosis

• Imaging:
○ Imaging studies are frequently diagnostic in advanced disease. Diagnosing early CP is difficult.
○ **Plain abdominal films** show calcifications in about 30% of patients with CP. This finding, combined with loss of pancreatic function, can be diagnostic of CP. Calcifications develop over 5–25 years and are most common with alcoholic and tropical CP.
○ **Transabdominal ultrasonography** and **computed tomography (CT)** are useful. The sensitivity of ultrasonography is 50–80%, and the specificity is 80–90%. CT has a sensitivity of 75–90% and specificity of >85% for the diagnosis of CP (see Chapter 27). Findings on CT include calcifications, ductal stones, abnormal size of the pancreas, a dilated pancreatic duct, and pseudocysts (Figure 19.2).
○ **Endoscopic retrograde cholangiopancreatography (ERCP)** is considered the gold standard among imaging procedures for the diagnosis of CP, with a sensitivity and specificity of 70–90% and 80–100%, respectively. ERCP reveals ductal abnormalities including stenoses, dilatation (normal diameter of the main pancreatic duct is 3 mm), and irregularities of the main pancreatic duct and its side branches. A "chain-of-lakes" or "beading" appearance of the pancreatic duct, indicating alternating areas of dilatation and stricture, is typical of advanced CP. ERCP also facilitates therapeutic interventions, such

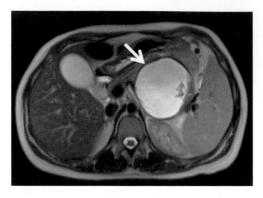

Figure 19.2 Magnetic resonance image (MRI) showing changes of chronic pancreatitis with a large pancreatic pseudocyst (arrow).

as placement of stents through stenoses or removal of ductal stones from the pancreatic duct.

- ○ **Magnetic resonance imaging (MRI) with magnetic resonance cholangiopancreatography (MRCP)** is noninvasive and has a sensitivity and specificity comparable to that of ERCP.
- ○ **Endoscopic ultrasonography (EUS)** is highly sensitive for detecting CP. Compared with ERCP, EUS has a lower risk of complications and can detect abnormalities suggestive of CP in the pancreatic parenchyma and ductal system that may not be not visible with other imaging modalities.
- Tests of pancreatic function:
  - ○ Exocrine pancreatic insufficiency can be identified directly by sampling duodenal contents for pancreatic secretions after administering a secretagogue such as secretin or cholecystokinin. Over a 1-hour intraduodenal collection, a bicarbonate concentration of <80 mEq/L is diagnostic of CP. This method is sensitive and can be useful in early CP, but it is not widely available and requires passing a duodenal tube by mouth and collecting pancreatic secretions for 1 hour.
  - ○ Indirect measures of exocrine dysfunction include serum trypsinogen, fecal chymotrypsin, and fecal elastase levels. Low levels indicate exocrine insufficiency, but these tests are unreliable until CP is advanced. Of the indirect tests, fecal elastase is widely available, requires only a single stool sample, and may be the most sensitive and specific of the fecal tests for diagnosing CP.
- Other laboratory studies:
  - ○ A 72-hour stool fat quantitation in patients with CP is typically greater than 7 g/day.

○ A vitamin B12 absorption test (Schilling test) may help in the diagnosis of CP; however, this test is not commonly used to diagnose CP and is generally not available.
○ Serum amylase and lipase levels may be slightly elevated in patients with symptomatic exacerbations of CP, but usually they are normal.

The diagnosis of CP depends largely on identifying characteristic clinical features by history, often in the setting of chronic alcohol abuse. Diagnostic tests for CP may be classified as those that detect abnormalities of pancreatic structure (imaging tests) and those tests that detect abnormalities of pancreatic function. Traditionally, ERCP has been considered the gold standard for assessing pancreatic ductal structure, and the secretin stimulation test has been viewed as the gold standard for assessing pancreatic function.

Treatment

- CP can cause a significant reduction in a patient's quality of life, and treatment should focus on alleviating symptoms (Figure 19.3).
- Patients should undergo imaging evaluation for the presence of complicating or concurrent factors, including pseudocysts, biliary stricture, or pancreatic cancer.
- General treatment recommendations include abstaining from alcohol and smoking and eating small, frequent meals to limit pancreatic enzyme secretion and to reduce symptoms of maldigestion.
  ○ Medical treatment for pain includes:
    - acetaminophen or nonsteroidal anti-inflammatory drugs (NSAIDS);
    - uncoated pancreatic enzymes, which suppress the release of cholecystokinin, the hormone that stimulates pancreatic secretion;
    - narcotics, tricyclic antidepressant drugs, or gabapentin; however, narcotic addiction is a major risk in patients with CP;
    - antioxidants, which limit free-radical damage to the pancreas but are of uncertain benefit.
  ○ Surgical or endoscopic treatments include celiac plexus block, endoscopic stenting of the pancreatic duct, pancreatic duct stone removal, sphincterotomy, and surgical resection or decompression of the pancreatic duct.
- Maldigestion and steatorrhea:
  ○ Pancreatic enzyme replacement with enterically coated formulations that contain at least 40000U of lipase with each meal is recommended.

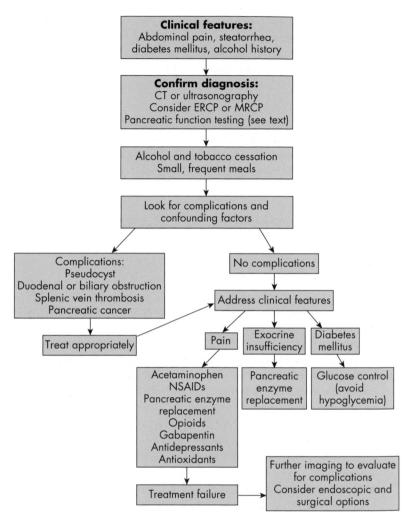

Figure 19.3 Algorithm for the diagnosis and treatment of chronic pancreatitis. (ERCP, endoscopic retrograde cholangiopancreatography; MRCP, magnetic resonance cholangiopancreatography; NSAIDs, nonsteroidal anti-inflammatory drugs.)

- ○ Non-enteric-coated pancreatic enzymes may be inactivated in the acidic environment of the stomach; therefore, a proton pump inhibitor or histamine H2 receptor antagonist is usually used in conjunction with such preparations.
- • Diabetes mellitus usually requires insulin in lower doses than those used for type I diabetes mellitus. Insulin regimens should be tailored to reflect the increased risk of hypoglycemia in patients with CP.

- Patients may require nutritional support with vitamins A, D, E, and K, as well as vitamin B12.

> In the duodenum, vitamin B12 is bound to R-proteins. Vitamin B12 normally is cleaved from R-proteins by proteases from the pancreas, thereby allowing the B12 to bind to intrinsic factor for absorption in the terminal ileum. Pancreatic insufficiency may cause vitamin B12 deficiency by leading to reduced cleavage of B12 from R-proteins.

Complications

- Pseudocysts:
  - Pseudocysts develop in 10–25% of patients with CP, most commonly in those with alcoholic CP.
  - Damage to pancreatic ducts leads to accumulation of pancreatic fluid inside or outside of the pancreas.
  - The pancreas and other adjacent structures, including the stomach, transverse colon, and omentum, form the walls of the pseudoscyst;
  - Many pseudocysts are asymptomatic, but as they increase in size, abdominal pain is more likely;
  - Other complications of pseudocysts may include obstruction of the bile duct, duodenum, or adjacent blood vessels, formation of fistulas, spontaneous infection, and abscess formation;
  - Enzymes in a pseudocyst may digest an adjacent arterial wall to create a pseudoaneurysm; the splenic artery is the most commonly affected vessel. A pseudoaneurysm may rupture, causing bleeding into the pseudocyst, adjacent viscera, or the peritoneal cavity. They may also bleed into the pancreatic duct, causing hemosuccus pancreaticus, which may present as gastrointestinal bleeding;
  - Ultrasonography, CT, and MRI are used to diagnose pseudocysts;
  - The indications for draining a pseudocyst include rapid enlargement, persistent pain, compression of surrounding structures, marked early satiety, and infection. Drainage may be achieved by a percutaneous, endoscopic, or surgical approach.
- Pancreatic ascites and pleural effusion:
  - Disruption of the pancreatic duct or rupture of a pseudocyst can lead to accumulation of pancreatic fluid in the pleural or peritoneal space;

- Diagnostic paracentesis or thoracentesis will reveal fluid with an elevated amylase level, usually higher than 1000 U/L;
- Treatment includes withholding oral feeding to minimize pancreatic secretions. Diuretics, serial paracentesis or thoracentesis, and somatostatin analogs are also used. Many patients benefit from endoscopic placement of a stent across a disrupted pancreatic duct. In some case surgical intervention is required.
- Biliary or duodenal obstruction:
  - Obstruction of the bile duct or the duodenum occurs at a rate of 10% and 5%, respectively. Obstruction may be caused by a pseudocyst or by fibrosis and inflammation in the pancreatic head.
  - Diagnostic studies include ERCP or MRCP for biliary obstruction and CT, upper endoscopy, or an upper gastrointestinal series for duodenal obstruction.
  - Treatment may include drainage of an obstructing pseudocyst, endoscopic stenting of a biliary or duodenal obstruction, or surgical gastrojejunostomy or choledochoenterostomy for relief of duodenal obstruction.
- Splenic vein thrombosis:
  - Pancreatic inflammation can cause thrombosis of the splenic vein, which courses along the posterior aspect of the pancreas.
  - Splenic vein thrombosis may lead to portal hypertension and isolated gastric varices.
  - Splenectomy is curative and is indicated if gastric variceal bleeding occurs.
- Pancreatic cancer:
  - Patients with CP are at an increased risk for developing pancreatic cancer. The risk is about 4% after 20 years.

Prognosis

- The quality of life of patients with CP is significantly worse than that of the general population. Tobacco use and ongoing alcohol use predict a worse prognosis.
- Abdominal pain often abates after 10 years or more of CP; frequently this coincides with the development of pancreatic insufficiency. The mortality ratio is approximately 3.6:1 when compared with patients without CP. Continued alcohol use increases the mortality rate by another 60%.
- The survival rate is about 70% at 10 years and 45% at 20 years. Most patients die from an associated condition, such as complications from continued alcohol use or smoking, or from pancreatic cancer or postoperative complications.

Pearls

The diagnosis of chronic pancreatitis requires a high index of clinical suspicion in a patient presenting with chronic abdominal pain.

Pain management is an important component of treatment of chronic pancreatitis.

Tobacco use and ongoing alcohol use predict a worse prognosis, and patients should be encouraged to stop smoking and alcohol consumption.

Questions

Questions 1 and 2 relate to the clinical vignette at the beginning of this chapter.

1. Which of the following is the next step in the management of this patient?
   A. Magnetic resonance cholangiopancreatography (MRCP)
   B. Endoscopic retrograde cholangiopancreatography (ERCP)
   C. Morphine for pain
   D. A lactose-free diet
   E. Alcohol and smoking cessation

2. Which of the following is the most appropriate additional therapy for this patient at this time?
   A. Narcotics
   B. Pancreatic enzyme replacement
   C. Percutaneous or endoscopic drainage of the pseudocyst
   D. Celiac plexus nerve block
   E. Surgical repair of the pseudocyst

3. A 55-year-old man with alcoholic chronic pancreatitis presents to the emergency department with hematemesis for the past hour. He has no history of peptic ulcer disease, and he does not take nonsteroidal anti-inflammatory drugs. He has no history of cirrhosis of the liver. His blood pressure is 92/63 mmHg, pulse rate 115/min, and respiratory rate 18/min, and he is afebrile. The history of chronic pancreatitis predisposes him to which of the following as an etiology of gastrointestinal bleeding?
   A. Esophageal varices
   B. Gastric varices
   C. Cameron lesion
   D. Gastric antral vascular ectasia (GAVE)

4. A 58-year-old woman presents for an evaluation of fatigue of 2 months' duration. She has a history of alcoholic chronic pancreatitis. She also has a history of osteoporosis for which she takes calcium, vitamin D, and a

(Continued)

bisphosphonate. She reports no cold intolerance, constipation, or weight gain. Laboratory studies reveal a hemoglobin level of 9 mg/dL and mean corpuscular volume of 110 fL. What is the most likely etiology of the macrocytic anemia?

A. Vitamin A deficiency

B. Hypothyroidism

C. Folate deficiency

D. Vitamin B12 deficiency

5. A 24-year-old woman presents with 3-month history of epigastric pain, nausea, and steatorrhea. Abdominal imaging shows pancreatic calcifications and a dilated pancreatic duct consistent with chronic pancreatitis. The patient moved to the US from southern India 2 months ago. What is the most likely etiology of her condition?

A. Hereditary pancreatitis

B. Alcoholic chronic pancreatitis

C. Tropical pancreatitis

D. Gallstone disease

E. Autoimmune pancreatitis

6. A 39-year-old man with alcoholic chronic pancreatitis would like to know if his life expectancy is shortened by his condition. Which of the following is the best response?

A. His life expectancy is unchanged by this diagnosis

B. If he abstains from alcohol, his life expectancy will be normal

C. If he abstains from both alcohol and tobacco, his life expectancy will be normal

D. His life expectancy is reduced, but abstaining from alcohol will decrease mortality

Answers

1. E

Patients with chronic pancreatitis who continue to consume alcohol and smoke cigarettes tend to have more severe symptoms and higher mortality than those who abstain from alcohol use. Referring the patient for ERCP or MRCP or prescribing narcotics for pain relief may be warranted in certain cases, but alcohol and smoking cessation, which alter the course of CP, should always be recommended.

2. B

Pancreatic enzyme replacement is therapeutic for both abdominal pain and steatorrhea associated with chronic pancreatitis. The other treatment options may be used, if indicated, in patients who do not improve with pancreatic enzyme replacement.

3. B

Pancreatic inflammation can cause thrombosis of the splenic vein, which courses along the posterior aspect of the pancreas. Splenic vein thrombosis causes gastric varices more frequently than esophageal varices. Splenectomy is the treatment of choice for bleeding gastric varices resulting from splenic vein thrombosis. Cameron lesions are linear erosions seen within a hiatal hernia and are not associated with chronic pancreatitis. Chronic pancreatitis does not predispose to GAVE.

4. D

Patients with chronic pancreatitis are prone to vitamin B12 deficiency. In the duodenum, vitamin B12 is bound to R-proteins. B12 is normally cleaved from R-proteins by proteases from the pancreas, thereby allowing the B12 to bind intrinsic factor for absorption in the ileum. The absence of such cleavage in patients with chronic pancreatitis leads to vitamin B12 deficiency. Folate does not require pancreatic enzymes for digestion or absorption. The patient's history is not consistent with hypothyroidism. Although vitamin A deficiency can occur with chronic pancreatitis, it does not cause macrocytic anemia.

5. C

The most common form of chronic pancreatitis in southern India and other tropical areas including Africa, southeast Asia, and Brazil, is tropical pancreatitis. Hereditary pancreatitis and autoimmune pancreatitis are possible diagnoses in this case, but because the patient is from southern India, tropical pancreatitis is more likely. She does not drink alcohol, making alcoholic chronic pancreatitis unlikely. Gallstones commonly cause acute, not chronic, pancreatitis.

6. D

The mortality rate is increased three- to fourfold in patients with chronic pancreatitis compared with that of persons without chronic pancreatitis, and continued alcohol use increases the mortality by another 60%. Smoking worsens the course of chronic pancreatitis. Therefore, abstaining from alcohol and smoking has the greatest influence on mortality but does not necessarily lead to a normal life expectancy.

Further Reading

Chauhan, S. and Forsmark, C.E. (2010) Pain management in chronic pancreatitis: a treatment algorithm. *Best Practice & Research. Clinical Gastroenterology*, 24, 323–335.

Domínguez-Muñoz J.E. (2011) Chronic pancreatitis and persistent steatorrhea: what is the correct dose of enzymes? *Clinical Gastroenterology and Hepatology*, 9, 541–546.

Forsmark, C.E. (2010) Chronic pancreatitis, in *Sleisenger and Fordtran's Gastrointestinal and Liver Disease: Pathophysiology/Diagnosis/Management*, 9th edn (eds M. Feldman, L.S. Friedman and L.J. Brandt), Saunders Elsevier, Philadelphia, pp. 985–1017.

Witt, H., Apte, M.V., Keim, V., et al. (2007) Chronic pancreatitis: challenges and advances in pathogenesis, genetics, diagnosis, and therapy. *Gastroenterology*, 132, 1557–1573.

Weblinks

http://emedicine.medscape.com/article/181554-overview
http://www.clevelandclinicmeded.com/medicalpubs/diseasemanagement/
gastroenterology/chronic-pancreatitis/

Bile Acid Metabolism

Nicole M. Griglione and Field F. Willingham

CHAPTER 20

Clinical Vignette

A 34-year-old man with Crohn's disease presents with chronic diarrhea since undergoing resection of his terminal ileum 4 months ago. He describes the stools as watery and small in volume but denies blood in the stool. He denies nausea, vomiting, fever, or abdominal pain. He does not take any prescription or over-the-counter medications and denies recent antibiotic use. Physical examination is unremarkable. Rectal examination reveals brown stool that is negative for occult blood. Laboratory tests including a complete blood count, comprehensive metabolic panel, stool culture for bacteria, stool examination for ova and parasites, and stool *Clostridium difficile* toxin assay are negative. A capsule endoscopy shows normal small intestinal mucosa and a normal appearing ileocolonic anastomosis.

Bile

- Bile is an alkaline, lipid-rich micellar solution that is isosmotic with plasma and consists of water, electrolytes, and organic solutes such as bile acids, phospholipids (e.g., phosphatidylcholine), cholesterol, proteins, and bile pigments (e.g., bilirubin).
- The liver secretes 500–600 mL of bile per day, which is delivered to the duodenum via the bile duct.

Bile Acids and Bile Salts

- Hepatocytes synthesize the primary bile acids, cholic acid and chenodeoxycholic acid (Figure 20.1), from cholesterol.

Essentials of Gastroenterology, First Edition. Edited by Shanthi V. Sitaraman, Lawrence S. Friedman.
© 2012 John Wiley & Sons, Ltd. Published 2012 by John Wiley & Sons, Ltd.

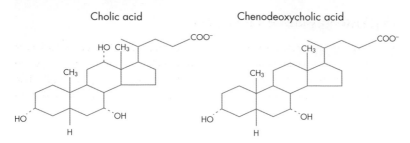

Figure 20.1 The primary bile acids, cholic acid and chenodeoxycholic acid.

- Prior to secretion into the bile canaliculi, primary bile acids are conjugated to glycine or taurine to form bile salts. Conjugation increases water solubility, preventing passive reabsorption from the small intestine.
  - Chenodeoxycholic acid is also epimerized to form the bile acid ursodeoxycholic acid, which is conjugated to taurine or glycine in hepatocytes.
  - Ursodeoxycholic acid represents less than 5% of the bile acid pool.
  - Ursodeoxycholic acid reduces cholesterol secretion into bile and improves biliary cholesterol solubility. Ursodeoxycholic acid has also been used as an oral therapy to dissolve small to medium-sized cholesterol gallstones.
- Primary bile acids and salts reach the small intestine, where they are converted by intestinal bacteria to secondary bile acids, deoxycholic acid and lithocholic acid, through dehydroxylation.
- The two major functions of bile acids and salts are:
  - Regulation of the total body pool of cholesterol:
    - bile acids and bile salts serve as the major excretory form of cholesterol;
    - factors that increase bile acid synthesis promote mobilization and excretion of cholesterol; factors that decrease bile acid synthesis increase the total body pool of cholesterol; factors that decrease reabsorption of bile acids increase synthesis of bile acids and therefore excretion of cholesterol.
  - Digestion and absorption of dietary lipid:
    - bile acids and salts facilitate the formation of micelles, which aid in the digestion and absorption of dietary lipid and fat-soluble vitamins from the small intestine.

The Enterohepatic Circulation

- Enterohepatic circulation refers to the circulation of bile acids and salts from the liver to the small intestine and back to the liver via the portal vein after reabsorption from the small intestine (Figure 20.2). The enterohepatic circulation helps to maintain an adequate bile acid pool

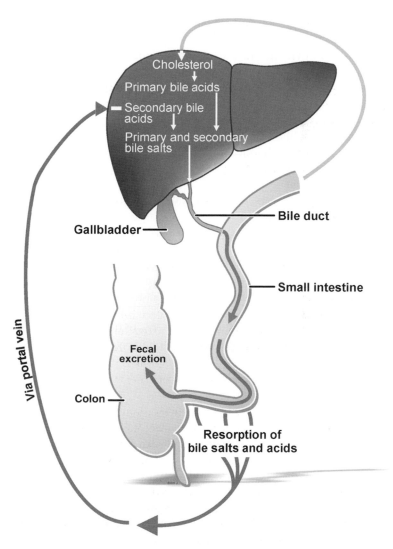

Figure 20.2 The enterohepatic circulation.

for digestion and absorption and minimizes the need for production of bile acids by hepatocytes.

- Hepatocytes synthesize approximately 600 mg of primary bile acids and salts per day:
  - in normal healthy persons, the total bile acid pool is 2–4 g;
  - on average, the bile acid pool cycles through the enterohepatic circulation two to four times per meal.
- During fasting, bile acids and salts are secreted into the bile ducts and stored and concentrated in the gallbladder.
- After a meal is ingested, the gallbladder contracts in response to cholecystokinin, and bile is secreted into the cystic duct, which drains into the duodenum via the bile duct. The gallbladder remains contracted during the meal.
  - This pattern of bile acid secretion and storage is maintained even after cholecystectomy, in which case the bile acids may be stored in the proximal small intestine.
- Reabsorption of bile acids and salts:
  - The majority of the bile acid pool in the small intestine is reabsorbed in the terminal ileum by active transport mediated by the ileal bile acid transporter.
  - A small fraction of the bile acids is absorbed throughout the small intestine by passive diffusion. About 600 mg per day of bile acids and bile salts are not absorbed and are excreted in the stool.
- Circulation of bile acids:
  - The bile acids absorbed in the terminal ileum enter the portal vein bound to albumin or high-density lipoprotein. The majority of the bile acids are taken up by hepatocytes and secreted back into bile canaliculi.
  - Depending on the type of bile acids, 10–50% of the bile acids returning to the liver via the portal vein are not taken up by the liver and instead are absorbed into the bloodstream. This fraction of bile acids is filtered by the kidneys. The bile acids are actively reabsorbed from the renal tubules, with less than 2% excreted in the urine.
- Hepatic uptake and secretion of bile acids:
  - The periportal hepatocytes primarily absorb and secrete recirculating bile acids; the pericentral hepatocytes predominantly secrete newly synthesized bile acids.
  - The secretion of recycled bile acids through the periportal hepatocytes induces hepatic bile flow, thus maintaining the enterohepatic circulation.
  - Secretion of bile acids into bile canaliculi occurs via the ATP-dependent bile acid efflux pump and is the rate-limiting step in the transport of bile acids from the portal system to the bile duct.

Disorders of Bile Acid Metabolism

Cholesterol Gallstones (see also Chapter 21)

- Up to 20% of women and 8% of men over age 40 develop cholesterol gallstones.
- These stones are comprised mostly of cholesterol monohydrate. Bile pigments, proteins, calcium salts, and fatty acids make up the remainder of the stone.
- Three main factors contribute to gallstone formation:
  - Increased biliary secretion of cholesterol:
    - When excess cholesterol is secreted into bile, adequate micelle formation with phospholipids and bile acids cannot occur. This results in precipitation of cholesterol crystals.
    - Increased biliary excretion of cholesterol is associated with obesity, high-fat diets, certain medications, increased 3-hydroxy-3-methylglutaryl-coenzyme A (HMG-CoA) reductase activity, and increased hepatic uptake of cholesterol from the bloodstream.
  - Nucleation, the formation of crystal nuclei in supersaturated bile:
    - Certain glycoproteins and mucin promote nucleation of cholesterol monohydrate crystals.
  - Gallbladder hypomotility:
    - Incomplete emptying of supersaturated and crystal-rich bile from the gallbladder allows stones to increase in size.
- Pregnancy predisposes to gallstone formation because of increased cholesterol saturation during the third trimester and sluggish postprandial gallbladder contraction.
- Women taking oral contraceptive pills have increased hepatic uptake of dietary cholesterol, stimulation of hepatic lipoprotein receptors, and biliary cholesterol secretion, which predispose to gallstone formation.
- Patients who experience rapid weight loss, as occurs after gastric bypass surgery, often develop cholesterol stones secondary to increased mobilization of tissue cholesterol and increased biliary secretion of cholesterol, as well as decreased enterohepatic circulation of bile acids.
- Biliary sludge can also lead to gallstone formation and can be seen in conditions that cause gallbladder hypomotility such as burns, surgery, pregnancy, total parenteral nutrition, and oral contraceptive use.

Bile Salt Diarrhea

- Impaired bile acid reabsorption due to surgical resection of the terminal ileum, loss of terminal ileal surface area (e.g., after radiation therapy or in Crohn's disease), or congenital defects in the ileal bile acid transporter may lead to diarrhea.

Table 20.1 Characteristic features of the two different mechanisms of bile salt diarrhea.

	Bile acid excess	Bile acid deficiency
Length of resection	<100 cm	≥100 cm
Compensatory hepatic synthesis of bile acid	Yes	No
Steatorrhea	No	Yes
Response to low-fat diet	No	Yes
Response to oral cholestyramine	Yes	No

- The nature of diarrhea and its management depend on the length of terminal ileum that is compromised (Table 20.1):
  - Secretory diarrhea results when excessive amounts of bile acids are delivered to the colon, thereby stimulating fluid and electrolyte secretion. Bile acid exposure may also increase colonic mucosal permeability and cause direct mucosal damage.
  - Steatorrhea occurs when greater than 100 cm of ileum is lost or diseased and the liver is unable to keep up with bile salt losses, thereby resulting in a lack of micelle formation and impaired dietary lipid digestion.

Cholecystectomy
- Cholecystectomy has little effect on bile acid secretion. However, patients may experience post-cholecystectomy diarrhea if the bile acid pool size exceeds the amount of bile acid absorbed by the ileal transport system. This state is usually only transient, and patients often respond to treatment with an oral bile acid sequestrant such as cholestyramine, colestipol, or colesevelam.

Small Intestinal Bacterial Overgrowth
- This can lead to deconjugation of bile acids in the proximal small intestine, thereby reducing intraluminal bile acid distribution, impairing formation of micelles, and in some cases leading to steatorrhea.

Pearls

Bile acids and salts serve as the major excretory pathway for cholesterol.

The enterohepatic circulation plays a vital role in dietary lipid and fat-soluble vitamin digestion as well as excretion of cholesterol and certain medications.

Interruption or impairment of the enterohepatic circulation occurs in certain conditions such as liver disease, terminal ileal resection, Crohn's disease, and small intestinal bacterial overgrowth and may lead to diarrhea, drug toxicity, or gallstone formation.

Questions

1. What is the most likely cause of diarrhea in the patient in the clinical vignette at the beginning of this chapter?
   A. Active Crohn's disease
   B. Bile acid-induced diarrhea
   C. Fat malabsorption
   D. Viral enteritis
2. Which of the following are the primary bile acids?
   A. Deoxycholic acid and lithocholic acid
   B. Glycocholic acid and taurocholic acid
   C. Hydrochloric acid and ursodeoxycholic acid
   D. Cholic acid and chenodeoxycholic acid
   E. Taurocholic acid and lithocholic acid
3. The secondary bile acids are produced in the:
   A. Liver
   B. Bile ducts
   C. Portal vein
   D. Small intestine
   E. Stomach
4. Absorption of bile acids occurs predominantly in which of the following segments of the gastrointestinal tract and by which mechanism?
   A. Duodenum via an active carrier-mediated process
   B. Jejunum via passive diffusion
   C. Terminal ileum via an active carrier-mediated process
   D. Ascending colon via passive diffusion

(Continued)

5. The rate-limiting step in transport of bile acids from the portal vein to the bile duct is:
   A. The ATP-dependent bile acid efflux pump located in the apical membrane of hepatocytes
   B. The ATP-dependent bile acid efflux pump located in the basolateral membrane of hepatocytes
   C. The ATP-dependent bile acid efflux pump located in the biliary canalicular membrane
   D. Passive diffusion of bile acids through the hepatocyte membrane
6. Which of the following is TRUE regarding the enterohepatic circulation?
   A. During fasting, bile acids are stored and concentrated in the gallbladder
   B. A fraction of bile salts is absorbed throughout the small intestine by passive diffusion
   C. Less than 10% of bile acids is excreted in the feces
   D. All of the above
7. Which of the following persons are predisposed to developing cholesterol gallstones?
   A. Pregnant women
   B. Persons with a history of gastric bypass surgery
   C. Thin white men
   D. A and B
   E. All of the above

Answers

1. B

   The patient likely has bile acid-induced diarrhea. He has undergone resection of the terminal ileum, which likely resulted in interruption of enterohepatic circulation. The liver compensates by increasing the synthesis of bile acids and bile salts, which overwhelm the already compromised reabsorption of bile acids and salts in the terminal ileum and leads to increased exposure of the colon to bile acids and salts, thereby resulting in the stimulation of fluid and electrolyte secretion. A trial of a bile acid sequestrant, such as cholestyramine, before meals may be helpful in this patient. Some patients with a greater portion of affected ileum may experience substantial bile acid losses in the feces. If the liver is unable to compensate by increasing production, intestinal fat malabsorption and steatorrhea can result. Diarrhea in these patients is less responsive to bile acid sequestrant medications and is best treated with a low-fat diet supplemented with medium-chain triglycerides.

2. D

Primary bile acids are cholic acid and chenodeoxycholic acid. They are synthesized in hepatocytes from cholesterol.

3. D

Primary bile acids and salts are converted by bacteria in the small intestine to secondary bile acids, deoxycholic acid and lithocholic acid, through dehydroxylation.

4. C

The majority of the bile acids are reabsorbed in the terminal ileum by active transport mediated by the ileal bile acid transporter.

5. A

6. D

7. D

Further Reading

Dawson, P.A. (2010) Bile secretion and the enterohepatic circulation, in *Sleisenger and Fordtran's Gastrointestinal and Liver Disease: Pathophysiology/Diagnosis/ Management*, 9th edn (eds M. Feldman, L.S. Friedman and L.J. Brandt), Saunders Elsevier, Philadelphia, pp. 1075–1088.

Greenberger, N.J. and Paumgartner, G. (2005) Diseases of the gallbladder and bile ducts, in *Harrison's Principles of Internal Medicine*, 16th edn (eds D.L. Kasper, E. Braunwald, A.S. Fauci, et al.), McGraw-Hill, New York, pp 1880–1882.

Robb, B.W. and Matthews, J.B. (2005) Bile salt diarrhea. *Current Gastroenterology Reports*, 7, 379–383.

Gallstones and Complications

Julia Massaad

CHAPTER 21

Clinical Vignette

A 46-year-old woman is seen in the office for a 4-month history of intermittent right upper quadrant pain. She reports a dull pain that usually begins shortly after a meal and radiates to the right shoulder. The pain lasts 1–2 hours and resolves spontaneously. These episodes have occurred three times in the past year. She denies any change in bowel habits, nausea, vomiting, jaundice, or fever. She has tried over-the-counter ranitidine for the pain with no improvement. Her past medical history is unremarkable. Her father has hypertension, and her mother has diabetes mellitus. She has six children who are healthy. She does not smoke cigarettes, drink alcohol, or use illicit drugs. On examination she is moderately obese (BMI 32). The physical examination is otherwise unremarkable. Laboratory tests including a complete blood count and comprehensive metabolic panel are unremarkable.

Gallstones (Cholelithiasis)

Pathogenesis

- Gallstones and their complications are among the most common gastrointestinal disorders with a prevalence of gallstones of 10–15% in western countries.
- Types of gallstones:
  - ○ Cholesterol stones: in western countries cholesterol is the principal constituent of 80% of gallstones. Cholesterol gallstones are composed mainly of cholesterol (70%), mixed with calcium salts, bile pigment, and glycoproteins.

Essentials of Gastroenterology, First Edition. Edited by Shanthi V. Sitaraman, Lawrence S. Friedman.
© 2012 John Wiley & Sons, Ltd. Published 2012 by John Wiley & Sons, Ltd.

- ○ Non-cholesterol stones:
  - black pigment stones, composed predominantly of calcium bilirubinate, are found in patients with cirrhosis or chronic hemolytic states;
  - brown pigment stones, composed of varying amounts of calcium bilirubinate, calcium phosphate, cholesterol, and organic material, are usually formed in the setting of biliary stasis, secondary to biliary stricture, or small bowel diverticula.
- Three principal defects are involved in the pathogenesis of gallstone formation: (1) supersaturation of bile with cholesterol; (2) accelerated nucleation; and (3) gallbladder hypomotility. The extent of cholesterol saturation in the bile stored in the gallbladder is the most important determinant of gallstone formation.

Risk Factors

- Age: approximately 50% of women will have gallstones by age 70
- Female sex (two- to threefold increased risk compared to males)
- Multiparity
- Diabetes mellitus
- Hypertriglyceridemia
- Total parenteral nutrition
- Ethnicity (70% of Pima Indian women have gallstones by age 25, and 50% of Scandinavian women have gallstones by age 50)
- Medications (ceftriaxone, octreotide, oral contraceptives)
- Diseases such as Crohn's disease involving the terminal ileum
- Rapid weight loss.

Natural History

- Eighty percent of persons with gallstones are asymptomatic.
- Complications of gallstones include biliary pain, cholecystitis, choledocholithiasis, cholangitis, and acute pancreatitis. Gallbladder carcinoma is a rare complication of chronic cholelithasis.
- The cumulative rate of complications in persons with asymptomatic cholelithiasis is estimated to be 1–4% at 10 years. Therefore, treatment of asymptomatic gallstones is not recommended except for persons who are at high risk for gallbladder cancer such as Native Americans and persons with a porcelain gallbladder (see later).
- In contrast, up to 50% of patients with gallstones and biliary pain will have recurrent pain, and the risk of biliary complications is estimated to be 1–2% per year. Therefore, cholecystectomy should be recommended for persons who have symptoms.

Clinical Features

- The typical symptom of gallstones is biliary pain, conventionally referred to as biliary colic. Biliary pain is characterized by severe, steady, epigastric or right upper quadrant pain that usually begins abruptly and peaks within 1 hour of onset. The pain may radiate to the right shoulder or scapula in approximately 50% of patients. Although termed "colic," the pain is steady and not intermittent.
  - Biliary pain is caused by intermittent obstruction of the cystic duct by a gallstone.
  - Biliary pain usually resolves gradually within 3 hours. Prolonged pain (>3 hours) should raise suspicion of a complication such as cholecystitis, cholangitis, or pancreatitis.

Diagnosis

- Laboratory tests (complete blood count, liver biochemical tests) are often normal in the setting of biliary pain, and a high index of suspicion is needed to confirm the diagnosis.
- The diagnosis of cholelithiasis is made by right upper quadrant ultrasonography, which has >95% sensitivity and specificity for the detection of gallstones that are larger than 2mm (see Chapter 27).

Treatment

- Symptomatic gallstone disease is treated surgically with laparoscopic cholecystectomy.
- Medical treatment of gallstone disease with oral ursodeoxycholic acid, with or without extracorporeal shock wave lithotripsy, is considered a treatment option in persons with small cholesterol stones who are not surgical candidates.

> Asymptomatic gallstones do not require treatment except in persons who are at high risk for gallbladder cancer such as Native Americans or persons with a porcelain gallbladder.

Common Gallstone Complications

Acute Cholecystitis

- Acute cholecystitis is the most common complication of gallstones. It is usually caused by prolonged obstruction of the cystic duct by an impacted stone (Table 21.1).

Table 21.1 Clinical manifestations, diagnosis, and treatment of gallstone diseases.

	Biliary pain	Acute cholecystitis	Choledocholithiasis	Acute cholangitis
Pathophysiology	Intermittent obstruction of the cystic duct	Continuing obstruction of the cystic duct	Intermittent obstruction of the BD	Continuing obstruction of the BD and infection
Symptoms	Infrequent epigastric/right upper quadrant pain <3 hours	Epigastric/right upper quadrant pain >3 hours, associated nausea and vomiting	Asymptomatic or similar to biliary pain (more frequent episodes)	Fever, jaundice, right upper quadrant pain (Charcot's triad)
Physical examination	Normal	Murphy's sign, fever, mild jaundice	Normal, possibly jaundice	Charcot's triad, + hypotension, altered mental status (Reynolds' pentad)
Laboratory tests (CBC, AST, ALT, ALP, bilirubin)	Normal	Leukocytosis, elevated bilirubin (<4mg/dL), mildly elevated AST, ALT, ALP	Elevated bilirubin, elevated AST, ALT, ALP	Leukocytosis, elevated AST, ALT, ALP
Imaging test(s)	Abdominal ultrasonography	Abdominal ultrasonography, HIDA scan	MRCP EUS ERCP PTC	MRCP EUS ERCP PTC
Treatment	Cholecystectomy	Antibiotics + cholecystectomy	ERCP followed by cholecystectomy; PTC if ERCP unsuccessful or unavailable	Antibiotics, ERCP followed by cholecystectomy; PTC if ERCP unsuccessful or unavailable

ALP, alkaline phosphatase; ALT, alanine aminotransferase; AST, aspartate aminotransferase; BD, bile duct; CBC, complete blood count; ERCP, endoscopic retrograde cholangiopancreatography; EUS, endoscopic ultrasonography; HIDA, hydroxy iminodiacetic acid; MRCP, magnetic resonance cholangiopancreatography; PTC, percutaneous transhepatic cholangiography.

- Acalculus cholecystitis: in 10% of patients, cholecystitis occurs in the absence of gallstones. Acalculus cholecystitis typically occurs in critically ill patients in the setting of major surgery, prolonged total parenteral nutrition, or extensive trauma.

Clinical Features
- Typical symptoms include a prolonged (>3 hours) episode of biliary pain that may be associated with nausea, vomiting, and fever.
- The physical finding that is nearly pathognomonic of acute cholecystitis is a positive Murphy's sign, which is the abrupt arrest of breathing during inspiration when the right costal margin is palpated and the inflamed gallbladder touches the examiner's hands.

Diagnosis
- Laboratory tests: leukocytosis as well as a mild elevation of the serum aminotransferase, alkaline phosphatase, and bilirubin (usually <4 mg/dL) levels may be seen.
- Imaging studies:
  - Right upper quadrant ultrasonography is the single best test to confirm acute cholecystitis. Findings on ultrasonography include gallbladder wall thickening, pericholecystic fluid, and a sonographic Murphy's sign (see Chapter 27).
  - Hepatobiliary scintigraphy (hydroxy iminodiacetic acid, or HIDA, scan) can be used to confirm or exclude acute cholecystitis with a high degree of sensitivity and specificity:
    - A HIDA scan is performed after the intravenous administration of a ^{99m}Tc-labeled HIDA.
    - A positive scan is defined by the lack of visualization of the gallbladder and normal excretion into the bile duct and small bowel within 30–60 minutes of the administration of the ^{99m}Tc-labeled HIDA.
  - Computed tomography (CT) is indicated if there is a concern for other complications of cholecystitis such as fistula or abscess.

Treatment
- Patients suspected of having acute cholecystitis should be admitted to the hospital, and fluid and electrolytes should be repleted.
- Broad-spectrum antibiotics should be initiated. A cephalosporin such as cefoxitin is effective in mild acute cholecystitis. In severely ill patients, ampicillin and an aminoglycoside or a third-generation cephalosporin and metronidazole are recommended.
- Cholecystectomy, preferably laparoscopic, is definitive treatment.

A prolonged (>3 hours) episode of biliary pain associated with nausea, vomiting, and fever should raise suspicion for acute cholecystitis.

Choledocholithiasis

- Choledocholithiasis is defined as the presence of gallstones in the bile duct (BD). BD stones usually have migrated from the gallbladder, but they can also form *de novo*.

Clinical Features

- Typically symptoms of choledocholithiasis include right upper quadrant pain with associated nausea and vomiting; however, the majority of persons with BD stones are asymptomatic.
- Physical examination is usually normal. If there is biliary obstruction, jaundice may be noted.

Diagnosis

- Laboratory tests: elevated serum alkaline phosphatase level and mild jaundice (serum bilirubin <5 mg/dL) are the most common laboratory findings.
- Imaging studies:
  - 50% of BD stones can be missed on ultrasonography. Therefore, ultrasonography is not the test of choice.
  - Endoscopic ultrasonography has >98% sensitivity and specificity for the detection of choledocholithiasis but requires an invasive endoscopic procedure.
  - Magnetic resonance cholangiopancreatography (MRCP) detects BD stones with >95% sensitivity and specificity.
  - Endoscopic retrograde cholangiopancreatography (ERCP) is the gold standard for the diagnosis of choledocholithiasis. Importantly, therapeutic interventions, including biliary decompression, stone extraction, and stent placement, can be performed with ERCP.
  - ERCP is the diagnostic test of choice when the suspicion for choledocholithiasis is high and an intervention is likely to be required, as in patients with jaundice secondary to BD stones. MRCP is generally the test of choice when the suspicion for choledocholithiasis is low or intermediate.

Treatment

- Treatment of asymptomatic choledocholithiasis is recommended due to the risk of life-threatening complications, including acute pancreatitis and cholangitis.

- Treatment includes ERCP with stone extraction as well as a cholecystectomy to prevent further stone formation and migration into the BD.
- ERCP alone is sufficient in patients who are considered to be at high risk for cholecystectomy.

> Choledocholithiasis is the most common cause of acute pancreatitis. Cholangitis is a life-threatening complication of choledocholithiasis. Therefore, choledocholithasis should be treated even in asymptomatic persons.

Acute Cholangitis

- Acute cholangitis is a life-threatening complication of gallstones usually caused by an impacted stone in the BD.
- The impacted stone predisposes to bacterial infection and septicemia.
  - The most common organisms include *Escherichia coli*, *Klebsiella* spp., *Pseudomonas*, and *Enterococcus*.

Clinical Features
- Typical symptoms, which comprise Charcot's triad, include fever, jaundice, and right upper quadrant pain.
  - A smaller proportion of patients (10–20%) also have altered mental status and hypotension (called Reynolds' pentad).

Diagnosis
- Laboratory tests: leukocytosis with a left shift, hyperbilirubinemia, and elevated serum alkaline phosphatase and aminotransferase levels are the typical laboratory findings.
- Imaging studies:
  - CT is more accurate than ultrasonography for the diagnosis of acute cholangitis. However, neither CT nor ultrasonography is good for excluding a BD stone.
  - ERCP is recommended as a diagnostic test and therapeutic modality.
  - As in choledocholithiasis, MRCP may be used for diagnosis.

Treatment
- A single intravenous broad-spectrum antibiotic, such as cefoxitin, is sufficient in mild cases. In severely ill patients, broad-spectrum antibiotics are indicated (e.g., ampicillin, gentamicin, and metronidazole or piperacillin-tazobactam). If resistant organisms are suspected, meropenem 1 g intravenously every 8 hours should be initiated.

- Urgent biliary decompression: the urgency of decompression depends on the patient's initial response to supportive therapy with fluid resuscitation and antibiotics. In patients who remain symptomatic, urgent ERCP is recommended.
  - In patients who are hemodynamically unstable, such as those with hypotension, ERCP cannot be performed; instead, a percutaneous cholecystostomy tube insertion is recommended to decompress the biliary system.
  - Cholecystectomy is recommended to prevent further gallstone formation or migration of a stone into the BD.

> Acute cholangitis is a life-threatening complication of gallstones that should be identified early and treated promptly.

Uncommon Gallstone Complications

Gallstone Ileus

- Gallstone ileus is defined as small bowel obstruction caused by a gallstone.
- The gallstone passes into the intestine through a cholecystoenteric fistula that forms after an episode of cholecystitis. Cholecystoenteric fistulas are typically seen in persons 65–75 years of age.
- The most common location of a cholecystoenteric fistula is the duodenum (termed Bouveret's syndrome), followed by the colon, stomach, and jejunum. The most common site of gallstone impaction is in the terminal ileum or ileocecal valve.
- Many patients with gallstone ileus may have serious concomitant medical illnesses such as coronary artery disease, diabetes mellitus, or pulmonary disease. Delayed diagnosis due to the intermittency of symptoms is not uncommon and leads to a high mortality rate (50%).

Diagnosis
- Gallstone ileus is diagnosed with a plain film of the abdomen: radiographic findings include pneumobilia (air in the biliary tree), dilated small bowel loops suggestive of partial or complete small bowel obstruction, and an impacted stone in the bowel (see Chapter 27).

Mirizzi's Syndrome

- Mirizzi's syndrome is a rare complication of prolonged cholelithiasis. It is defined as jaundice caused by obstruction of the common hepatic duct secondary to an impacted gallstone in the cystic duct.

- A stone impacted in the cystic duct can lead to pressure necrosis and obstruction of, or even a fistula to, the common hepatic duct (type I and type II Mirizzi syndrome, respectively).
- The diagnosis can be made by CT, ERCP, or MRCP. The characteristic extrinsic compression of the common hepatic duct is usually evident on ERCP or MRCP.
- Open cholecystectomy is the treatment of choice; however, ERCP with endoscopic stenting is being used increasingly as a primary therapeutic modality.

Porcelain Gallbladder

- Porcelain gallbladder is defined as intramural calcification of the gallbladder wall and is not a complication of gallstones. It is associated with an increased risk of gallbladder carcinoma, which can occur in up to 20% of individuals.
- The incidence of gallbladder cancer depends on the pattern of gallbladder wall calcification, with selective mucosal calcification causing a significant cancer risk compared with diffuse intramural calcification, which does not seem to increase the risk of gallbladder cancer.
- Patients are usually asymptomatic, and laboratory tests are normal. The diagnosis is made with a plain abdominal X-ray or CT showing calcifications in the gallbladder wall.
- Prophylactic cholecystectomy is indicated to prevent gallbladder carcinoma.

Emphysematous Cholecystitis

- Persons with emphysematous cholecystitis have a clinical presentation similar to those with acute cholecystitis.
- The etiology of emphysematous cholecystitis is related to cystic duct ischemia secondary to atherosclerosis. Therefore, elderly persons (without gallstones) and persons with diabetes mellitus are at increased risk of developing emphysematous cholecystitis.
- Gas-forming organisms infect the gallbladder wall and lead to gas pockets that are evident on abdominal imaging.
- The risk of gallbladder perforation is high. Therefore, emergent treatment with broad-spectrum antibiotics that include anaerobic coverage and early cholecystectomy is recommended.

Gangrenous Cholecystitis

- Gangrenous cholecystitis is a severe form of acute cholecystitis that results in gallbladder wall necrosis and perforation. It is associated with high mortality and morbidity.

- Persons who are at high risk of gangrenous cholecystitis are elderly men with multiple comorbidities.
- The clinical presentation is similar to that of acute nongangrenous cholecystitis; gangrene is often not suspected preoperatively.
- Treatment is with broad-spectrum antibiotic coverage and emergent, usually open, cholecystectomy.

Pearls

The most common type of gallstones are cholesterol stones; women are affected much more commonly than men.

Asymptomatic gallstones generally do not require treatment except in persons at high risk of gallbladder cancer.

Prolonged biliary pain (>3 hours) suggests acute cholecystitis.

Even asymptomatic choledocholithiasis should be treated. Acute cholangitis requires immediate antibiotic therapy and urgent bile duct decompression.

Questions

Question 1 relates to the clinical vignette at the beginning of this chapter.
1. Which of the following is the best test to confirm the diagnosis?
   A. Right upper quadrant ultrasonography
   B. Computed tomography
   C. Magnetic resonance cholangiopancreatography
   D. Endoscopic retrograde cholangiopancreatography
2. A 54-year-old woman with a history of hypertension and type 2 diabetes mellitus presents to the office for evaluation of a 6-month history of occasional right upper quadrant pain. The pain occurs every 2 months or so, is severe and constant, radiates to the back, and is often precipitated by a fatty meal. She denies nausea, vomiting, fevers, chills, or jaundice. Laboratory tests, including a complete blood count and comprehensive metabolic panel, are normal except for a mildly elevated serum alkaline phosphatase level. Right upper quadrant ultrasonography shows cholelithiasis. Which of the following is the next step in the management of this patient?
   A. Upper endoscopy
   B. Laparascopic cholecystectomy
   C. Magnetic resonance cholangiopancreatography (MRCP)
   D. Reassurance
3. A 24-year-old African American man with sickle cell disease is admitted to the hospital for fevers, chills, right upper quadrant pain, and jaundice of 2

(Continued)

days' duration. Laboratory tests show a white blood cell count of 24 000/ mm³ with 89% neutrophils, serum aspartate aminotransferase level 125 U/L, alanine aminotransferase 214 U/L, and bilirubin 5 mg/dL. Right upper quadrant ultrasonography shows cholelithasis, with no evidence of chole- cystitis, and a dilated bile duct with intraductal stones. The next step in the management of this patient is which of the following?

A. Emergent cholecystectomy

B. Broad-spectrum antibiotics and endoscopic retrograde cholangiopan- creatography (ERCP)

C. Broad-spectrum antibiotics and percutaneous transhepatic cholangiog- raphy (PTC)

D. Broad-spectrum antibiotics only

4. Risk factors for gallstone formation include all of the following EXCEPT:

A. Diabetes mellitus

B. Hypertriglyceridemia

C. Hypercholesterolemia

D. Total parenteral nutrition

E. Older age

5. A 79-year-old man is admitted to the hospital with fever, abdominal pain, jaundice, and altered mental status of 1 day duration. Laboratory tests show a white blood cell count of 18 000/mm³, serum alkaline phosphatase level 400 U/L, aspartate aminotransferase 200 U/L, alanine aminotrans- ferase 216 U/L, and bilirubin 4 mg/dL. Right upper quadrant ultrasono- graphy is unremarkable. Blood cultures are positive for *E. coli*. He continues to be febrile despite treatment with broad-spectrum antibiotics for 24 hours. Which of the following is the next best step in the management of this patient?

A. Computed tomography (CT) of abdomen and pelvis

B. Urgent endoscopic retrograde cholangiopancreatography (ERCP)

C. Magnetic resonance imaging and magnetic resonance cholangiopan- creatography (MRI/MRCP)

D. An intravenous antifungal agent

6. A 63-year-old woman is admitted to the hospital with a 2-day history of right upper quadrant pain and fever. Laboratory tests show mild leukocy- tosis and elevated serum alkaline phosphatase and bilirubin levels. Ultrasonography shows mild gallbladder wall thickening but no other signs of cholecystitis. Which of the following tests will confirm the diagnosis of acute cholecystitis in this patient?

A. Repeat ultrasonography in 24–48 hours

B. HIDA scan

C. Magnetic resonance cholangiopancreatography (MRCP)

D. Endoscopic retrograde cholangiopancreatography (ERCP)

7. A 56-year-old woman is seen in the office for follow up of vague, constant right upper quadrant pain of 2 years' duration. Laboratory tests, including a complete blood cell count and comprehensive metabolic panel are normal. Abdominal ultrasonography shows evidence of intramural calcifications in the gallbladder wall. Upper endoscopy is negative. Which of the following is the most appropriate next step in the management of this patient?
   A. Magnetic resonance imaging and magnetic resonance cholangiopancreatography (MRI/MRCP)
   B. Repeat abdominal ultrasonography in 4 weeks
   C. Cholecystectomy
   D. Reassurance

8. A 32-year-old woman is seen for follow up of a right upper quadrant ultrasonography that was ordered to evaluate hepatomegaly noted on a routine annual physical examination. The patient is asymptomatic. The ultrasonography shows evidence of gallstones but no other abnormality. Laboratory tests including serum aminotransferase, alkaline phosphatase, and bilirubin levels are normal. Which of the following is the next best step in the management of this patient?
   A. Reassurance
   B. Repeat ultrasonography in 1 year
   C. Cholecystectomy
   D. Treatment with ursodeoxycholic acid

Answers

1. A
   The patient describes symptoms consistent with biliary pain, likely from cholelithiasis. Her age, sex, and parity are risk factors for cholelithiasis. The differential diagnosis includes choledocholithiasis, cholecystitis, pancreatitis, gastroesphageal reflux disease, and peptic ulcer disease. Ultrasononography is the best test to confirm cholelithiasis.

2. B
   The clinical presentation is suggestive of biliary pain. The differential diagnosis includes choledocholithiasis, cholecystitis, pancreatitis, gastroesophageal reflux disease, and peptic ulcer disease. Ultrasonography has >95% sensitivity and specificity for the detection of gallstones or cholecystitis and is a cost-effective test compared with MRCP. The treatment of choice of symptomatic cholelithiasis is cholecystectomy. Upper endoscopy is not indicated at this time.

3. B
   This patient has classic symptoms of acute cholangitis (Charcot's triad – right upper quadrant pain, fever, and jaundice). Acute cholangitis is caused

(Continued)

by a stone impacted in the bile duct, with secondary bacterial proliferation. It is likely that this patient has black pigment stones given his history of sickle cell disease. Irrespective of the type of gallstone, the treatment of choice for acute cholangitis is broad-spectrum antibiotics followed by biliary decompression. The preferred method of biliary decompression is ERCP. PTC is reserved for cases in which ERCP is not available or not possible, given the lower risk of complications with an ERCP. A cholecystectomy is not required urgently but should be considered once the acute cholangitis resolves.

4. C

Hypercholesterolemia is not a risk factor for gallstone formation. Hypertriglyceridemia, on the other hand, and low high density lipoprotein (HDL) levels are strong predictors of gallstone formation. All the other conditions increase the risk of gallstone formation.

5. B

The patient has acute cholangitis as evidenced by fever, abdominal pain, jaundice, and altered mental status. He has bacteremia and is not responding to intravenous antibiotic treatment. Cholangitis is a life-threatening condition and requires urgent biliary decompression. The next best step in the management of this patient is biliary decompression and removal of the bile duct (BD) stone by ERCP. If the patient is hemodynamically unstable, percutaneous cholecystostomy should be performed. Ultrasonography that is negative for gallstones does not alter the management of cholangitis. CT and MRI are better diagnostic modalities than ultrasonography for visualizing BD stones, but they do not have any therapeutic potential and will only delay treatment.

6. B

A HIDA scan confirms cystic duct obstruction based on lack of visualization of the gallbladder within 30–60 minutes of intravenous administration of ^{99m}Tc-labeled hydroxy iminodiacetic acid. Repeating the ultrasonography will only delay the diagnosis and might not provide further evidence of acute cholecystitis. MRCP is an expensive test with a much higher sensitivity for bile duct stones and dilatation than ultrasonography. ERCP is an invasive modality that is not indicated in the diagnosis or treatment of acute cholecystitis.

7. C

Intramural calcifications in the gallbladder wall are characteristic of porcelain gallbladder, a condition that predisposes to carcinoma of the gallbladder in 20% of cases. Porcelain gallbladder is an indication for cholecystectomy even if the patient is asymptomatic. MRI/MRCP is not indicated, since the diagnosis of porcelain gallbladder is already made by ultrasonography. Repeating ultrasonography is not necessary and will only delay treatment.

> **8. A**
> Treatment of asymptomatic gallstone disease is not recommended given the low risk of complications. The patient is asymptomatic and does not need any further therapy or follow-up of her stones unless symptoms of biliary disease occur.

Further Reading

Abou-Saif, A. and Al-Kawas, F. (2002) Complications of gallstone disease: Mirizzi syndrome, cholecystocholedochal fistula, and gallstone ileus. *American Journal of Gastroenterology*, 97, 249–254.

Ahmed, A., Cheung, R. and Keeffe, E. (2000) Management of gallstones and their complications. *American Family Physician*, 61, 1673–1680.

Hanau, L. and Steigbigel, N. (2000) Acute cholangitis. *Infectious Disease Clinics of North America*, 14, 521–546.

Portincasa, P., Moschetta, A. and Palasciano, G. (2006) Cholesterol gallstone disease. *Lancet*, 368, 230–239.

Stephen, A. and Berger, D. (2001) Carcinoma in the porcelain gallbladder: a relationship revisited. *Archives of Surgery*, 129, 699–703.

Wang, D. and Afdhal, N. (2010) Gallstone disease, in *Sleisenger and Fordtran's Gastrointestinal and Liver Disease: Pathophysiology/Diagnosis/Management*, 9th edn (eds M. Feldman, L.S. Friedman and L.J. Brandt), Saunders Elsevier, Philadelphia, pp. 1089–1119.

> **Weblink**
>
> http://www.aafp.org/afp/20000315/1673.html

Common Problems in Gastroenterology

Jan-Michael A. Klapproth and Shanthi V. Sitaraman

Acute Gastrointestinal Bleeding

Tanvi Dhere

CHAPTER 22

Clinical Vignette

A 63-year-old man presents to the emergency department (ED) with hematemesis that started 2 hours ago. He was working at his computer, began to feel nauseated, and vomited two cups of bright red blood. He vomited once more in the ED. He also noted passage of black tarry stool. He takes ibuprofen 1g daily for osteoarthritis of his knees. He drinks up to six to eight beers a day, does not smoke cigarettes, and has no history of illicit drug use. Vital signs show a blood pressure of 145/86mmHg supine and 100/65mmHg upright; pulse rate 112/min supine and 130/min upright; respiratory rate 14/min; and oxygen saturation 94% on room air. The abdomen is soft and nontender, and bowel sounds are normal. The liver edge cannot be palpated. The spleen tip is palpable in the left upper quadrant. There is fluid wave and shifting dullness suggesting the presence of ascites. A few spider angiomas are noted on the chest. Rectal examination shows maroon stools. Laboratory tests show a white blood cell count of 7200/mm^3, hemoglobin level 10g/dL, platelet count 100000/mm^3, and mean corpuscular volume 99fL. A comprehensive metabolic panel shows a sodium of 128mEq/L, potassium 4.2mEq/L, blood urea nitrogen 45mg/dL, creatinine 1.3mg/dL, alanine aminotransferase 45U/L, aspartate aminotransferase 92U/L, alkaline phosphatase 90U/L, and total bilirubin 1.5mg/dL. The prothrombin time is 13.4 seconds and international normalized ratio is 1.4.

General

- Acute gastrointestinal (GI) bleeding accounts for >350000 hospital admissions in the US each year.

Essentials of Gastroenterology, First Edition. Edited by Shanthi V. Sitaraman, Lawrence S. Friedman.
© 2012 John Wiley & Sons, Ltd. Published 2012 by John Wiley & Sons, Ltd.

Table 22.1 GI bleeding nomenclature.

Presentation	Definition	Association with	
		UGIB	LGIB
Coffee ground emesis	Dark gastric contents; usually signifies prolonged exposure to gastric acid	+	–
Hematemesis	Emesis of bright red color	+	–
Melena	Black, tarry stool with a characteristic smell	+	+
Hematochezia	Passage of bright blood per rectum; may be admixed with stool	+	+

LGIB, lower gastrointestinal bleeding; UGIB, upper gastrointestinal bleeding.

- The overall mortality rate for upper GI bleeding is 5–10% and has not changed since the 1970s. The mortality rate for lower GI bleeding is approximately 4%.

Definitions

- The ligament of Treitz, a suspensory ligament located between the duodenum and jejunum and connecting to the diaphragm, is the key landmark separating **upper GI** (UGIB) from **lower GI** bleeding (LGIB). UGIB refers to hemorrhage proximal to, whereas LGIB refers to hemorrhage distal to, the ligament of Treitz.
- Hematemesis, coffee ground emesis, or melena typically indicates UGIB (Table 22.1).
- **Melena** is black, tarry, malodorous stool that usually indicates hemorrhage proximal to the ligament of Treitz. Occasionally, bleeding from a source in the small bowel or right colon may also cause melena. The black color is caused by oxidation of the iron in hemoglobin by gastric acid or by bacteria. A volume of approximately 100–200 mL of blood in the upper GI tract is needed to cause melena. Melena may persist for several days after bleeding has ceased.
- Black stool that does not contain occult blood may result from ingestion of iron, bismuth, or various foods and should not be mistaken for melena.

Etiology

- UGIB constitutes 75% of all cases of acute GI bleeding. Causes of UGIB (Table 22.2) include:
  - **Peptic ulcer disease**: Duodenal and gastric ulcers, gastropathy, and duodenitis (see Chapter 3) are the most common causes of UGIB and account for 40–50% of all cases of UGIB. Less common causes of peptic ulcer include Cushing ulcer (gastric and duodenal ulcers associated with increased intracranial pressure) and Curling ulcer (acute ulcer of the duodenum associated with severe burns).
  - **Esophageal and gastric varices** account for 20–30% of cases of UGIB.
  - **Mallory–Weiss tears** account for 5–15% of cases of UGIB; they are tears at the gastroesophageal junction in the mucosa due to retching, repeated vomiting, or coughing.
  - **Erosive esophagitis** accounts for 10% of cases of UGIB.
    - Common causes of erosive esophagitis in immunocompetent patients include gastroesophageal reflux disease and radiation therapy.
    - In immunosuppressed persons, erosive esophagitis is typically caused by infections, such as *Candida* spp., cytomegalovirus, herpes simplex virus, or human immunodeficiency virus or may be idiopathic.
  - **Vascular lesions** account for less than 5% of cases of UGIB. Examples of vascular lesions include Dieulafoy's lesion (a superficial submucosal arteriole), arteriovenous malformations, telangiectasias (as in hereditary hemorrhagic telangiectasia, or Osler–Weber–Rendu disease), and gastric vascular antral ectasia (GAVE, or "watermelon" stomach), which may be associated with chronic renal failure, portal hypertension, or collagen vascular disease.
  - **Neoplasms** of the esophagus, stomach, or duodenum may cause UGIB.
  - Uncommon causes:
    - **Hemobilia** (bleeding into the biliary tree) may occur in patients who have undergone liver biopsy or experienced trauma or hepatobiliary manipulation.
    - **Hemosuccus pancreaticus** (bleeding into the pancreatic duct) may occur with acute or chronic pancreatitis, pancreatic cancer, or pancreatic duct manipulation.
    - **Aortoenteric fistula** (communication between the abdominal aorta, usually an aneurysm, and third portion of the duodenum). Bleeding from an aortoenteric fistula often presents as a brief "herald" bleed followed by an acute massive bleed and is associated with a high mortality rate.

Table 22.2 Differential diagnosis of upper gastrointestinal bleeding (UGIB).

Cause (% of all cases of UGIB)	Pathogenic factors	Presentation	Course	Treatment
PUD (40–50%)	NSAIDs *H. pylori* infection Curling ulcer, Cushing ulcer	Melena Hematemesis Coffee ground emesis Hematochezia	Self-limited in 80% of cases Endoscopic therapy needed in 20% of cases	Intravenous PPI Endoscopic hemostasis
Esophageal/gastric varices (20–30%)	Chronic liver disease Splenic vein thrombosis (gastric varices)	Severe hypovolemia Melena Hematemesis Hematochezia	In 80–90% of cases, bleeding ceases following urgent endoscopic intervention performed within 12 hrs Mortality rate 15–40%	Octreotide Antibiotics Endoscopic hemostasis Sengstaken-Blakemore tube TIPS Splenectomy for splenic vein thrombosis
Mallory–Weiss tear (5–15%)	Retching Heavy alcohol ingestion Coughing	Hematemesis Coffee ground emesis	Resolves spontaneously in >95% of cases <10% have continued bleeding	Supportive Endoscopic hemostasis if ongoing bleeding

Erosive esophagitis (10%)	GERD Alcohol NSAIDs Infection Radiation	Hematemesis Coffee ground emesis Melena	<5% risk of rebleeding	PPI Sucralfate Treatment of infection
Vascular malformation (<5%)	Angiodysplasias associated with CKD Anticoagulation Osler–Weber–Rendu disease Dieulafoy's lesion GAVE Portal hypertensive gastropathy	Hematemesis Coffee ground emesis Melena Iron-deficiency anemia	Dieulafoy's lesion may result in significant blood loss Recurrent GI bleeding can occur in a third of patients with Osler–Weber–Rendu disease, most commonly above age 40 Patients with bleeding diatheses have worse outcomes than those without diatheses Bleeding from angiodysplasias in the setting of aortic stenosis may improve with aortic valve replacement	Endoscopic ablation
Neoplasms (1%)	Family history Smoking Age >65 H. pylori infection	Iron deficiency + FOBT Weight loss Dyspepsia	Majority present with advanced disease	Chemotherapy, radiation, surgery

CKD, chronic kidney disease; FOBT, fecal occult blood test; GAVE, gastric antral vascular ectasia; GERD, gastroesophageal reflux disease; H. pylori, Helicobacter pylori; NSAIDs, nonsteroidal anti-inflammatory drugs; PPI, proton pump inhibitor; PUD, peptic ulcer disease; TIPS, transjugular intrahepatic portosystemic shunt.

> A clue to esophageal or gastric malignancy as a cause of UGIB is the presence of iron-deficiency anemia in the setting of acute GI bleeding.

- Causes of LGIB (Table 22.3) include:
  - ○ **Diverticulosis** accounts for 25–40% of cases of LGIB. Right-sided diverticula bleed more frequently than left-sided diverticula. They are more common in persons >65 years of age and in those with chronic constipation.
  - ○ **Angiodysplasia** accounts for 3–37% of cases of LGIB.
    - ▪ Angiodysplasias (or angioectasias) are ecstatic thin-walled venules or capillaries in the mucosa or submucosa. Their development is age-related.
    - ▪ They are typically seen in the cecum or ascending colon but may occur anywhere in the GI tract, including the small bowel. Although angiodysplasias can bleed spontaneously, bleeding is associated with the use of anticoagulants and aspirin or other nonsteroidal anti-inflammatory drugs (NSAIDs). They may also bleed in the setting of uremia due to platelet dysfunction from uremia.
    - ▪ Bleeding from angiodysplasia may be associated with aortic stenosis (Heyde's syndrome).
  - ○ **Neoplastic disease** accounts for 15% of cases of LGIB. Most present as chronic occult blood loss and iron-deficiency anemia rather than acute blood loss.
  - ○ **Colitis** accounts for 10% of cases of LGIB. Causes of colitis include ischemia, infection, radiation therapy, and inflammatory bowel disease.
  - ○ **UGIB** may present as LGIB. 11% of patients suspected initially of having a LGIB are found to have an UGI source of bleeding.
  - ○ **Internal hemorrhoids**. Bleeding from internal hemorrhoids is typically intermittent, small in quantity, and self-limited but can be massive, resulting in hemodynamic compromise.
  - ○ Uncommon causes of LGIB include intestinal intussusception, colonic varices, solitary rectal ulcer syndrome, and aortoenteric fistula.

> Hematochezia in the setting of UGIB is an ominous sign because it signifies that the patient is bleeding at a rapid rate.

Table 22.3 Differential diagnosis of lower gastrointestinal bleeding (LGIB).

Cause (% of all cases of LGIB)	Pathogenic factors	Presentation	Course	Treatment
Diverticulosis (25–40%)	Constipation Older age Low fiber intake	Abrupt onset of painless maroon stools or bright red blood per rectum	>60% cease spontaneously within 12 hours of onset Rebleeding in 25–35% of cases	Colonoscopy Angiography with embolization Surgery
Angiodysplasia (3–37%)	CKD Anticoagulation Aortic stenosis	Intermittent melena Iron-deficiency anemia Painless hematochezia	>80% success rate of endoscopic treatment	Endoscopic hemostasis Estrogen Octreotide
Internal hemorrhoids (10%)	Constipation	Painless intermittent bloody stools	Majority present with small-volume bleeding	Suppositories Band ligation Hemorrhoidectomy

(Continued)

Table 22.3 (*Continued*)

Cause (% of all cases of LGIB)	Pathogenic factors	Presentation	Course	Treatment
Neoplasms (15%)	Family history Older age Polyposis syndromes Lynch syndrome (HNPCC) IBD	Iron deficiency	40% mortality rate	Chemotherapy, radiation, surgery
Colitis (10%)	Ischemia IBD Infection (e.g., *Shigella*, *Salmonella*, CMV) Radiation	Bloody stools Bright red blood per rectum	Most cases of ischemic colitis resolve with no complications 20% of patients with extensive colitis due to IBD require surgery	Supportive treatment for ischemic colitis Glucocorticoids, infliximab, cyclosporine, surgery for IBD Antibiotics/antiviral agents for infections Argon plasma coagulation for radiation proctitis
UGIB (11%)	NSAIDs *H. pylori* infection	Brisk hematochezia	Mortality rate can be up to 30%	Endoscopic hemostasis Angiography Surgery

CKD, chronic kidney disease; CMV, cytomegalovirus; *H. pylori*, *Helicobacter pylori*; IBD, inflammatory bowel disease; HNPCC, hereditary nonpolyposis colorectal cancer; NSAIDs, nonsteroidal anti-inflammatory drugs; UGIB, upper gastrointestinal bleed.

Risk Factors for GI Bleeding

- Older age
- Prior history of GI bleed
- Chronic liver disease
- Coagulation disorders
- Use of medications such as anticoagulants, aspirin and other NSAIDs, and antiplatelet agents such as clopidogrel.

Clinical Features

History

- The onset, duration, severity, and character of emesis (bright red blood, coffee ground), quantity of emesis, and presence of melena or hematochezia and associated nausea, retching, and abdominal pain should be determined.
- Associated symptoms including long-standing heartburn, chronic constipation, diarrhea, and nosebleeds should be ascertained.
- A history of chronic liver disease should be elicited. The history should also include an assessment for risk factors for liver disease such as a history of illicit drug use, alcohol abuse, blood transfusions, and unprotected sex as well as a family history of liver disease.
- Key features of the past medical history include previous GI bleeding, abdominal surgery, and concomitant medical conditions.
- A thorough medication history should be obtained. Use of NSAIDs, anticoagulants, and antiplatelet agents such as clopidrogrel should be determined. Gingko biloba, a herbal supplement, may also increase the risk of bleeding. Prior ingestion of a caustic agent should be determined.
- The social history should include alcohol, tobacco, and illicit drug use.
- The family history should include liver disease, bleeding disorders, cancer, and inflammatory bowel disease.

Physical Examination

- The assessment of hemodynamic stability is of utmost importance in patients with acute GI bleeding. Patients should be evaluated immediately for symptoms and signs of shock, and those without overt tachycardia or hypotension should be examined for orthostatic hemodynamic changes.
- Orthostatic changes in pulse rate and blood pressure are indicative of hypovolemia in the setting of GI bleeding. An increase in the pulse rate of 20/min and a drop in blood pressure of 20 mmHg systolic or 10 mmHg diastolic from the supine to standing position indicate

roughly 700 mL of blood loss. Lightheadedness or dizziness when standing from a sitting position is a sensitive marker for the presence of orthostasis.

- Patients should be examined for stigmata of chronic liver disease (e.g., spider angiomas, ascites, palmar erythema, splenomegaly, caput medusae). Peritoneal signs (abdominal rebound tenderness, guarding or rigidity) may indicate a perforated ulcer, perforated colon (from ischemic colitis, inflammatory bowel disease), or toxic megacolon (due to inflammatory bowel disease).

Treatment

General
- Regardless of the source of bleeding, fluid resuscitation is the first and most important step in the management of GI bleeding, especially in patients with hemodynamic compromise. Measures include the following:
  - Placement of two large-bore (16- or 18-gauge) intravenous (IV) lines or a central venous line.
  - Immediate volume expansion with IV fluids.
  - Transfusion of packed red blood cells.
  - Correction of coagulopathy. Transfuse fresh frozen plasma to normalize a prolonged prothrombin time (international normalized ratio <1.5) and platelets to maintain the platelet count >50 000/mm³.
  - Vasopressors may be indicated in some patients if volume expansion alone does not stabilize the blood pressure.
- Hemodynamic instability or evidence of significant ongoing blood loss (active hematemesis, melena, or at least moderately severe hematochezia) is an indication for admission to an intensive care unit for close monitoring.
- Laboratory tests including a complete blood count, comprehensive metabolic panel, prothrombin time, and partial prothrombin time should be obtained in all patients. Blood should be typed and cross-matched.
- All anticoagulants should be withheld. Antihypertensive medications should be used with caution.

UGIB
- If UGIB is suspected, an urgent consultation with a gastroenterologist and surgeon should be obtained.
  - The hemoglobin level at the time of presentation of acute GI bleeding may be higher than the patient's actual hemoglobin level due to hemoconcentration.

- ○ A 2–3% decrease in the hematocrit value reflects blood loss of ~500 mL.
- ○ A blood urea nitrogen-to-creatinine ratio >36 may be found in patients with UGIB (without underlying renal insufficiency) due to prerenal azotemia and absorption of digested blood during intestinal transit.
- ○ In addition to a low hemoglobin level, patients with cirrhosis may have low white blood cell and platelet counts and a prolonged prothrombin time.

> Use of a nasogastric (NG) tube is controversial. NG lavage may be negative in 10% of patients with UGIB, and a clear aspirate does not necessarily rule out UGIB. NG lavage may be useful, however, in the setting of hematochezia resulting in hemodynamic compromise where an UGIB may be the source. If the NG lavage shows bilious return (indicating no blood in stomach and duodenum), then an upper source is unlikely, and management for LGIB can proceed as noted in Figure 22.1. If the aspirate is clear and not bilious, bleeding from the duodenum cannot be ruled out definitively, and esophagoduodenoscopy (EGD) should be performed.

- • Variceal UGIB (see Chapter 16):
  - ○ In patients with suspected variceal bleeding, octreotide should be administered intravenously in a dose of 50 μg bolus followed by 50 μg/hr. Octreotide is preferred to intravenous vasopression plus nitroglycerin.
  - ○ Antibiotics should be administered in all cases of suspected variceal bleed. Antibiotics reduce the incidence of spontaneous bacterial peritonitis associated with acute variceal bleeding. Ceftriaxone 1 g IV or norfloxacin 400 mg orally twice daily for 7 days is recommended.
  - ○ EGD can be diagnostic as well as therapeutic and should be performed once a patient is hemodynamically stable (Table 22.4):
    - ■ For active bleeding from esophageal varices upper-endoscopic band ligation or sclerotherapy can be used to stop bleeding; where available, band ligation is preferred.
    - ■ Gastric varices are not amenable to these endoscopic treatments in most cases; where available, injection of cyanoacrylate may be an option.
    - ■ Insertion of a Sengstaken–Blakemore or Minnesota tube may be necessary for massive variceal hemorrhage. These tubes have gastric and esophageal balloons that can be inflated to tamponade varices.

Table 22.4 Endoscopic predictors of peptic ulcer rebleeding.

Endoscopic finding	Frequency	Risk of rebleeding without endoscopic hemostasis	Treatment
Arterial spurting	10%	90%	PPI + endoscopic hemostasis
Nonbleeding visible vessel	25%	50%	PPI + endoscopic hemostasis
Adherent clot	10%	25–30%	PPI +/− endoscopic hemostasis
Oozing without visible vessel	10%	10–20%	PPI +/− endoscopic hemostasis
Pigmented spot	10%	7–10%	PPI Consider discharge from ED
White-based ulcer	35%	3–5%	PPI Consider discharge from ED

ED, emergency department; PPI, proton pump inhibitor.

- A transjugular intrahepatic portosystemic shunt (TIPS) may be placed to manage patients with variceal bleeding that does not respond to medical or endoscopic treatment. TIPS reduces elevated portal pressure by creating a communication between the hepatic vein and an intrahepatic branch of the portal vein.
- Nonvariceal UGIB:
  - If peptic ulcer disease is suspected, a proton pump inhibitor (PPI) should be given either intravenously (esomeprazole or pantoprazole 80 mg bolus followed by 8 mg/hr or lansoprazole 60 mg bolus followed by 6 mg/hr for 72 hours) or orally (twice daily dosing) if an intravenous formulation is not available. Once endoscopic treatment is performed or if there is no rebleeding within 24 hours, the patient can be transitioned to an oral PPI once daily.
  - EGD can be diagnostic as well as therapeutic and should be performed once the patient is hemodynamically stable (Table 22.4).

○ For active bleeding from a gastric or duodenal ulcer, endoscopic hemostatic modalities such as injection of epinephrine plus electrocautery or placement of hemoclips may be used.
○ Angiography may be used when endoscopic control of bleeding cannot be achieved.
○ Surgery is indicated in patients with ongoing bleeding despite medical and endoscopic treatment (see Chapter 4).

LGIB
• UGIB should be ruled out before attempting to localize the source of presumed LGIB that results in hemodynamic compromise. NG lavage may be useful but may be negative in 10% of cases. EGD may be necessary to rule out an UGIB.
• Colonoscopy is generally considered the test of choice for diagnosis and potential therapy (Figure 22.1).

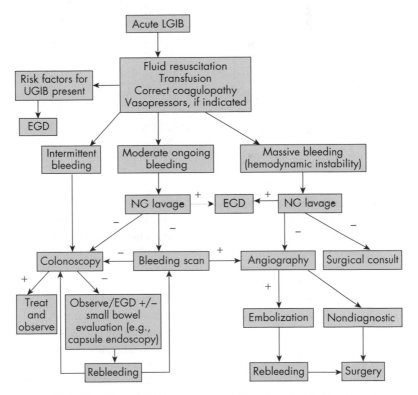

Figure 22.1 Algorithm for the management of lower gastrointestinal bleeding (LGIB). (EGD, esophagogastroduodenoscopy; NG, nasogastric; UGIB, upper GI bleeding.)

- ○ If bleeding stops spontaneously, subsequent colonoscopy is recommended. Colonoscopy identifies the source of bleeding in >70% of patients.
  - ○ In patients who are hemodynamically stable but continue to bleed, colonoscopy can be performed after a rapid purge with polyethylene glycol solution administered through a NG tube. If the source is not found, a bleeding scan can be considered.
- A bleeding (tagged red blood cell) scan utilizes technetium sulfur colloid-labeled autologous red blood cells, which are infused back into the patient to detect the site of bleeding.
  - ○ The study detects GI bleeding that occurs at a rate of >0.1 mL/min and is more sensitive than angiography.
  - ○ A bleeding scan does not localize the site of bleed precisely and is not therapeutic.
- In patients who continue to bleed and are hemodynamically unstable, multidetector computed tomography angiography may be diagnostic and angiography may be diagnostic and therapeutic (with embolization or intraarterial infusion of vasopressin).
  - ○ The study detects GI bleeding that occurs at a rate of 0.5–1.5 mL/min.
  - ○ The diagnostic yield is variable and depends on the timing of the procedure, patient selection, and experience and skill of the radiologist.
  - ○ Complications of angiography include acute kidney injury, cholesterol emboli, and bowel infarction.
- Surgery may be required for uncontrolled bleeding or recurrent diverticular bleeding, which can occur in up to 35% of cases.
- Although colonoscopy is the diagnostic test of choice for LGIB, a plain abdominal X-ray and/or computed tomography (CT) may be used to diagnose ischemic colitis.
  - ○ Irregular thickening of the mucosal folds may lead to classic "thumbprinting" on plain film.
  - ○ The presence of pneumatosis (air in the wall of the colon) and portomesenteric venous gas may be an ominous sign indicating transmural infarction.
  - ○ CT may show a thickened colonic wall.
- Capsule endoscopy, a noninvasive modality to image the small bowel, can be used to identify the source of bleeding when EGD, colonoscopy, and other modalities fail to reveal a source.

Pearls

Regardless of the source of bleeding, fluid resuscitation is the first and most important step in the management of GI bleeding.

Upper endoscopy is the diagnostic test of choice for UGIB.

Bleeding from esophageal or gastric varices carries a mortality rate of 50% if untreated.

An UGI source of bleeding should be ruled out in patients with hemodynamically significant LGIB.

The diagnostic test of choice for LGIB depends on the rapidity of bleeding; colonoscopy is often the preferred initial test.

Questions

Questions 1 and 2 relate to the clinical vignette at the beginning of this chapter.

1. Which of the following should be the first step in the management of this patient?
    A. A proton pump inhibitor
    B. Angiography
    C. Fluid resuscitation
    D. Intravenous octreotide
    E. Consultation with a gastroenterologist or surgeon
2. Which of the following medications is preferred in the treatment of this patient's acute GI bleeding?
    A. A proton pump inhibitor and octreotide
    B. Octreotide alone
    C. Vasopressin and nitroglycerin
    D. Vasopressin alone
3. A 27-year-old man presents to the emergency department with three episodes of bright red blood per rectum the day after completing a marathon. The bleeding has resolved. He notes cramping lower abdominal discomfort prior to bowel movements. His vital signs include a blood pressure of 95/50 mmHg and pulse rate 112/min. The hemoglobin level is 14 g/dL. The remainder of the laboratory tests are normal. Which of the following is the next best step in the management of this patient?

(Continued)

    A. Perform a rapid purge with polyethylene glycol for immediate colonoscopy

    B. Provide supportive care with intravenous fluids and perform an elective colonoscopy

    C. Perform a bleeding scan

    D. Consult a surgeon for possible colectomy

4. A 23-year-old woman presents to the emergency department with an episode of vomiting bright red blood. She has had flu-like symptoms and nausea for the past week and has been retching and vomiting straw-colored fluid. She denies rectal bleeding or melena. She denies use of nonsteroidal anti-inflammatory drugs (NSAIDs) or anticoagulants. The past medical history is unremarkable. Vitals signs include a blood pressure of 123/76 mmHg and pulse rate 95/min. Rectal examination shows brown stool that is negative for occult blood. The hemoglobin value is 15.2 g/L. Which of the following would you recommend?

    A. Reassure the patient and provide anti-emetics for nausea

    B. Computed tomography (CT) scan

    C. Nasogastric (NG) lavage

    D. Angiography

5. A 25-year-old man presents with a moderate amount of bright red blood in his bowel movements. He reports diarrhea (four to six loose stools per day) over the past 6 months and notes that many bowel movements have been mixed with blood in the past month. He has urgency and tenesmus. He also reports cramping lower abdominal pain that is relieved by a bowel movement but has no nausea, vomiting, or melena. He reports an unintentional weight loss of 18 lb (8 kg) over the past 6 months. Physical examination reveals a blood pressure of 120/80 mmHg, pulse rate 80/min, and temperature 100.3 °F (38 °C). The remainder of the examination is unremarkable except for maroon stool on rectal examination. Laboratory tests show a hemoglobin level of 7.8 g/dL with a mean corpuscular volume of 68 fL. The white blood cell count is 14 200/mm^3 and platelet count 556 000/mm^3. The remainder of the blood tests are normal. Which of the following is the most likely diagnosis?

    A. Ulcerative colitis

    B. Diverticulosis

    C. Portal hypertensive gastropathy

    D. Colonic arteriovenous malformation

    E. Hemorrhoids

6. A 68-year-old man presents to the emergency department with bright red blood per rectum that started 4 hours ago. He denies abdominal pain, nausea, vomiting, hematemesis, or melena. He has no prior history of gastrointestinal bleeding. He is otherwise healthy. He takes no prescription or over-the-counter medications. He does not drink alcohol or smoke

cigarettes. Vital signs include a blood pressure of 82/46 mmHg and pulse rate 124/min. Physical examination is unremarkable. There are no stigmata of chronic liver disease. Rectal examination shows clots. The patient refuses an NG tube. Laboratory tests, including a complete blood count and comprehensive metabolic panel, are normal except for a hemoglobin level of 6.8 g/dL. Colonoscopy is performed after a rapid purge and is normal. Which of the following tests should be considered next?

A. Capsule endoscopy
B. Bleeding scan
C. Esophagogastroduodenoscopy (EGD)
D. Repeat colonoscopy
E. Angiography

Answers

1. C

2. A

This patient has an acute UGIB and is hemodynamically unstable, as suggested by tachycardia and orthostasis. Fluid resuscitation with two large-bore intravenous lines should be the first step in the management of this patient. Although the patient appears to have signs of liver disease, a bleeding peptic ulcer cannot be excluded. Therefore, continuous infusion of a proton pump inhibitor (in case of an ulcer) and octreotide (in case of varices) is warranted. Once the patient is hemodynamically stable, esophagogastroduodenoscopy (EGD) should be performed to determine the source of bleeding. Angiography has no role in the initial management of an UGIB. Vasopressin and nitrates may be used in variceal bleeding as an alternative to octreotide.

3. B

This patient has LGIB, likely due to intestinal ischemia, a not uncommon occurrence in marathon runners. The bleeding has ceased, and the patient does not require a rapid purge for immediate colonoscopy or a bleeding scan. Hypotension and tachycardia indicate hypovolemia, which requires fluid resuscitation. A colonoscopy can be performed electively during the same hospital admission after adequate fluid resuscitation and blood transfusion.

4. A

This patient presents with classic symptoms of a Mallory–Weiss tear, as indicated by several episodes of retching and nonbloody emesis prior to hematemesis. The diagnosis of a Mallory–Weiss tear can often be made by history alone. Bleeding is self-limited in 90% of patients with a Mallory–Weiss tear. Endoscopic therapy in indicated if there is evidence of ongoing

(Continued)

bleeding. Reassuring the patient and providing anti-emetics to help relieve nausea related to an acute viral illness would be the most appropriate management.

5. A

The patient is young and is presenting with chronic diarrhea that has become bloody. The presentation is suggestive of ulcerative colitis. He has significant weight loss and elevated white blood cell and platelets counts as well as anemia. He has no stigmata of liver disease, and therefore portal hypertensive gastropathy is unlikely. Diverticulosis and colonic arteriovenous malformation are unlikely given the patient's age. Hemorrhoids present with bright red blood per rectum without weight loss, microcytic anemia, or other systemic features.

6. C

Approximately 10% of cases of LGIB are due to an upper GI source; therefore, an EGD should be performed. A bleeding scan and angiography may be considered if the EGD is negative and the patient has ongoing bleeding. Repeat colonoscopy is not indicated at this time. Capsule endoscopy may be considered if the EGD is negative and the patient is hemodynamically stable.

Further Reading

Adler, D.G., Leighton, J.A., Davila, R.E., *et al.* (2004) Standards of Practice Committee ASGE Guideline: the role of endoscopy in acute non-variceal hemorrhage. *Gastrointestinal Endoscopy*, 60, 497–504.

Barkun, A.N., Bardou, M., Kuipers, E.J., *et al.* (2010) International consensus upper gastrointestinal bleeding conference group. International consensus recommendations on the management of patients with nonvariceal upper gastrointestinal bleeding. *Annals of Internal Medicine*, 152, 101–113.

Davila, R.E., Rajan, E., Adler, D.G., et al. (2005) Standards of Practice Committee ASGE Guideline: the role of endoscopy in the patient with lower-GI bleeding: the role of endoscopy in the patient with lower gastrointestinal hemorrhage. *Gastrointestinal Endoscopy*, 62, 656–660.

Garcia-Tsao, G., Sanyal, A.J., Grace, N.D., *et al.* (2007) Practice Guidelines Committee of the American Association for the Study of Liver Diseases; Practice Parameters Committee of the American College of Gastroenterology: Prevention and management of gastroesophageal varices and variceal hemorrhage in cirrhosis. *Hepatology*, 46, 922–938.

Weblinks

http://www.nature.com/nrgastro/journal/v7/n5/full/
  nrgastro.2010.42.html
http://www.merckmanuals.com/professional/sec02/ch010/ch010a.html

Abdominal Pain

Kamil Obideen

CHAPTER 23

Clinical Vignette 1

A 65-year-old man presents with a 2-month history of constant epigastric abdominal pain associated with nausea, early satiety, and a 6-lb (2.7-kg) weight loss. His past medical history is significant for hypertension and degenerative joint disease of both knees. His medications include amlodipine and ibuprofen. He does not drink alcohol or smoke cigarettes. On physical examination, he is afebrile with a blood pressure of 105/85 mmHg, pulse rate 105/min, and respiratory rate 15/min. Abdominal examination reveals epigastric tenderness on deep palpation. Laboratory tests reveal a hemoglobin level of 10 g/dL.

Clinical Vignette 2

A 31-year-old woman is seeking a second opinion for abdominal pain of 10 years' duration. Her symptoms began at age 20. The abdominal pain occurs daily, is usually diffuse, constant, dull, or cramping in nature, and unrelated to eating, having a bowel movement, physical activity, or her menstrual cycle. The pain has increased in intensity and duration over the past 5 years. She denies blood in the stool, diarrhea, constipation, anemia, weight loss, or nocturnal pain but occasionally sees mucus in the stool. She has missed a substantial number of days at work because of abdominal pain and has had several visits to the emergency department. She is usually treated with morphine and phenargan and discharged with a prescription for narcotics. A review of her

(Continued)

Essentials of Gastroenterology, First Edition. Edited by Shanthi V. Sitaraman, Lawrence S. Friedman.
© 2012 John Wiley & Sons, Ltd. Published 2012 by John Wiley & Sons, Ltd.

medical records indicates extensive diagnostic testing that has been negative for major medical disorders. Tests performed include two colonoscopies, three esophagogastroduodenoscopies, multiple computed tomographies of the abdomen and pelvis, and magnetic resonance imaging of the abdomen. All the tests were normal. She underwent cholecystectomy 6 years ago. A laparoscopy done 3 years ago showed some adhesions but was otherwise normal. She is currently under the care of a psychiatrist who diagnosed posttraumatic stress disorder resulting from a childhood history of physical abuse and family deprivation. She takes paroxetine 20 mg daily. She is single and has one daughter from a previous marriage. She lives with her mother. On examination, she appears to be in moderate pain and "wincing" while holding her abdomen. She is afebrile with a blood pressure of 110/60 mmHg and pulse rate 80/min. Abdominal examination is unremarkable when she is distracted.

General

- Abdominal pain is a complex sensation, the manifestations of which depend on an interplay between pathophysiologic and psychosocial factors.
- Abdominal pain is one of the most common causes of visits to a primary care provider, accounting for 2.5 million visits to office-based physicians per year. It is the most frequent reason for a gastroenterology consultation.

Classification

Abdominal pain can be classified based on neurologic origin or clinical presentation.
- Based on **neurologic** origin of the pain, abdominal pain can be divided into three types:
  - **Visceral pain**: stimulation of visceral nerves produces dull, poorly localized pain felt in the midline. Pain is perceived in the abdominal region corresponding to the affected organ's embryonic origin (Table 23.1). Ischemia, inflammation, distention of a hollow organ, or capsular stretching of a solid organ produces visceral pain.
  - **Somatoparietal pain**: pain arises from stimulation of the parietal peritoneum and is generally more intense and more precisely localized than visceral pain.
  - **Referred pain** is felt in areas far from the affected organ (e.g., gallbladder disease may be experienced as pain in the right subscapular area). Referred pain is the result of convergence of visceral afferent neurons and somatic afferent neurons from different anatomic

Table 23.1 Localization of visceral pain based on embryonic origin.

Location of pain	Organ	Embryonic origin	Nerves stimulated
Epigastrium	Stomach First two portions of the duodenum Liver Gallbladder Pancreas	Foregut	Vagus nerve (parasympathetic) Greater thoracic splanchnic nerve (sympathetic)
Periumbilical	Third and fourth portions of the duodenum Jejunum Ileum Cecum Appendix Ascending and proximal two thirds of the transverse colon	Midgut	Vagus nerve (parasympathetic) Greater thoracic splanchnic nerve (sympathetic)
Hypogastrium	Distal one third of the transverse colon, descending colon, sigmoid colon, and rectum Upper portion of the anal canal Ovaries, fallopian tubes, and uterus Seminal vesicles and prostate gland Ureters and urinary bladder	Hindgut	Pelvic splanchnic nerve (parasympathetic) Lesser thoracic splanchnic nerve (sympathetic)

regions on second-order neurons in the spinal cord at the same
spinal segment.
- Based on **clinical** presentation, abdominal pain can be divided into
acute, subacute, or chronic:
  - **Acute**: pain of less than a few days' duration that has worsened
progressively until the time of presentation (see Chapter 25).

○ **Subacute**: pain that lasts a few days to less than 6 months.
○ **Chronic**: pain that has remained unchanged for months to years.

Etiology

- Chronic abdominal pain may be "functional" (no identifiable structural disease) or "organic" (identifiable structural disease) (Table 23.2). Neuromusculoskeletal disorders such as anterior cutaneous nerve entrapment, myofascial pain syndromes, and thoracic nerve radiculopathy may present as abdominal pain.
- The most common cause of chronic abdominal pain is a functional disorder such as irritable bowel syndrome (see Chapter 7) or functional abdominal pain syndrome (FAPS).

Approach to Diagnosis

History and Physical Examination

- Initial work-up of a patient with chronic abdominal pain should focus on differentiating functional from organic causes. The history is critical.

Clinical features that suggest an organic etiology include weight loss, fever, change in appetite, nocturnal awakening with pain, association of pain with bowel movements, dehydration, electrolyte abnormalities, symptoms or signs of gastrointestinal blood loss, anemia, and signs of malnutrition.

- On the basis of the history there often is no need for an extensive diagnostic work-up, if the characteristics of the abdominal pain fit Rome III criteria for irritable bowel syndrome (Chapter 7), functional dyspepsia, or FAPS.
- FAPS is considered a biopsychosocial disorder in which symptoms can be attributed to brain–gut dysfunction or abnormal perception of normal gut function. The cognitive and emotional centers of the central nervous system are the primary modulator of pain in FAPS. Psychosocial factors including major depression, anxiety disorder, somatoform disorder, and life stresses such as physical, sexual, or emotional abuse are common in patients with FAPS. FAPS is usually associated with loss of daily functioning including work or school absenteeism and limitations in social activities.

Table 23.2 Some causes of chronic abdominal pain.

	Structural disorders	Functional gastrointestinal disorders
Chronic intermittent pain	*Inflammatory* Chronic appendicitis Chronic or relapsing pancreatitis Fibrosing mesenteritis Inflammatory bowel disease *Vascular* Mesenteric ischemia *Metabolic* Diabetic neuropathy Familial Mediterranean fever Porphyria Uremia *Musculoskeletal* Anterior cutaneous nerve entrapment syndrome Myofascial pain syndrome *Others* Gallstones Intermittent bowel obstruction (hernia, intussuception, adhesion, volvulus) Peptic ulcer disease	Biliary pain (sphincter of Oddi dysfunction) Functional abdominal pain syndrome Functional dyspepsia Irritable bowel syndrome Levator ani syndrome Pelvic floor dysfunction Severe gastroparesis
Chronic constant pain	Abscess Chronic pancreatitis Inflammatory bowel disease Malignancy Pelvic inflammatory disease	Functional abdominal pain syndrome Functional dyspepsia

Rome III criteria for the diagnosis of FAPS: all the following must be present in the previous 3 months with symptom onset at least 6 months before diagnosis: (1) continuous or nearly continuous abdominal pain; (2) no or only occasional relationship of pain with physiologic events (e.g., eating, defecation, or menses); (3) some loss of daily functioning; (4) the pain is not feigned (i.e., not malingering); (5) insufficient symptoms to meet criteria for another functional gastrointestinal disorder that would explain the pain.

- A thorough physical examination should be performed. The abdominal examination should include inspection, auscultation (for bruits), percussion, and palpation (for organomegaly, masses, and ascites). The patient should be evaluated for signs of malnutrition (e.g., muscle wasting).

Diagnostic Tests

The following laboratory measurements are recommended in most patients with suspected organic chronic abdominal pain. Judicious use of laboratory and imaging tests is recommended in patients suspected of having functional abdominal pain.

- Complete blood count with differential cell count.
- Comprehensive metabolic profile.
- Serum amylase and lipase levels.
- Urinalysis.
- Imaging and endoscopic studies should be guided by symptoms and signs:
  - ultrasonography is recommended for patients presenting with right upper quadrant pain; ultrasonography is sensitive and specific for the detection of gallstones and their complications;
  - computed tomography of the abdomen and pelvis;
  - endoscopy (esophagogastroduodenoscopy, colonoscopy, capsule endoscopy).
- Other specialized tests include magnetic resonance imaging, magnetic resonance cholangiopancreatography, endoscopic ultrasonography, gastric emptying scan, and mesenteric angiography.
- If the diagnosis is not clear after initial assessment and testing, watchful waiting with close monitoring is appropriate.

Pearls

Chronic abdominal pain in patients over 50 years of age or in immunocompromised persons requires work-up for an organic illness.

Laboratory and diagnostic imaging evaluation must be tailored to answer specific questions arising from a carefully derived differential diagnosis based on a detailed history and physical examination. Unnecessary laboratory testing is costly and often clouds the diagnostic picture.

Questions

Questions 1 and 2 relate to the clinical vignettes at the beginning of this chapter.

1. What is the most appropriate next step in the management of the patient presented in Clinical Vignette 1?
   A. *Helicobacter pylori* serology
   B. Trial of a proton pump inhibitor
   C. Abdominal ultrasonography
   D. Upper endoscopy

2. What is the most appropriate next step in the management of the patient presented in Clinical Vignette 2?
   A. Abdominal ultrasonography
   B. Computed tomography of abdomen and pelvis
   C. Colonoscopy
   D. No further testing

3. A 29-year-old woman presents with a 6-month history of right lower quadrant pain associated with diarrhea. She reports a 5-lb (2.3-kg) weight loss during this time. On physical examination, she appears thin and pale; she has mild right lower quadrant tenderness on palpation but has no rebound tenderness or guarding. Laboratory tests are remarkable for a hemoglobin level of 9 g/dL. Stool cultures and tests for ova and parasites and *Clostridium difficile* toxin are negative. Which of the following tests is most likely to establish the diagnosis?
   A. Small bowel follow through
   B. Ultrasonography
   C. Computed tomography (CT)
   D. Colonoscopy

4. A 64-year-old man presents with a 9-month history of diffuse, postprandial abdominal pain, nausea, and constipation. He reports sitophobia (fear of eating) and a weight loss of 25 lb (11.4 kg) over the past 6 months. His past

(Continued)

medical history is significant for hypertension, transient ischemic attacks, and a prior carotid endarterectomy. His medications include hydrochloro-thiazide and aspirin. Physical examination reveals a thin man with tempo-ral wasting. He has bilateral carotid bruits. The remainder of the examination is unremarkable. Laboratory tests show a hemoglobin level of 11.2 g/dL. Computed tomography of the abdomen is unremarkable, except for athero-sclerosis of the aorta. Upper endoscopy and colonoscopy are normal. Which of the following is the next best step in the management of this patient?

A. Abdominal ultrasonography
B. Small bowel follow through
C. Mesenteric angiography
D. Capsule endoscopy
E. Laparotomy

Answers

1. D

The patient is over 50 years of age and has "alarm" symptoms, including anemia, early satiety, and weight loss. Upper endoscopy is the best initial test to evaluate the patient's epigastric pain.

2. D

The patient is young and presents with symptoms typical of chronic func-tional abdominal pain and no alarm symptoms (e.g., weight loss, anemia, fever, nocturnal pain). She already has had extensive diagnostic testing. She meets the Rome III criteria for functional abdominal pain syndrome. Therefore, no further testing is indicated.

3. D

The patient has chronic abdominal pain associated with diarrhea, weight loss, and anemia. Her clinical presentation is suspicious for inflammatory bowel disease, and colonoscopy is the best initial test to confirm the diagnosis.

4. C

This patient presents with classic symptoms of chronic mesenteric ischemia ("abdominal angina"). Mesenteric angiography will confirm the diagnosis. All other tests listed are not indicated.

Further Reading

Millham, F.H. (2010) Acute abdominal pain, in *Sleisenger and Fordtran's Gastrointestinal and Liver Disease: Pathophysiology/Diagnosis/Management*, 9th edn (eds M. Feldman, L.S. Friedman and L.J. Brandt), Saunders Elsevier, Philadelphia, pp. 151–162.

Penner, R. and Majumdar, S. (2010) Diagnostic approach to abdominal pain in adults. http://www.uptodate.com/contents/diagnostic-approach-to-abdominal-pain-in-adults. (Accessed 21 June 2011)

Yarze, J.C. and Friedman, L.S. (2010) Chronic abdominal pain, in *Sleisenger and Fordtran's Gastrointestinal and Liver Disease: Pathophysiology/Diagnosis/ Management*, 9th edn (eds M. Feldman, L.S. Friedman and L.J. Brandt), Saunders Elsevier, Philadelphia, pp. 163–172.

Weblinks

http://www.webmd.com/digestive-disorders/abdominal-pain

http://www.merckmanuals.com/professional/sec02/ch011/ch011b.html

http://www.nature.com/ajg/journal/v105/n4/full/ajg201068a.html

Jaundice

Nader Dbouk and Preeti A. Reshamwala

CHAPTER 24

Clinical Vignette

A healthy neonate delivered 3 days ago is scheduled for discharge. During feeding the mother notices that the baby's eyes are yellow and notifies the nurse. The mother and baby are otherwise well, and the pregnancy had been uneventful. The pediatrician notes no abnormalities on physical examination except for jaundice; he orders several laboratory studies. Results reveal a serum total bilirubin level of 18 mg/dL, direct bilirubin 1.0 mg/dL, and indirect bilirubin 17 mg/dL. A complete blood count is normal, and there is no evidence of hemolysis on the peripheral blood smear. On further questioning, the infant's father recalls that he had an older brother who died at age 3 years. The infant remains in the hospital for phototherapy due to frank jaundice, while the pediatrician obtains a genetic counselor to consult on the case.

Definition

- Jaundice (also known as icterus) is the clinical manifestation of hyper-bilirubinemia and is characterized by yellow discoloration of the skin, mucous membranes, and conjunctivae.

Bilirubin Metabolism

- Bilirubin, a hydrophobic and potentially toxic compound, is the end-product of heme degradation (Figure 24.1). In healthy adults, 70–80% of bilirubin is derived from the breakdown of senescent erythrocytes. Most of the remaining 20–30% is derived from the breakdown of

Essentials of Gastroenterology, First Edition. Edited by Shanthi V. Sitaraman, Lawrence S. Friedman.
© 2012 John Wiley & Sons, Ltd. Published 2012 by John Wiley & Sons, Ltd.

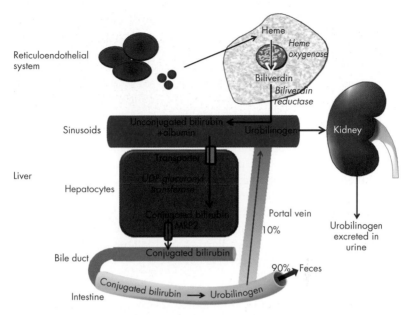

Figure 24.1 Bilirubin metabolism. (MRP2, multi-drug associated protein 2; UDP, uridine diphosphate.)

hemoproteins such as catalase and cytochrome oxidases in the liver, and a minor component arises from the premature destruction of erythrocytes in the bone marrow or circulation.

• Bilirubin is formed in the reticuloendothelial system, predominantly in the spleen. Heme is metabolized to biliverdin by the enzyme heme oxygenase; biliverdin is then converted to unconjugated bilirubin by the enzyme biliverdin reductase.

• Unconjugated bilirubin is a hydrophobic molecule that circulates in the plasma noncovalently bound to albumin.

• Unconjugated bilirubin passes through the sinusoids into the space of Disse, where the bilirubin dissociates from albumin and is taken up by the hepatocytes by a transporter (an organic anion transporter that has not been fully characterized). Unconjugated bilirubin is converted to a water-soluble form through conjugation to glucuronic acid, which is mediated by the enzyme uridine diphosphate (UDP) glucuronyl transferase.

• The majority (up to 98%) of conjugated bilirubin is then secreted into the bile through an apically located active transport process mediated by the multidrug resistance-associated protein 2 (MRP2).

• Bilirubin is detected by the van den Bergh reaction. Bilirubin is cleaved to form a colored compound that can be assayed by spectrophotometry. Conjugated bilirubin is cleaved rapidly and is referred to as direct bilirubin, whereas unconjugated bilirubin is cleaved slowly and is referred to as indirect bilirubin.

- A small amount of conjugated bilirubin is secreted into the hepatic sinusoids, enters the circulation, and is filtered by renal glomeruli and detected in the urine. (A small amount of conjugated bilirubin may be bound to albumin ["delta bilirubin"] and not filtered by the glomeruli.) With hyperbilirubinemia, filtered bilirubin gives the urine a classic tea-colored appearance. In contrast, unconjugated bilirubin is hydrophobic, bound to serum albumin, and not filtered by the glomeruli; therefore, it is not detected in the urine.
- The normal serum bilirubin level is 1–1.5 mg/dL. The conjugated fraction constitutes <15% of the total bilirubin (normal value <0.3 mg/dL).
- Jaundice develops at bilirubin concentrations of ≥3 mg/dL. Other symptoms such as pruritus, diarrhea, and fatigue also may develop when the serum bilirubin level is ≥3 mg/dL.

In general, total serum bilirubin correlates with poor outcomes in patients with alcoholic hepatitis and chronic liver disease. Serum bilirubin is a critical component of the Model for End-Stage Liver Disease (MELD) score, which is used to assess survival of patients with end-stage liver disease (see Chapter 16).

Differential Diagnosis

Clinically, causes of jaundice may be classified as: 1) isolated disorders of bilirubin metabolism; 2) liver disease; and 3) obstruction to bile flow.

Isolated Disorders of Bilirubin Metabolism
Isolated unconjugated hyperbilirubinemia can be due to increased bilirubin production, decreased hepatocellular uptake, or decreased conjugation.

- Increased bilirubin production can be seen in patients with the following conditions:
  - hemolytic anemias, which can be hereditary (e.g., hereditary spherocytosis, sickle cell disease) or acquired (e.g., autoimmune hemolytic anemia);
  - large hematomas: the increase in bilirubin occurs during the resorption phase of the hematoma;
  - repeated blood transfusions;
  - ineffective erythropoeisis (e.g., thalassemia).

- Decreased hepatocellular uptake can be seen in patients taking certain drugs such as rifampin or cyclosporine A.
- Impaired conjugation of bilirubin can be seen in Gilbert's syndrome, Crigler–Najjar syndrome, and physiologic jaundice of the newborn (see later).
  - Gilbert's syndrome:
    - most common inherited cause of hyperbilirubinemia;
    - autosomal recessive disorder, with a prevalence of 10% among Caucasians;
    - a mutation in the TATAA region in the 5′ promoter region of UDP glucuronyl transferase results in reduced levels of UDP glucuronyl transferase;
    - serum bilirubin levels may increase two- to threefold with fasting, dehydration, alcohol ingestion, or acute illness;
    - Gilbert's syndrome has a benign course, and affected persons are asymptomatic. Elevated levels of unconjugated bilirubin generally are detected as an incidental finding on routine laboratory testing and are associated with reduced mortality because bilirubin is an antioxidant.
  - Crigler–Najjar syndrome type I:
    - autosomal recessive disorder;
    - UDP glucuronyl transferase activity is absent, and patients often die in the neonatal period due to kernicterus;
    - phototherapy can prevent kernicterus, and liver transplantation is curative.
  - Crigler–Najjar syndrome type II:
    - autosomal recessive disorder;
    - intermediate UDP glucuronyl transferase activity;
    - patients are usually asymptomatic in the neonatal period but present with jaundice in early childhood;
    - phenobarbital increases UDP glucuronyl transferase activity and reduces bilirubin levels and should be administered to help prevent neurologic complications.

Isolated conjugated hyperbilirubinemia is seen in two other disorders associated with reduced excretion of bilirubin into the bile canaliculi and inherited in an autosomal recessive pattern, Dubin–Johnson syndrome and Rotor's syndrome.

- Patients with Dubin–Johnson syndrome have mutations in the *MRP2* gene and characteristic black pigmentation in their liver that is not present in Rotor's syndrome. The genetic defect in Rotor's syndrome is not yet identified.
- Both of these syndromes have a benign course and do not cause impairment in liver function.

Liver Disease

Jaundice associated with liver disease is characterized by an increase in the serum bilirubin level that usually occurs in association with elevated liver biochemical test (serum aminotransferase, alkaline phosphatase) levels and prolongation of the prothrombin time. Bilirubin is predominantly conjugated in liver disease. Hyperbilirubinemia can occur with acute liver injury, chronic liver disease, or liver disease associated with cholestasis. Jaundice is typically an initial presentation of acute liver disease. In contrast, jaundice develops in late stages of chronic liver disease (e.g., cirrhosis).

- Acute liver disease:
  - Jaundice is typically the initial clinical presentation in patients with acute or subacute liver injury. These conditions are associated with markedly elevated serum aminotranferase levels out of proportion to the bilirubin and alkaline phosphatase levels (see Chapter 12). Examples of acute liver injury include:
    - viral hepatitis (e.g., hepatitis A, B, C, D and E and Epstein–Barr virus infection);
    - drugs and hepatotoxins (e.g., alcohol, acetaminophen);
    - ischemic hepatitis;
    - Reye's syndrome;
    - acute fatty liver of pregnancy;
    - pre-eclampsia.
- Chronic liver disease:
  - In chronic liver disease, jaundice is seen late in the course when cirrhosis is present and is an ominous sign of hepatic decompensation (see Chapters 13, 14, and 15). Examples of chronic liver disease include the following:
    - chronic viral hepatitis (hepatitis B, C, and D);
    - chronic exposure to toxins, particularly alcohol;
    - alpha-1 antitrypsin deficiency;
    - autoimmune hepatitis;
    - nonalcoholic fatty liver disease;
    - hereditary hemochromatosis;
    - Wilson disease.
- Liver disease with prominent cholestasis:
  - Cholestasis signifies impairment of bile flow from the liver. This can be due either to hepatocyte dysfunction and impaired transport of bilirubin to the bile canaliculi (intrahepatic cholestasis) or obstruction of the extrahepatic bile ducts (extrahepatic cholestasis, discussed later). Cholestatic disorders are typically associated with predominant elevation of serum bilirubin and alkaline phosphatase

levels relative to aminotransferase levels (see Chapter 12). Major causes of intrahepatic cholestasis include:

- Infiltrative diseases:
  - granulomatous disorders of the liver: these can be caused by infections (tuberculosis, syphilis, parasites, fungal diseases, leprosy, *Mycobacterium avium* complex infection, and brucellosis), drugs (allopurinol, sulfonamides, and quinidine), and systemic disorders (sarcoidosis, Wegner's granulomatosis, and Hodgkin's lymphoma);
  - systemic amyloidosis, which can present with hepatomegaly and jaundice: other findings may include macroglossia, heart failure, renal failure, and intestinal malabsorption.
- Disorders involving the biliary ductules:
  - primary biliary cirrhosis is characterized by inflammation of the small intrahepatic bile ducts and occurs primarily in middle-aged women (see Chapter 15);
  - graft-versus-host disease occurs in up to 10% of bone marrow transplant recipients;
  - drug-induced cholestasis: may be accompanied by other symptoms including arthralgias, fever, and rash, in addition to peripheral eosinophilia. Numerous medications can cause cholestasis, including estrogen, anabolic steroids, erythromycin, mirtazapine, trimethoprim–sulfamethoxazole, terbinafine, amoxicillin–clavulinic acid, oral contraceptives, clopidogrel, and tricyclic antidepressants, as well as total parenteral nutrition.

Obstruction to Bile Flow

Obstruction of the bile ducts can be due to intrinsic disorders of the bile ducts, extrinsic compression, or occlusion of the bile duct lumen.

- Diseases of the bile ducts:
  - congenital disorders such as choledochal cysts and biliary atresia;
  - inflammatory disorders such as primary sclerosing cholangitis (see Chapters 8 and 15);
  - infectious disorders such as acquired immunodeficiency syndrome (AIDS) cholangiopathy;
  - cholangiocarcinoma.
- Extrinsic compression of the bile ducts (e.g., by neoplasms such as pancreatic carcinoma, hepatocellular carcinoma, ampullary adenoma, and lymphoma or by pancreatitis or an aneurysm)
- Choledocholithiasis (see Chapter 21).
  - The most common of cause of bile duct obstruction is gallstones.

Chronic cholestasis may lead to various complications including hypercholes-terolemia, fat-soluble vitamin deficiencies, osteopenia, pruritus, and steator-rhea. Patients should be screened routinely with bone densitometry, and supplementation with calcium and vitamin D should be recommended. Serum levels of fat-soluble vitamins (A, D, E, and K) should be measured and sup-plemented in case of deficiency.

Clinical Features

- The history should include the onset and duration of jaundice. Important associated symptoms include fatigue, abdominal pain, nausea, vomiting, pruritus, fever or chills, weight loss, and arthralgias or arthritis.
- Conjugated hyperbilirubinemia can cause darkening of the urine, which may precede the onset of jaundice. Tea-colored urine, therefore, may be a more accurate indicator of the onset of hyperbilirubinemia than skin yellowing.
- Potential risk factors for liver disease or other systemic disorders that may be associated with jaundice should be identified. Assessment for risk factors for liver disease should include a history of illicit drug use, alcohol abuse, blood transfusions, and unprotected sex and a family history of liver or pancreatic disease.
- A meticulous medication history, including prescription, over-the-counter, and herbal agents, should be obtained (see Chapter 12).
- The past medical and surgical history should identify disorders associ-ated with jaundice such as hepatobiliary disease, hemolytic anemia (e.g., sickle cell disease), AIDS, inflammatory bowel disease, and pre-vious biliary surgery.
- The physical examination should focus on signs of systemic infection (fever, tachycardia, tachypnea), chronic liver disease (ascites, spider angiomas, palmar erythema, gynecomastia and testicular atrophy in men, hepatosplenomegaly, and cognitive impairment), and heart failure.

The characteristic symptom of hyperbilirubinemia is jaundice (yellowing of the skin, conjunctivae, and mucous membranes). Jaundice develops at bilirubin concentrations of $\geq 3\,mg/dL$. Both conjugated and unconjugated hyperbiliru-binemia result in jaundice.

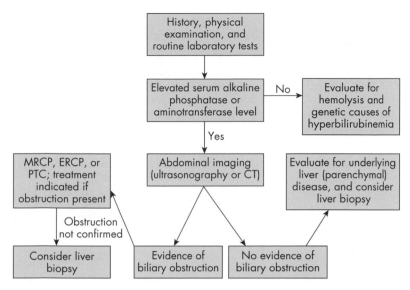

Figure 24.2 Algorithm for the approach to the patient with jaundice (CT, computed tomography; ERCP, endoscopic retrograde cholangiopancreatography; MRCP, magnetic resonance cholangiopancreatography; PTC, percutaneous transhepatic cholangiography.)

Diagnosis

- Simple laboratory tests provide clues to the etiology of jaundice. These tests include a complete blood count and liver biochemical tests including serum total bilirubin, alkaline phosphatase, alanine aminotransferase (ALT), and aspartate aminotransferase (AST) levels and the prothrombin time (Figure 24.2).
- Patients with an elevated serum bilirubin level but otherwise normal liver enzyme levels and liver function should be evaluated for evidence of hemolysis and genetic disorders associated with hyperbilirubinemia. In these disorders, most often, the majority of the elevated bilirubin is unconjugated.
- Patients with abnormal liver enzymes should undergo abdominal imaging (ultrasonography or computed tomography) to look for evidence of liver disease or biliary obstruction.
- Patients suspected of having liver disease should undergo a work-up to identify the specific cause of liver disease (see Chapters 12, 13, and 15). Screening laboratory studies may include viral serologies (including those for hepatitis B and C), serum levels of iron, transferrin, and ferritin (for hemochromatosis), serum ceruloplasmin (for Wilson

disease), antimitochondrial antibodies (for primary biliary cirrhosis), and antinuclear antibodies, smooth muscle antibodies, and serum protein electrophoresis or serum immunoglobulins (for autoimmune hepatitis).

- Patients with biliary obstruction should undergo further evaluation with magnetic resonance cholangiopancreatography (MRCP), endoscopic retrograde cholangiopancreatography (ERCP), or percutaneous transhepatic cholangiography (PTC) to visualize the bile ducts. ERCP and PTC also offer the potential for therapeutic intervention to relieve the obstruction when the index of suspicion for obstruction is high (see Chapter 21).
- A liver biopsy may be necessary in patients with abnormal liver enzymes without evidence of biliary obstruction on imaging.

Treatment

- The management of the patient with jaundice depends on the cause. When jaundice is caused by liver disease, management should be directed towards the underlying cause.
- Elevation of unconjugated bilirubin in neonates and infants has the potential to cause kernicterus with irreversible brain injury and should be treated promptly. Phototherapy reduces the risk of neurotoxicity by rendering bilirubin more water soluble.
- If drug-induced cholestasis is suspected, all potential culprits should be discontinued and the patient observed for resolution of symptoms.
- Patients with biliary tract obstruction due to choledocholithiasis or malignancy often require endoscopic or surgical intervention to restore adequate biliary drainage (see Chapter 21).
- Pruritus can be treated with antihistamines, cholestyramine or other bile acid-binding resins, and rifampin.
- Steatorrhea is common in patients with advanced cholestatic liver disease and can be managed by a reduction in oral fat intake and substitution of dietary fat with medium-chain triglycerides (see Chapter 6).

Special Patient Populations

- Jaundice in the **postoperative patient** is often multifactorial. Predisposing factors include drug-induced liver toxicity from inhalational anesthetics, intraoperative or perioperative hypotension with ischemic liver injury, blood transfusions, total parenteral nutrition, and sepsis.
- Jaundice in the **critically ill patient** is often a manifestation of liver dysfunction occurring in a patient with sepsis and multiorgan

dysfunction syndrome. Other potential etiologies include drug-induced hepatocellular injury or cholestasis, blood transfusions, and hypotension causing ischemic injury (ischemic hepatitis or ischemic cholangiopathy).

- Jaundice in **pregnancy** can be due to intrahepatic cholestasis of pregnancy, which usually presents in the third trimester and resolves within 2 weeks of delivery. Other less common conditions include acute fatty liver of pregnancy, which also occurs in the third trimester and is a life-threatening condition that necessitates urgent delivery. HELLP (hemolysis, elevated liver enzymes, low platelets) syndrome, a complication of pre-eclampsia, is characterized by hemolysis and elevated liver enzymes and is also treated by urgent delivery.
- **Neonatal** jaundice occurs in 60% of term and 80% of pre-term infants. Physiologic jaundice occurs due to increased hemolysis of fetal erythrocytes coupled with reduced hepatic conjugation of bilirubin due to a developmental delay in the expression of UDP glucuronyl transferase, thus leading to unconjugated hyperbilirubinemia. Bilirubin levels usually peak at around 72 hours, and 5–10% of infants develop serum bilirubin levels >10 mg/dL. In such cases phototherapy can be used to reduce the risk of neurologic damage. Pathologic jaundice usually presents within the first 24 hours and can be due to infections, inherited enzyme deficiencies such as glucose-6-phosphate dehydrogenase (G6PD) deficiency, congenital deficiencies of bilirubin conjugating enzymes and bile acid transporters, fetal–maternal ABO incompatibility, breast-milk jaundice, and dehydration.

Pearls

Jaundice is a clinical manifestation of both unconjugated and conjugated hyperbilirubinemia and usually indicates a total bilirubin level of ≥3 mg/dL.

Normally, conjugated bilirubin in the serum constitutes <15% of the total bilirubin. Small increases in serum conjugated bilirubin levels should raise suspicion of liver injury.

A thorough history, physical examination, and simple laboratory tests should provide clues to the etiology of jaundice.

Isolated hyperbilirubinemia is unlikely to be due to liver disease or biliary obstruction and generally indicates increased bilirubin production (e.g., hemolysis), impaired hepatic uptake (e.g., rifampin), or impaired conjugation (e.g., Gilbert's syndrome).

Liver disease and biliary obstruction are associated with predominantly conjugated hyperbilirubinemia.

Imaging studies are helpful in evaluating a jaundiced patient for extrahepatic biliary obstruction and the presence of chronic liver disease.

Questions

Question 1 relates to the clinical vignette at the beginning of this chapter.

1. Which of the following is the most likely diagnosis?
   A. Gilbert's syndrome
   B. Dubin–Johnson syndrome
   C. Crigler–Najjar syndrome type I
   D. Crigler–Najjar syndrome type II
   E. Rotor syndrome

2. Cholestasis may be a consequence of which of the following conditions?
   A. Biliverdin reductase deficiency
   B. Hemolysis
   C. Organic anion transporter deficiency
   D. Bile duct obstruction by gallstones
   E. All of the above

3. A 20-year-old male college student is referred to you for evaluation of hyperbilirubinemia noted on routine laboratory testing. He has no complaints and feels well. His total bilirubin level is 3 mg/dL (unconjugated bilirubin 2.7 mg/dL). Liver biochemical tests are otherwise normal. He does not drink alcohol and is on no medications. There is no family history of liver disease. He states that he recalls being told in the past that he had a slightly elevated bilirubin level, but the elevation resolved spontaneously on follow up. Which of the following should be done next?
   A. Percutaneous liver biopsy
   B. Magnetic resonance image
   C. Endoscopic retrograde cholangiopancreatography
   D. Check a urine drug screen for barbiturates and a serum blood-alcohol level
   E. Reassurance

4. A 15-year-old African American boy presents with jaundice. He has no other symptoms. His past medical history is unremarkable. He does not take any prescription or over-the-counter medications. Physical examination is unremarkable. Laboratory tests including a complete blood count and serum electrolyte, creatinine, aminotransferase, and alkaline phosphate levels are normal except for a hemoglobin of 5.8 g/dL, mean corpuscular volume 78 fL, total bilirubin 16 mg/dL, and direct bilirubin 2 mg/dL. Which of the following is most likely to be found on further laboratory investigation?
   A. IgM antibody to hepatitis A virus
   B. Low serum ceruloplasmin level
   C. Crescent shaped erythrocytes on peripheral blood smear
   D. Elevated serum level of angiotensin-converting enzyme
   E. None of the above

Answers

1. C

    Crigler–Najjar syndrome types I and II are autosomal recessive disorders associated with absent and reduced levels of UDP glucuronyl transferase, respectively. Patients with Crigler–Najjar syndrome present with marked unconjugated hyperbilirubinemia and little, if any, direct, or conjugated, bilirubin. Crigler–Najjar syndrome type I is a lethal disease; patients present in the neonatal period with jaundice, and mortality is due to kernicterus (the accumulation of unconjugated bilirubin in the brain). Liver transplantation is curative because it replaces the UDP glucuronyl transferase that has been deleted by the autosomal recessive mutation that causes the disease. Phototherapy is life-saving and serves as a bridge to liver transplantation. Crigler–Najjar syndrome type II presents in childhood. Because some activity of UDP glucuronyl transferase is present, the disease is not lethal and can be treated with phenobarbital. Gilbert's syndrome is a benign condition that is usually not detected until childhood or adolescence. Dubin–Johnson and Rotor syndromes are associated with direct hyperbilirubinemia and are not lethal.

2. D

    Cholestasis is a condition in which the flow of bile from the liver is impaired. This can occur because of hepatocyte dysfunction and impaired transport of bilirubin to the bile canaliculi (intrahepatic cholestasis) or obstruction of the extrahepatic bile ducts (extrahepatic cholestasis). Cholestatic disorders are typically associated with a serum elevation of direct bilirubin (conjugated fraction) and alkaline phosphatase levels relative to the aminotransferase levels. Choices B and C are associated with isolated hyperbilirubinemia. Biliverdin reductase deficiency results in a decreased production of bilirubin.

3. E

    The patient has Gilbert's syndrome, a benign condition characterized by elevation of unconjugated bilirubin levels, often triggered by physiologic stress or fasting, in an otherwise healthy person.

4. C

    The patient is an African American who has isolated unconjugated hyperbilirubinemia and microcytic anemia; therefore, the most likely cause of his marked hyperbilirubinemia is hemolytic anemia due to sickle cell disease. Hemolytic anemia is a common cause of indirect, or unconjugated, hyperbilirubinemia, and sickle cell disease is a leading cause of hemolysis. Note that patients with sickle cell disease may also present with cholestasis due to pigmented gallstones (see Chapter 21), in which case elevated conjugated bilirubin levels along with elevated alkaline phosphatase levels may be

(Continued)

seen. Acute hepatitis A, diagnosed by an antibody to hepatitis A virus in serum, presents with elevated aminotransferase levels and, in some cases, jaundice (see Chapter 13). A low serum ceruloplasmin level may be indicative of Wilson disease, a disorder in which copper accumulates in the liver and hemolytic anemia and indirect hyperbilirubinemia may occur. This disease is found primarily in Caucasians, and the red blood cells do not display the typical crescent, or sickle, shape seen in sickle cell disease (see Chapter 15). The angiotensin-converting enzyme level is a test used to aid in the diagnosis of granulomatous hepatitis, which typically is associated with jaundice and cholestasis, as may occur in patients with sarcoidosis. Because the alkaline phosphatase level is normal and the patient has hemolytic anemia, this diagnosis is unlikely.

Further Reading

Lidofsky, S.D. (2010) Jaundice, in *Sleisenger and Fordtran's Gastrointestinal and Liver Disease: Pathophysiology/Diagnosis/Management*, 9th edn (eds M. Feldman, L.S. Friedman and L.J. Brandt), Saunders Elsevier, Philadelphia, pp. 323–336.

Zollner, G. and Trauner, M. (2008) Mechanisms of cholestasis. *Clinics in Liver Disease*, 12, 1–26.

Weblink

http://www.merckmanuals.com/professional/sec03/ch022/ch022d.html

Abdominal Emergencies

Mohammad Wehbi

CHAPTER 25

Clinical Vignette 1

A 55-year-old woman presents to the emergency department with severe, constant, periumbilical pain that began 5 hours earlier. Her past medical history is significant for coronary artery disease and laparoscopic appendectomy 10 years ago, complicated by postoperative right lower extremity deep venous thrombosis. On physical examination, the blood pressure is 120/95 mmHg, pulse rate 120/min, and respiratory rate 12/min. She is afebrile but in moderate distress. Abdominal examination shows mild diffuse tenderness to palpation. There is no guarding or rebound tenderness. Bowel sounds are normal. A plain abdominal radiograph, complete blood count, comprehensive metabolic panel, and erythrocyte sedimentation rate are normal.

Clinical Vignette 2

A 60-year-old man presents to the emergency department with the abrupt onset of severe diffuse abdominal pain a few hours earlier. He has a long-standing history of rheumatoid arthritis and has been using a combination of aspirin and other nonsteroidal anti-inflammatory drugs to control his pain. For the past 3 weeks he has had intermittent dyspepsia relieved by food or the ingestion of milk products. He denies rectal bleeding, nausea, or vomiting. His past medical history is otherwise unremarkable, and his family history is noncontributory. He does not drink alcohol, smoke cigarettes, or use illicit drugs. On physical examination, the patient is in moderate distress and lying still on the examining table, refusing to move. The blood pressure is 90/55 mmHg and pulse rate 130/min. There is rigidity, guarding, and rebound tenderness on abdominal examination. Bowel sounds are absent. The patient refuses a rectal examination. Laboratory investigations reveal a white blood count of $16\,500/mm^3$, hemoglobin $15\,g/dL$, and platelet count $460\,000/mm^3$.

Essentials of Gastroenterology, First Edition. Edited by Shanthi V. Sitaraman, Lawrence S. Friedman.
© 2012 John Wiley & Sons, Ltd. Published 2012 by John Wiley & Sons, Ltd.

General

- Acute abdominal pain (an "acute abdomen") refers to the sudden onset of severe abdominal pain that is less than a few days in duration.
- Acute abdominal pain constitutes 5–10% of all visits to an emergency department. Up to 10% of patients are estimated to have a life-threatening cause or require surgery.

Etiology

- Acute abdominal pain represents a spectrum of diseases that may range from benign self-limited conditions to surgical emergencies.
- Common causes of acute abdominal pain are outlined in Table 25.1.

Clinical Features

- A focused history and physical examination are the cornerstones of identifying the cause of acute abdominal pain and guiding diagnostic testing and treatment. Patients who have a surgical abdomen (e.g., peritoneal signs, hemodynamic instability) should be identified promptly, and tests to confirm the etiology and a surgical consultation should be obtained expeditiously.

History

- The history should include details of the location, radiation, onset, duration, severity, and quality of the pain and any exacerbating and alleviating factors.

> Patients at the extremes of age, those who are immunocompromised, pregnant women, and patients in an intensive care unit with an acute abdominal process often have nonspecific symptoms and can deteriorate rapidly.

- Elucidation of the onset of pain may be helpful in identifying the cause and directing emergent intervention:
  - Sudden or abrupt onset (maximal pain reached in seconds): perforated viscus, mesenteric infarction, ruptured aneurysm, ovarian torsion, acute myocardial infarction, pulmonary embolism.
  - Rapid onset (maximal pain reached in minutes to hours): strangulated hernia, volvulus, intussusception, biliary pain, diverticulitis, renal colic.

Table 25.1 Causes of acute abdominal pain and suggested evaluation.

Type of pain	Differential diagnosis	Laboratory tests	Imaging tests	Additional tests
Surgical	Acute mesenteric ischemia or infarction Bowel obstruction Perforated bowel Ruptured aortic aneurysm or aortic dissection Ruptured ectopic pregnancy Strangulated hernia Volvulus	Complete blood count with differential Serum electrolytes, glucose, blood urea nitrogen, and creatinine Serum pregnancy test (women) Coagulation studies (prothrombin time and partial thromboplastin time) Liver biochemical tests Serum amylase and lipase Blood and urine cultures Cardiac enzymes Electrocardiogram Type and screen	Supine and upright plain abdominal radiograph Chest X-ray Abdominal ultrasonography Computed tomography of the abdomen and pelvis	Surgical consultation Mesenteric angiography for suspected acute intestinal ischemia

(Continued)

Table 25.1 (*Continued*)

Type of pain	Differential diagnosis	Laboratory tests	Imaging tests	Additional tests
Nonsurgical	**Intra-abdominal causes** Acute appendicitis Cholecystitis, cholangitis Diverticulitis Enteritis and/or colitis Gynecologic causes (pelvic inflammatory disease, ovarian cyst) Mesenteric lymphadenitis Metabolic conditions such as sickle cell crisis, porphyria, heavy metal poisoning Pancreatitis Pyelonephritis, renal colic **Extra-abdominal causes** Myocardial infarction Metabolic disorders (e.g., diabetic ketoacidosis) Pulmonary embolism Infections (e.g., pneumonia)	Consider any of the above tests based on clinical suspicion	Consider any of the above tests based on clinical suspicion	Magnetic resonance imaging Magnetic resonance cholangiopancreatography Upper endoscopy, colonoscopy HIDA scan Endoscopic retrograde cholangiopancreatography Mesenteric angiography Small bowel follow through Transvaginal ultrasonography

HIDA, hydroxy iminodiacetic acid.

○ Gradual onset (maximal pain reached in hours): acute appendicitis, acute pancreatitis, peptic ulcer disease, mesenteric lympadenitis, cystitis, salpingitis, prostatitis.

• Associated symptoms such as fevers and chills, nausea and vomiting, diarrhea or constipation, hematochezia, melena, jaundice, and a change in the color of urine or stool should be elicited.

Abdominal pain that is of sudden or abrupt onset and associated with peritoneal signs on physical examination is a surgical emergency. Investigation of the cause should be performed expeditiously, and a surgical consultation should be obtained (see Table 25.1).

• A complete medication history, past medical history, and family history should be obtained.

• The review of systems should include changes in diet, bowel habits, and urination. In a female patient, an obstetric and gynecologic history, including the pattern of menstrual cycles, is of utmost importance.

Physical Examination

• The physical examination, particularly the abdominal examination, should be repeated serially in a patient with abdominal pain.

• The patient's general appearance and demeanor may help to narrow the differential diagnosis of abdominal pain; patients with peritonitis tend to lie still, whereas those with colic cannot find a comfortable position.

• Changes in vital signs that indicate a potentially life-threatening condition include fever, tachycardia, and hypotension.

• The physical examination should be guided by the location of the pain. Rectal and pelvic examinations must be performed in patients with left lower quadrant pain or pelvic pain.

• Certain signs are highly predictive of some diseases (Table 25.2).

In a patient with acute abdominal pain, fever, protracted vomiting, syncope or presyncope, and evidence of gastrointestinal blood loss are ominous signs of an emergent or surgical condition.

Diagnostic Tests

• Laboratory tests: an elevated peripheral white blood cell count is suggestive of infection or inflammation. Up to 25% of patients with acute abdominal pain may have a normal white blood cell count;

Table 25.2 Signs on the examination of the abdomen associated with specific conditions.

Sign	Description	Associated condition
Carnett	Pain elicited when a supine patient tenses the abdominal wall by lifting the head and shoulders off the examination table	Abdominal wall conditions (e.g., myositis)
Chandelier	Manipulation of the cervix causes the patient to lift the buttocks off the table	Pelvic inflammatory disease
Cullen	Bluish discoloration around the periumbical region	Retroperitoneal hemorrhage (e.g., pancreatitis, ruptured abdominal aneurysm, intra-abdominal bleeding from anticoagulants)
Grey-Turner	Discoloration of the flanks	Retroperitoneal hemorrhage (causes as for Cullen sign above)
Iliopsoas	Abdominal pain with hyperextension of the right hip	Appendicitis, Crohn's disease
Kehr	Severe left shoulder pain	Splenic rupture
McBurney	Tenderness in the right lower quadrant located two thirds of the distance between the iliac crest and umbilicus	Appendicitis
Murphy	Abrupt inspiratory arrest on palpation of the right upper quadrant	Acute cholecystitis
Obturator	Abdominal pain with internal rotation of right hip	Appendicitis, Crohn's disease
Rovsing	Right lower quadrant pain when left lower quadrant is palpated	Appendicitis

therefore, a normal white blood cell count should not deter further evaluation. Serum amylase and lipase levels should be obtained in patients with acute epigastric pain. A urinalysis should be obtained in all patients with acute abdominal pain. A pregnancy test (urine or blood) should be obtained in all affected women of child-bearing age.

- Imaging: ultrasonography is sensitive for detecting gallstones and is recommended in patients with right upper quandrant pain. Transvaginal ultrasonography should be considered in patients suspected of having an ectopic pregnancy. In all other patients, computed tomography (CT) with intravenous contrast is recommended. In patients in whom contrast dye is contraindicated, ultrasonography or magnetic resonance imaging may be considered.

Treatment

- The patient should undergo aggressive fluid resuscitation and repletion of electrolytes and, if necessary, blood. Broad-spectrum antibiotic therapy should be initiated if indicated.
- Surgical emergencies should be identified promptly, and a surgical consultation should be obtained expeditiously.
- Treatment is guided by the etiology.

Acute Appendicitis

General
- Acute appendicitis is the most common cause of abdominal pain requiring surgical intervention.
- The incidence of appendicitis is 11 per 10000 population, with an estimated 250000 cases annually.
- The overall lifetime risk for men is 8.6% and for women 6.7%.

Pathophysiology
- Obstruction of the appendiceal lumen by a fecolith, foreign body, lymphoid hyperplasia, or worms, bacterial overgrowth, ischemia, and inflammation.

Clinical and Laboratory Features
- Steady, severe epigastric or periumbilical pain with rebound tenderness:
  - pain frequently shifts to the right lower quadrant;
  - aggravation of pain with walking or moving indicates perforation;

  ○ McBurney sign, obturator sign, Rovsing sign, or iliopsoas sign (see Table 25.2) are highly specific for appendicitis; however, these signs are present in <50% of patients.
- Nausea and vomiting, anorexia, and fever are typical.
- Symptoms can be mild or nonspecific in pregnant women and the elderly.
- Leukocytosis.

Diagnosis
- CT with intravenous and oral (± rectal) contrast (see Chapter 27):
  ○ diagnostic accuracy 95–98%;
  ○ findings:
    ▪ dilated appendix with wall thickening and adjacent inflammatory reaction;
    ▪ possibly abscess formation.
- Graded compression ultrasonography is an alternative imaging modality for children, adolescents, and pregnant women (see Chapter 27):
  ○ diagnostic accuracy 78–96%;
  ○ findings:
    ▪ appendiceal diameter >6 mm;
    ▪ muscular wall thickening ≥3 mm;
    ▪ presence of a complex mass.

Treatment
- Urgent initiation of antibiotic therapy.
- Laparoscopic appendectomy:
  ○ prompt intervention is the key to avoiding lethal complications such as perforation;
  ○ if perforation is present, an open surgical approach is the standard of care.

Intestinal Obstruction

General
- Intestinal obstruction accounts for 15% of all cases of abdominal pain presenting to an emergency department and >300 000 hospitalizations per year in the US.

Classification
- Small bowel (SBO) or large bowel obstruction (LBO).
- Partial or complete.

Etiology
- SBO in adults:
  ○ postoperative adhesions cause 70–75% of all cases;
  ○ incarcerated hernia;
  ○ tumors.
- SBO in children:
  ○ intussusception;
  ○ intestinal atresia;
  ○ meconium ileus.
- LBO:
  ○ colon cancer causes a majority of cases of LBO (60%);
  ○ strictures from chronic diverticular disease (20%);
  ○ colonic vovulus (5%);
  ○ Crohn's disease;
  ○ intussusception;
  ○ extrinsic tumor compression;
  ○ fecal impaction.

Clinical and Laboratory Features
- Symptoms common in both SBO and LBO:
  ○ acute onset of cramping abdominal pain with progressive obstipation;
  ○ dehydration resulting in tachycardia, orthostatic hypotension, dry mucous membranes.
- Symptoms common in SBO:
  ○ Nausea and vomiting.
- Physical examination may reveal abdominal distention with tympany. Bowel sounds are initially hyperactive and become progressively hypoactive.
- Laboratory test results in both SBO and LBO are nonspecific. Leukocytosis and electrolyte abnormalities may be present.

Complications
- Bowel ischemia, necrosis, perforation, peritonitis.

Diagnosis

> Delayed diagnosis increases mortality, especially with increasing age and comorbidities.

- Plain abdominal X-ray in the supine and upright position (see Chapter 27).

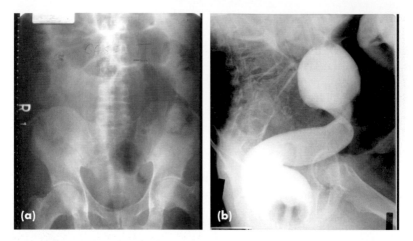

Figure 25.1 Sigmoid volvulus. (a) Abdominal radiograph showing massively dilated sigmoid colon that almost fills the entire abdomen. (b) Film from a single-contrast barium enema showing a "twist" of the sigmoid colon. (Images courtesy of Dr. Pradeep Mittal, Department of Radiology, Emory University, Atlanta, GA, USA.)

- ○ Diagnostic in 50–70% of cases:
  - ▪ SBO: dilated proximal small bowel loops and collapsed, gasless distal small bowel loops, with air-fluid levels at different heights;
  - ▪ LBO: sensitivity 84%, specificity 72%; water soluble enemas increase sensitivity and specificity to 96% and 98%, respectively;
  - ▪ LBO due to sigmoid volvulus: appearance of "bent inner tube" in right upper quadrant (Figure 25.1);
  - ▪ LBO due to cecal volvulus: appearance of "coffee bean" in left upper quadrant (Figure 25.2);
  - ▪ Paralytic LBO: massively dilated cecum >10 cm in diameter
- • CT: gold standard:
  - ○ sensitivity 92%, specificity 93% for diagnosing bowel obstruction.

Treatment
- • Partial SBO:
  - ○ conservative therapy with rehydration, antiemetics, bowel rest, and nasogastric tube for decompression;
  - ○ surgical intervention if lack of improvement with conservative management or if mesenteric ischemia is suspected.
- • Complete SBO and LBO:
  - ○ surgical intervention; the exact type of surgery depends on the location of the obstruction.

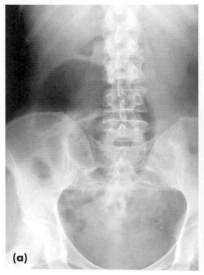
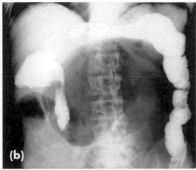

(a)

(b)

Figure 25.2 Cecal volvulus. (a) Abdominal radiograph showing dilated cecum that has assumed the shape of a "kidney" and has rotated toward the midabdomen and left upper quadrant. (b) Film from a single-contrast barium enema showing barium-filled colon that can be traced proximally to the right upper quadrant, where there is an abrupt cutoff. The dilated cecum lies in the mid-abdomen. (Images courtesy of Dr. Pradeep Mittal, Department of Radiology, Emory University, Atlanta, GA, USA.)

Diverticulitis

General
* Diverticulits accounts for 4% of all patients who present with acute abdominal pain to an emergency department.
* Ten to twenty-five percent of patients with diverticulosis develop diverticulitis.
* Eighty percent of persons with diverticulitis are age 50 years or older.
* Risk factors for diverticulosis include low dietary fiber intake, obesity, and lack of physical activity.

Pathophysiology
* Diverticula are most commonly present in the sigmoid colon, where the luminal diameter of the colon is the smallest and intracolonic pressure is highest.
* A fecolith obstructs a diverticulum.
* Microperforation is common.

Clinical and Laboratory Features
- Typical symptoms include left lower quadrant pain, fever, and nausea.
- Physical examination may reveal left lower quadrant tenderness to palpation. The presence of diffuse tenderness and rebound tenderness indicate perforation and a surgical emergency.
- Leukocytosis is frequent.

Complications
- Abscess
- Fistulas
- Colonic stricture
- Peritonitis.

Diagnosis
- CT with intravenous, oral, and rectal contrast.

Treatment
- Antibiotic therapy with coverage for Gram-negative rods and anaerobes (e.g., ciprofloxacin plus metronidazole).
- Urgent surgical intervention if there are peritoneal signs.
- Elective surgery may be considered for repeated attacks; resection is generally performed 6 weeks after the initial presentation. A primary colocolonic anastomosis is usually performed.

Gastrointestinal Tract Perforation

General
- The incidence of gastrointestinal tract perforation in the US is 100 per 100 000 population per year.
- The mortality rate is 30–50%.

Etiology and Pathophysiology
- Penetrating foreign body: endoscopy, ingestion of foreign bodies, gunshot.
- Extrinsic compression of lumen: tumor, hernia, adhesions, volvulus.
- Intrinsic compression of lumen: tumor, stricturing Crohn's disease.
- Damage to gastrointestinal wall: peptic ulcer.
- Gastrointestinal ischemia: thromboembolism.
- Infection: cytomegalovirus, *Salmonella typhi* infection.

Clinical and Laboratory Features
- Sudden or abrupt onset of abdominal pain. Peritoneal signs (guarding and rebound tenderness) are typically present on physical examination. Bowel sounds may be absent.

- Marked leukocytosis (typically the white blood cell count is >20 000/ mm^3), thrombocytosis, elevated serum lactate level, serum electrolyte abnormalities.

Diagnosis
- Imaging: chest and upright and supine abdomen X-rays or helical CT (sensitivity 95%, specificity 97%).

Treatment
- Broad-spectrum antibiotics, adjusted depending on location of perforation and operative findings to cover Gram-positive and negative bacteria and anaerobes.
- Surgery.

Acute Mesenteric Ischemia

Classification and Etiology
- Superior mesenteric artery embolus (SMAE): usually an embolus results from a cardiac arrhythmia.
- Superior mesenteric artery thrombus (SMAT): occlusion due to underlying artherosclerosis, hypercoagulable state, vasculitis, or aneurysm.
- Non-occlusive mesenteric ischemia (NOMI): during a low-flow state, as in severe heart failure or shock.
- Mesenteric venous thrombus (MVT): usually affects superior mesenteric vein; caused by a hypercoagulable state, abdominal infection, inflammation, or portal hypertension.

Clinical Features
- Persistent, poorly localized pain out of proportion to findings on abdominal examination.
- Hypovolemic shock may be present in 25% of patients.

Diagnosis and Treatment
- Plain abdominal radiograph: thumbprinting, pneumatosis intestinalis, portal venous gas bubbles.
- SMAE, SMAT: angiography with intra-arterial papaverine or laparotomy with resection and embolectomy.
- NOMI: angiography with intra-arterial papaverine.
- MVT: CT, anticoagulation.

Ruptured Abdominal Aortic Aneurysm

General

- An abdominal aortic aneurysm (AAA) is a localized dilatation of the abdominal aorta exceeding the normal diameter by more than 50%; it is the most common form of aortic aneurysm.
- Approximately 90% of AAAs occur infrarenally.

Pathophysiology

- The basic pathophysiologic mechanism underlying AAA development and rupture is thought to be degradation of the tunica media by proteolytic enzymes, particularly matrix metalloproteinases.

Clinical Features

- Sudden or abrupt onset of acute abdominal (mid-abdominal, paravertebral, or flank) pain.
- Classic triad: shock, pulsatile abdominal mass, and abdominal pain.

Diagnosis and Treatment

- Emergent surgical referral:
  - Imaging intervention results in a delay in surgery and may prove fatal.

Pearls

Evaluation of acute abdominal pain at the extremes of age (infants and the elderly) is a challenge due to difficulty in obtaining the history and potentially misleading laboratory data. Therefore, a carefully obtained history, thorough physical examination, and high index of suspicion are needed to make a diagnosis and institute appropriate treatment.

During evaluation of acute abdominal pain, conditions of the abdominal wall, such as muscle strain or herpes zoster infection, should be considered.

Serum amylase and lipase levels should be obtained in patients with acute abdominal pain. These tests are not included in a comprehensive metabolic panel in most laboratories.

Surgical consultation should be obtained early, especially in persons who have peritoneal signs and those who are hemodynamically unstable (tachycardia and hypotension).

Questions

Questions 1 and 2 relate to clinical vignette 1 at the beginning of this chapter.

1. Which of the following is the most appropriate diagnostic test?
   A. Doppler ultrasonography of the portal, splenic, and superior mesenteric veins
   B. Doppler ultrasonography of the celiac, superior mesenteric, and inferior mesenteric arteries
   C. Computed tomography (CT)
   D. Mesenteric arteriography
   E. Exploratory laparotomy

2. Which of the following is the most likely diagnosis?
   A. Mesenteric ischemia
   B. Small bowel obstruction
   C. Appendicitis
   D. Cholecystitis
   E. Perforated peptic ulcer

Questions 3 and 4 relate to clinical vignette 2 at the beginning of this chapter.

3. Which of the following is the most likely diagnosis?
   A. Bowel obstruction
   B. Perforated peptic ulcer
   C. Cholelithiasis
   D. Hepatic abscess
   E. Renal colic

4. Which of the following should be done next?
   A. Magnetic resonance imaging (MRI)
   B. Abdominal ultrasonography
   C. Plain film of the abdomen
   D. Mesenteric arteriography

5. Which of the following is the most common cause of large bowel obstruction?
   A. Colon stricture
   B. Crohn's disease
   C. Colon cancer
   D. Volvulus

6. A 47-year-old man presents to the emergency department with a two-day history of progressive left lower quadrant abdominal pain. The pain is constant and associated with low-grade fever, nausea, and constipation. Physical examination is remarkable for a temperature of 101.5 °F (38.6 °C), blood

(Continued)

pressure 110/70 mmHg, and pulse rate 112/min. Abdominal examination reveals guarding in the left lower quandrant and tenderness to palpation. There is no rebound tenderness. Bowel sounds are present. Laboratory test results are remarkable for a white blood cell count of 15 000/mm^3. Which of the following is the best next step in the management of this patient?

A. Colonoscopy

B. Ultrasonography

C. Plain film of the abdomen

D. Barium enema

E. Intravenous antibiotics

Answers

1. C
2. A

The patient's severe persistent periumbilical pain in the face of minimal findings on physical examination and normal laboratory test results and a history of coronary artery disease are concerning for mesenteric ischemia. All other diagnoses listed are possible, but mesenteric ischemia must be ruled out because it is a life-threatening emergency. CT is an appropriate test to perform, and if the index of suspicion for mesenteric ischemia is high, mesenteric arteriography can be diagnostic and therapeutic.

3. B

Physical examination in this patient (peritoneal signs, absent bowel sounds) is most concerning for a perforated viscus. Given the use of nonsteroidal anti-inflammatory drugs, a perforated peptic ulcer is a likely possibility. Bowel obstruction causes colicky pain and bowel sounds are generally present, although they may be high pitched or absent in advanced obstruction. Abdominal pain associated with cholelithiasis or hepatic abscess and renal colic do not cause peritonitis.

4. C

A plain film of the abdomen along with an upright chest X-ray or a CT has the highest sensitivity and specificity to detect free air in the abdomen. All other tests are not indicated in this patient.

5. C
6. E

This patient's clinical presentation is suspicious for diverticulitis. Because he is febrile and has an elevated white blood cell count, it is reasonable to administer antibiotics immediately. Computed tomography (not ultrasonography) is the diagnostic test of choice. Colonoscopy is contraindicated when diverticulitis is suspected because of the risk of perforation. A plain film of the abdomen will have a poor diagnostic yield. CT is superior to barium enema for the diagnosis of diverticulitis and its complications.

Further Reading

Cappell, M.S. (2008) Common gastrointestinal emergencies. *Medical Clinics of North America*, 92, xi–xiv.

Diaz, J.J., Bokhari, F., Mowery, N.T., *et al.* (2008) Guidelines for management of small bowel obstruction. *Journal of Trauma*, 64, 1651–1664.

Jacobs, D.O. (2007) Diverticulitis. *New England Journal of Medicine*, 357: 2057–2066.

Shanley, C.J. and Weinberger, J.B. (2008) Acute abdominal vascular emergencies. *Medical Clinics of North America*, 92, 627–647.

Silen, W. (2010) The principles of diagnosis in acute abdominal disease, in *Cope's Early Diagnosis of the Acute Abdomen*, 22nd edn. (ed W. Silen), Oxford University Press, New York, pp. 3–17.

Weblink

http://www.upmc.com/healthatoz/pages/
healthlibrary.aspx?chunkiid=179512

Picture Gallery

Shanthi Srinivasan and Shanthi V. Sitaraman

Classic Pathology

Neal R. Patel, Meena Prasad, Douglas C. Parker,
Charles W. Sewell, and Henry C. Olejeme

CHAPTER 26

Esophageal Squamous Cell Carcinoma

Esophageal squamous cell carcinoma most commonly occurs in adults over age 45. It affects men four times as frequently as women and is nearly sixfold more common in African Americans than Caucasians. Risk factors include alcohol and tobacco use, poverty, caustic esophageal injury, achalasia, and tylosis (genetic hyperkeratosis of the palms and soles). Persons with esophageal squamous cell cancer typically present with progressive dysphagia for solid food and weight loss.

Morphology

- Fifty percent of squamous cell carcinomas occur in the middle third of the esophagus.
- Early lesions appear as small, gray–white, plaque-like thickenings. Over time they grow into tumor masses that may be polypoid or exophytic and protrude into and obstruct the lumen.
- Some tumors ulcerate or diffusely infiltrate and spread within the esophageal wall and cause thickening, rigidity, and luminal narrowing (Figure 26.1a).

Microscopic Features

- Squamous cell carcinoma is characterized by irregular nests of infiltrating, atypical squamous cells displaying abundant eosinophilic cytoplasm.
- A characteristic lesion in squamous cell carcinoma is condensation of keratin in the shape of a whorl, known as a keratin "pearl" (Figure 26.1b).

Essentials of Gastroenterology, First Edition. Edited by Shanthi V. Sitaraman, Lawrence S. Friedman.
© 2012 John Wiley & Sons, Ltd. Published 2012 by John Wiley & Sons, Ltd.

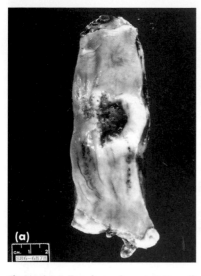
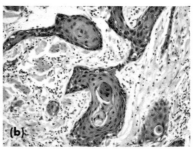

Figure 26.1 Esophageal squamous cell carcinoma. (a) Gross image showing an ulcerated tumor and luminal narrowing in the mid-esophagus.
(b) Photomicrograph showing infiltrating nests of atypical epithelial cells with an intraepithelial keratin "pearl." Hematoxylin and eosin, 400×.

Barrett's Esophagus and Esophageal Adenocarcinoma

Barrett's esophagus is a complication of chronic gastroesophageal reflux disease (GERD) (see Chapter 1). It is characterized by intestinal metaplasia of the esophageal squamous mucosa. Barrett's esophagus is estimated to occur in approximately 10% of persons with GERD and is most common in white men over 50 years of age. Barrett's esophagus is considered a premalignant lesion. Esophageal adenocarcinoma arises from Barrett's epithelium and is preceded by dysplasia.

Morphology
- The diagnosis of Barrett's esophagus requires both endoscopic evidence of abnormal mucosa above the gastroesophageal junction and intestinal metaplasia documented by histologic examination.
- Barrett's esophagus can be recognized endoscopically as one or several tongues or patches of salmon-colored mucosa extending proximally from the gastroesophageal junction (Figure 26.2a).
- Esophageal adenocarcinoma usually occurs in the distal third of the esophagus and may invade the adjacent gastric cardia. It is almost always seen in association with Barrett's esophagus. Esophageal

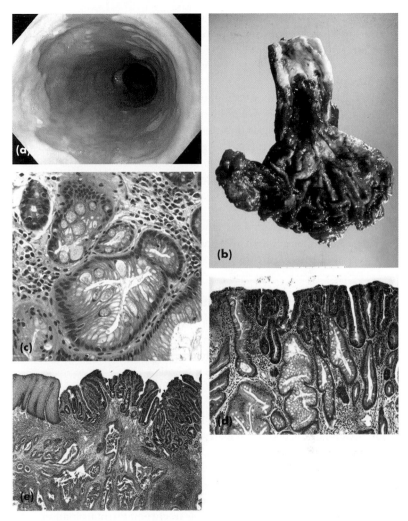

Figure 26.2 Barrett's esophagus and esophageal adenocarcinoma.
(a) Endoscopic image of Barrett's esophagus showing salmon-colored mucosa
extending superiorly from the gastroesophageal junction. (b) Gross image of an
esophageal adenocarcinoma showing an ulcerated lesion in the distal
esophagus. (c) Photomicrograph of Barrett's esophagus showing intestinal-type
columnar epithelium with goblet cells. Hematoxylin and eosin, 200×.
(d) Photomicrograph of Barrett's esophagus showing epithelial dysplasia
characterized by cells displaying hyperchromatic nuclei with pleomorphism and
increased nuclear-to-cytoplasmic ratio. Hematoxylin and eosin, 200×.
(e) Photomicrograph of esophageal adenocarcinoma arising from Barrett's
epithelium showing atypical glandular epithelium invading into the lamina
propria. Hematoxylin and eosin, 100×.

adenocarcinoma may appear as flat or raised patches initially, but over time large masses may develop. Tumors may infiltrate diffusely, ulcerate, and invade deeply (Figure 26.2b).

Microscopic Features
- Intestinal-type columnar epithelium with goblet cells displaying distinct mucin vacuoles is generally considered necessary for the diagnosis of Barrett's esophagus (Figure 26.2c).
- When dysplasia is present, the gland architecture is abnormal and shows budding, irregular shape, and cellular crowding. Dysplastic epithelium exhibits irregular stratification, nuclear pleomorphism with hyperchromasia, and an increased nuclear-to-cytoplasmic ratio (Figure 26.2d).
- Invasive esophageal adenocarcinomas show atypical intestinal-type glandular epithelium with invasion into the underlying lamina propria or deeper layers (Figure 26.2e).

Herpes Virus and Cytomegalovirus Esophagitis

Herpes virus and cytomegalovirus (CMV) infections typically occur in immunocompromised persons but may occur in healthy persons. Patients with viral esophagitis present with dysphagia and odynophagia and may have superimposed candida esophagitis.

Morphology
- Endoscopy may provide a clue to the type of viral esophagitis. Herpes virus causes punched-out (clearly demarcated) ulcers, whereas CMV causes shallow ulcers.

Microscopic Features
- Microscopic features of herpes esophagitis are seen in epithelial cells and include nuclear molding, nuclear chromatin margination, and multinucleated cells (Figure 26.3a). These changes are usually seen at the periphery of an ulcer.
- CMV esophagitis is characterized by eosinophilic nuclear and cytoplasmic viral inclusions within epithelial, endothelial, and stromal cells (Figure 26.3b).

Gastric Adenocarcinoma

The incidence of gastric adenocarcinoma varies widely with geographic region. The highest incidence is seen in Japan, Chile, Costa Rica, and Eastern Europe. The incidence of gastric adenocarcinoma in the US

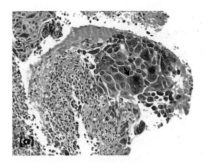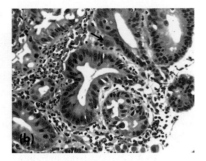

Figure 26.3 Viral esophagitis. (a) Photomicrograph of herpes esophagitis showing squamous epithelial cells at the periphery of an ulcer with characteristic multinucleated giant cell (arrow). Hematoxylin and eosin, 400×. (b) Photomicrograph of cytomegalovirus esophagitis showing intranuclear and intracytoplasmic viral inclusions in the epithelial, stromal (arrow), and endothelial cells. Hematoxylin and eosin, 400×.

dropped by 85% during the twentieth century. Common symptoms of gastric adenocarcinoma include weight loss, early satiety, nausea, and vomiting. The most common risk factor for gastric adenocarcinoma is *Helicobacter pylori* infection.

Morphology
- There are two major types of gastric adenocarcinoma: intestinal type and diffuse (infiltrative) type:
  - Intestinal-type gastric cancer tends to form a bulky tumor, exophytic mass, or ulcerated tumor.
  - Diffuse-type tumors grow along the gastric wall. They frequently evoke a desmoplastic reaction that stiffens the gastric wall; such a rigid, thickened wall may impart a leather-bottle appearance to the stomach, termed "linitis plastica" (Figure 26.4a).

Microscopic Features
- The neoplastic cells of intestinal-type gastric cancer typically grow in a cohesive fashion to form irregular glands of atypical epithelium that contain apical mucin vacuoles. Abundant mucin may be present in the lumens of the glands.
- The neoplastic cells of diffuse-type gastric cancer are composed of diffusely infiltrating dyshesive cells that generally do not form glands and contain large mucin vacuoles that expand the cytoplasm and displace the nucleus to the periphery, creating a "signet-ring cell" morphology (Figure 26.4b).

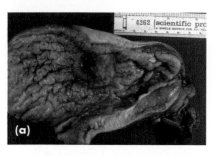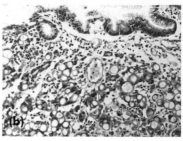

Figure 26.4 Gastric adenocarcinoma. (a) Gross image of a diffuse-type gastric adenocarcinoma. Note that the gastric wall is markedly thickened, imparting a leather-bottle appearance to the stomach (linitis plastica), and rugal folds are partially lost. (b) Photomicrograph of diffuse-type gastric adenocarcinoma. Signet-ring cells can be recognized by their large intracytoplasmic mucin vacuoles and peripherally displaced, crescent-shaped nuclei. Hematoxylin and eosin, 200×.

Helicobacter pylori Gastritis

H. pylori is a Gram-negative microaerophilic bacterium that colonizes the surface of epithelial cells of the antrum (see Chapter 3). In the US the estimated prevalence of *H. pylori* is 20% in persons younger than 30 years and 50% in those older than 60 years. *H. pylori* is the most common cause of chronic gastritis. Seventy percent of gastric ulcers and 80–95% of duodenal ulcers are attributed to *H. pylori* infection. In a subset of patients, the gastritis progresses to involve the gastric body and fundus, thereby resulting in pangastritis, which is associated with multifocal mucosal atrophy, reduced acid secretion, intestinal metaplasia, and an increased risk of gastric adenocarcinoma.

Morphology
- When viewed endoscopically, *H. pylori* gastritis appears erythematous (Figure 26.5a); sometimes the antrum has a nodular appearance.

Microscopic Features
- *H. pylori* shows tropism for gastric epithelia, and the bacteria are concentrated within the superficial mucus overlying gastric epithelial cells in the surface and neck regions.
- Organisms are often demonstrated in routine hematoxylin and eosin-stained section and can be highlighted with a variety of special stains such as the Steiner stain (Figure 26.5b).

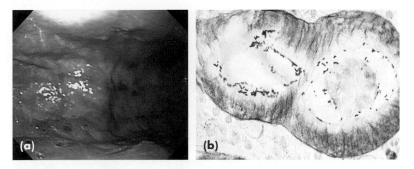

Figure 26.5 *Helicobacter pylori* gastritis. (a) Endoscopic image showing erythema, subepithelial hemorrhages, and erosions of the gastric antrum. (b) Photomicrograph showing abundant spiral-shaped *H. pylori* on the surface of mucous neck cells. Steiner's stain, 600×.

- The characteristic inflammatory infiltrate in *H. pylori* gastritis includes intraepithelial neutrophils, which form pit abscesses, and plasma cells in the lamina propria.

Crohn's Disease

Crohn's disease is a chronic relapsing and remitting inflammatory bowel disease that is characterized by transmural inflammation that can occur anywhere in the gastrointestinal tract from the mouth to anus (see Chapter 8).

Morphology

- Transmural inflammation with associated thickening of the bowel wall and constriction of the lumen are characteristic pathologic findings in Crohn's disease (Figure 26.6a).
- Areas of active disease are sharply demarcated from normal tissue. Multiple distinct areas of affected mucosa with intervening normal mucosa are known as "skip lesions" (Figure 26.6b).
- Linear mucosal ulceration occurs on the luminal surface, and there is frequently a characteristic "cobblestone" appearance to the mucosal surface.
- Mesenteric fat extends around the serosal surface, a phenomenon known as "creeping fat."
- Fissures may also develop between mucosal folds and form into fistulous tracts (Figure 26.6c) or areas of perforation with abscess formation.

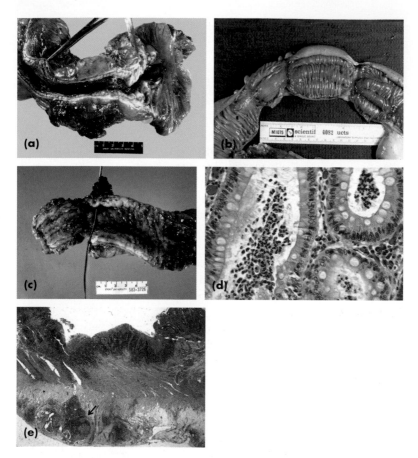

Figure 26.6 Crohn's disease. (a) Gross image of the terminal ileum showing transmural thickening. (b) Gross image of diseased (scarred) segment of the bowel (demarcated by brackets) with normal appearing bowel on either side ("skip lesion"). (c) Gross image of a fistula in the bowel wall.
(d) Photomicrograph of a crypt abscess. Hematoxylin and eosin, 400×.
(e) Photomicrograph showing transmural inflammation, crypt distortion, and a noncaseating granuloma in the serosa (arrow). Hematoxylin and eosin, 40×.

Microscopic Features

- Typically, there is significant destruction and distortion of normal villous and crypt architecture secondary to inflammation.
- Crypt abscesses are frequently present and are characterized by neutrophilic aggregates within the crypts (Figure 26.6d). Crypt abscesses are also seen in other colitides including infectious colitis and ulcerative colitis.

- In the subserosa, lymphoid aggregates and noncaseating granulomas are typical findings in Crohn's disease (Figure 26.6e).

Celiac Disease

Celiac disease is an autoimmune enteropathy that develops in a genetically predisposed person (see Chapter 6). Over 95% of persons who develop celiac disease carry human leukocyte antigen (HLA) alleles DQ2 or DQ8. The prevalence of celiac disease is 0.5–1% in the US, and the disorder occurs predominantly in Caucasians. Classic symptoms of celiac disease include fatigue, bloating, and chronic diarrhea; however, a majority of patients, especially adults, are asymptomatic. Celiac disease is associated with other autoimmune diseases including autoimmune hypothyroidism, type 1 diabetes mellitus, primary biliary cirrhosis, and microscopic colitis. The diagnosis is made by detecting tissue transglutaminase antibodies in serum and characteristic findings on distal duodenal biopsy specimens.

Morphology
- Endoscopy may show "scalloping" of the small intestinal mucosal folds (Figure 26.7a), a paucity of mucosal folds, a nodular pattern to the mucosa, or a mosaic pattern, termed "cracked-mud" appearance.

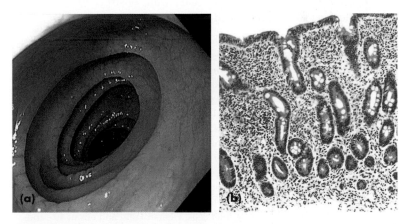

Figure 26.7 Celiac disease. (a) Endoscopic image showing scalloping of the jejunal mucosa. (b) Photomicrograph showing marked villous atrophy. Intraepithelial lymphocytes with dense nuclei are present in the surface epithelium. Hematoxylin and eosin, 100×.

Microscopic Features

- Microscopic features of celiac disease are categorized according to the Marsh classification:
  - Marsh stage 0: normal mucosa;
  - Marsh stage 1: increased number of intraepithelial lymphocytes, usually exceeding 20 per 100 enterocytes;
  - Marsh stage 2: proliferation of the crypts of Lieberkühn;
  - Marsh stage 3: partial or complete villous atrophy (Figure 26.7b);
  - Marsh stage 4: hypoplasia of the small bowel architecture.
- The histologic changes are reversible on a gluten-free diet.

Tubular Adenoma and Adenocarcinoma of the Colon

Adenomatous polyps, also known as adenomas, are intraepithelial neoplasms that have the propensity to progress to adenocarcinoma (see Chapter 10). Adenomas that are >1 cm, have villous architecture, or have high-grade dysplasia are more likely to progress to adenocarcinoma.

Morphology

- Endoscopically adenomas appear as polypoid lesions that protrude into the lumen (Figure 26.8a). Adenomas may be sessile (flat) or pedunculated (with a stalk) (Figure 26.8b).
- Endoscopically adenocarcinoma may appear as a mass lesion that can be circumferential, infiltrate the colon wall, obstruct the lumen, or have ulcerations (Figure 26.8c,d).

---▶

Figure 26.8 Colonic adenoma and adenocarcinoma. (a) Endoscopic view of a tubular adenoma. (b) Gross image of the colon showing two pedunculated adenomas. (c) Endoscopic image of two colonic adenocarcinomas that are semi-circumferential (ci) and ulcerated and obstructing the lumen (cii). (d) Gross image of a colonic adenocarcinoma. Note the elevated, nodular margin surrounding the central area of ulceration. The tumor encircles and infiltrates into the bowel wall. Normal mucosa is seen on either side of the tumor. (e), (f) Photomicrographs of a pedunculated tubular adenoma showing well differentiated glands in a crowded arrangement overlying normal colonic mucosa. The glands of the polyp display increased density with hyperchromatic nuclei and a reduced number of goblet cells. Hematoxylin and eosin, 40× and 100×. (g) Photomicrograph of a moderately differentiated adenocarcinoma displaying glandular morphology with atypical epithelium characterized by pleomorphic, hyperchromatic nuclei, and abnormal mitosis. Hematoxylin and eosin, 400×.

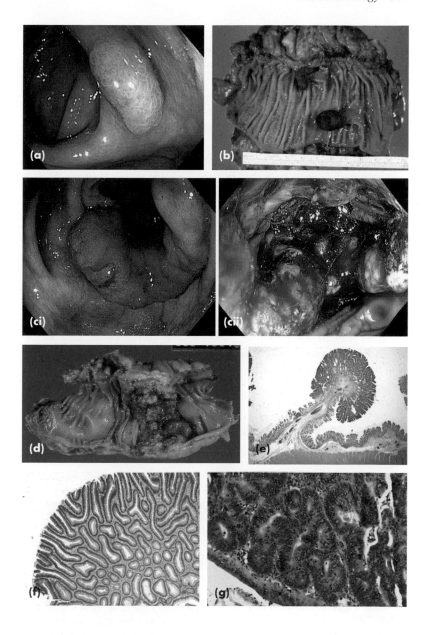

Microscopic Features

- Adenomas may be tubular, villous, tubulovillous, or serrated. Tubular adenomas have more than 75% tubular architecture, and villous adenomas have more than 50% villous architecture. Tubulovillous adenomas are adenomas with 25–50% villous architecture. Serrated adenomas have mixed hyperlastic epithelium and tubular architecture. The majority of adenomas are of tubular morphology.
- Adenomatous epithelium is characterized by hypercellularity of colonic crypts with cells that possess variable amounts of mucin and pleomorphic, hyperchromatic nuclei (Figure 26.8e,f).
- Most adenocarcinomas are at least moderately differentiated and show atypical, mucin-producing columnar cells. These cells display palisaded, large, oval nuclei that exhibit hyperchromasia, pleomorphism, and excessive mitosis (Figure 26.8g).

Carcinoid Tumor

The majority of carcinoid tumors are found in the gastrointestinal tract; about 40% occur in the small intestine, 25% in the colon, 25% in the appendix, and less than 10% in the stomach. These tumors are typically well differentiated and have a slow, indolent course.

Morphology

- Carcinoid tumors are nodular or polypoid in appearance (Figure 26.9a) and yellow or tan in color. Endoscopically they appear as submucosal polyps.

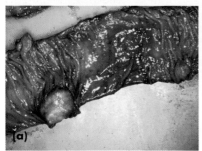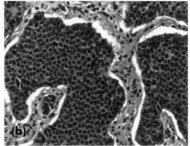

Figure 26.9 Carcinoid tumor. (a) Gross image of the ileum showing a submucosal, tan-colored polypoid tumor. (b) Photomicrograph showing an irregular nest of relatively uniform, small neuroendocrine cells with round nuclei and eosinophilic cytoplasm. Hematoxylin and eosin, 40×.

Microscopic Features
- Carcinoid tumors are characterized by relatively uniform trabecula or gland-like nests of cells with eosinophilic cytoplasm and a central round-to-oval, stippled nucleus (Figure 26.9b).
- The microscopic appearance of the nucleus is often described as a "salt-and-pepper" pattern due to the fine and coarse clumps of chromatin present.

Pseudomembranous Colitis

The most common cause of pseudomembranous colitis is *Clostridium difficile* infection (see Chapter 5). Risk factors for developing *C. difficile* colitis include recent antibiotic use, recent hospitalization, inflammatory bowel disease, chemotherapy, and older age. Clinical symptoms include watery diarrhea, leukocytosis, fever, abdominal pain, and dehydration. The diagnosis is made by detecting *C. difficile* toxin in the stool. Flexible sigmoidoscopy or colonoscopy is usually not required to make the diagnosis but, when performed, may reveal characteristic "pseudomembranes" that appear as yellow, gray, or white plaques 2–5 mm in diameter.

Morphology
- Tan-colored pseudomembranes are present at sites of mucosal injury. An adherent layer of inflammatory cells and debris forms the superficial pseudomembrane layer.

Microscopic Features
- The characteristic histopathologic finding resembles a "volcano-like eruption" in the mucosal epithelium (Figure 26.10). This "eruption" is characterized by damaged crypts that are distended by neutrophils and mucopurulent exudates that cover the mucosal surfaces as the pseudomembranous layer.

Acute Liver Failure Caused by Acetaminophen Toxicity

Approximately half of all cases of acute liver failure in the US are secondary to acetaminophen toxicity. Acetaminophen is metabolized by hepatocytes largely by conjugation with sulfate and glucuronide derivatives and excreted renally. The remainder is converted to a toxic intermediate by the cytochrome P-450 system. The toxic intermediate subsequently undergoes reduction by glutathione into a nontoxic metabolite. When toxic levels of acetaminophen are ingested, its metabolism by the

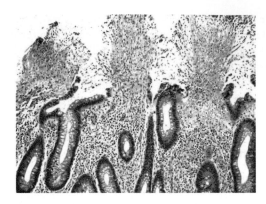

Figure 26.10 Pseudomembranous colitis. Photomicrograph showing the classic "volcano-like eruption" of mucopurulent exudates extending from the damaged crypts. A predominantly neutrophilic inflammatory infiltrate is seen in the lamina propria. Hematoxylin and eosin, 200×.

cytochrome P-450 pathway is increased. In the settings of alcohol use, malnourishment, fasting, viral illness with dehydration, or ingestion of other substances or medications that are known to induce the activity of the cytochrome P-450 oxidative enzymes, glutathione levels are depleted, resulting in hepatocyte injury and death and liver failure. N-acetylcysteine is an antidote for acetaminophen toxicity.

Microscopic Features

- The classic histologic feature of acetaminophen toxicity is hepatocyte necrosis in a centrilobular pattern (zone 3 of the hepatic acinus) (Figure 26.11). Severe toxicity causes massive necrosis. The zone 3 necrosis can also be seen in ischemic hepatitis and as a result of several other toxins.
- Inflammatory infiltration is usually minimal. This is in contrast to other etiologies (e.g., viral hepatitis) in which marked inflammation and massive necrosis are common.

Hereditary Hemochromatosis

Hereditary hemochromatosis (HH) comprises several inherited disorders of iron homeostasis characterized by increased intestinal absorption of iron that results in deposition of iron in the liver, pancreas, heart, and other organs (see Chapter 15). HH is caused most commonly by a gene mutation in the *HFE* gene that results in unregulated iron absorption.

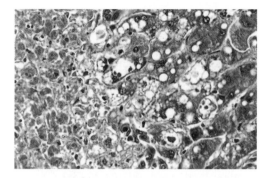

Figure 26.11 Acute liver failure caused by acetaminophen toxicity. Photomicrograph of a liver biopsy specimen showing necrotic hepatocytes on the left and early stages of cell injury and death, including ballooning, steatosis, and apoptosis, on the right. Note the relative absence of an inflammatory infiltrate. Hematoxylin and eosin, 400×.

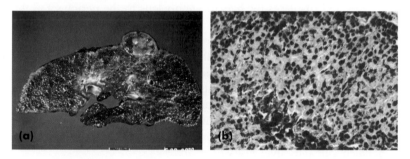

Figure 26.12 Hereditary hemochromatosis. (a) Gross image of the liver, which appears dark brown due to extensive iron deposition. Hepatocellular carcinoma is seen protruding above the capsule. (b) Photomicrograph showing extensive hemosiderin deposition highlighted with Perls' Prussian blue stain. Hematoxylin and eosin, 200×.

Morphology
- In hemochromatosis, the liver is typically enlarged due to iron accumulation.
- The dark brown color of the liver is due to extensive iron deposition (Figure 26.12a).

Microscopic Features
- The extensive iron deposition within the liver in HH is highlighted by staining with Perls' Prussian blue (Figure 26.12b). The intense blue granules correspond to ferritin and hemosiderin deposition within the siderosomes (iron-laden lysosomes).

Alcoholic Liver Disease

Alcoholic liver disease consists of an overlapping spectrum of three entities: hepatic steatosis (fatty liver), alcoholic hepatitis, and cirrhosis (see Chapter 14). Alcoholic steatosis is reversible with cessation of alcohol. Although alcoholic hepatitis is reversible with abstinence, repeated episodes lead to irreversible fibrosis and cirrhosis.

Morphology
- If concurrent hepatic steatosis is present, the gross liver specimen may be enlarged, yellow, and greasy (Figure 26.13a).
- Alcoholic cirrhosis is typically micronodular in appearance (Figure 26.13b).

Microscopic Features
- Steatosis is typically macrovesicular, in which lipid accumulation compresses and displaces the hepatocyte nucleus to the periphery of the cell (Figure 26.13c).
- The histologic features of alcoholic hepatitis include a neutrophilic infiltrate with hepatocyte swelling and necrosis (Figure 26.13d) and Mallory bodies (or Mallory hyaline). Mallory (or Mallory–Denk) bodies (Figure 26.13e) are eosinophilic intracytoplasmic inclusions of keratin filaments that are characteristic of alcoholic liver disease. However, Mallory bodies are not specific for alcoholic liver disease and may be present in Wilson disease, primary biliary cirrhosis, and nonalcoholic fatty liver disease.
- With repeated bouts of alcoholic hepatitis, sinusoidal stellate cells and portal tract fibroblasts may be activated, resulting in fibrosis and cirrhosis. Alcohol-associated cirrhosis is typically micronodular and characterized by regenerative nodules with surrounding fibrous tissue that bridges portal tracts (Figure 26.13f). Steatosis and Mallory bodies in some remaining hepatocytes may be a clue to the etiology.

Cholestasis

Cholestasis occurs secondary to impaired bile flow, causing accumulation of bile salts within hepatocytes. Causes of cholestasis include bile duct obstruction (e.g., gallstones, primary sclerosing cholangitis, primary biliary cirrhosis) and medications (see Chapters 20 and 21).

Microscopic Features
- Brown bile pigments collect in the cytoplasm of hepatocytes and result in a fine, foamy appearance, termed feathery degeneration (Figure 26.14).

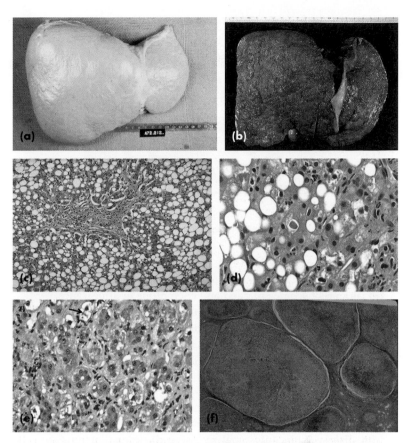

Figure 26.13 Alcoholic liver disease. (a) Gross image of hepatic steatosis (fatty liver). Note the yellowish shiny appearance of the liver. (b) Gross image of a liver with predominantly micronodular cirrhosis. (c) Photomicrograph of hepatic steatosis showing lipid vacuoles compressing and displacing the hepatocyte nucleus to the periphery of the cell. Hematoxylin and eosin, 100×. (d) Photomicrograph of alcoholic hepatitis showing hepatocyte swelling and necrosis with a surrounding inflammatory infiltrate containing neutrophils. Hematoxylin and eosin, 400×. (e) Photomicrograph of alcoholic hepatitis showing a Mallory body, with the characteristic twisted-rope appearance (arrow) seen within a degenerating hepatocyte. Hematoxylin and eosin, 200×. (f) Photomicrograph of a cirrhotic liver showing regenerative nodules of hepatocytes surrounded by dense fibrous connective tissue. Masson's trichrome, 40×.

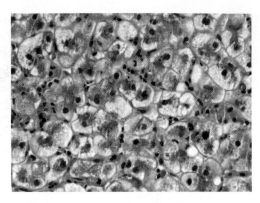

Figure 26.14 Cholestasis. Photomicrograph showing brown bile pigment in the cytoplasm of hepatocytes. Feathery degeneration of hepatocytes is present. Hematoxylin and eosin, 200×.

- Hepatocytes become enlarged and edematous in appearance.
- There may be associated proliferation of bile duct epithelial cells, edema of the portal tracts, and neutrophilic infiltration. Bile plugs may develop in dilated bile canaliculi.
- Unrelieved obstruction can lead to portal tract fibrosis and eventually to cirrhosis.

Wilson Disease

Wilson disease is an autosomal recessive disorder that results in the accumulation of copper in the liver, brain, and eye (see Chapter 15).

Microscopic Features
- Hepatic damage in Wilson disease can range from mild changes such as steatosis to massive necrosis.
- Histologic features include vacuolated nuclei, mild to moderate fatty changes, and focal hepatocyte necrosis (Figure 26.15). Cytochemical staining for copper and copper binding protein may be helpful in establishing the diagnosis.

Primary Biliary Cirrhosis

Primary biliary cirrhosis is a cholestatic liver disease that results in destruction of intrahepatic bile ducts by an autoimmune inflammatory process (see Chapter 15). It predominantly affects middle-aged women.

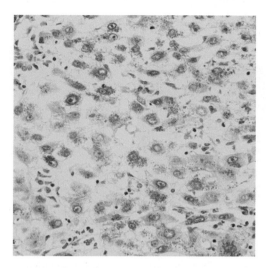

Figure 26.15 Wilson disease. Photomicrograph showing accumulation of copper (reddish granules) within hepatocytes. Orceine stain, 200×. (Courtesy of Dr. Matthew Lim, Department of Pathology, Emory University, Atlanta, GA, USA.)

Morphology
- In primary biliary cirrhosis the severity of disease varies in different areas of the liver.
- Early in the course of the disease the liver appears normal; however, as the disease progresses the liver appears green because of bile stasis (Figure 26.16a).

Microscopic Features
- Early in the disease, lymphocytes, macrophages, and plasma cells infiltrate the portal tracts (Figure 26.16b). Inflammatory cells accumulate around the bile ducts.
- Loss of interlobular bile ducts is a cardinal feature. Noncaseating granulomas, called "the florid duct lesion" (Figure 26.16b), and lymphocytic infiltration are seen in the portal tracts.
- Endstage primary biliary cirrhosis is indistinguishable from other causes of cirrhosis.

Alpha-1 Antitrypsin Deficiency

Alpha-1 antitrypsin deficiency is an autosomal recessive disorder that results in precocious emphysema and liver disease (see Chapter 15). Liver disease occurs in persons who are ZZ homozygotes as a result of

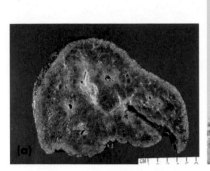
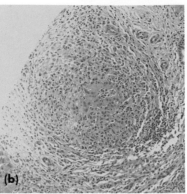

Figure 26.16 Primary biliary cirrhosis. (a) Gross image showing a cirrhotic liver with cholestasis. (b) Photomicrograph showing a dense chronic inflammatory infiltrate with a granuloma in the portal tract and loss of bile ductules. Hemotoxylin and eosin, 200×. (Courtesy of Dr. Matthew Lim, Department of Pathology, Emory University, Atlanta, GA, USA.)

accumulation of abnormal alpha-1 antitrypsin in hepatocytes, which leads to an autophagocytic response, mitochondrial dysfunction, and an inflammatory response leading to hepatocyte damage.

Morphology
- The liver may exhibit a range of findings from cholestasis to fibrosis to cirrhosis.

Microscopic Features
- The hallmark of alpha-1 antitrypsin deficiency is the presence of eosinophilic cytoplasmic globules in hepatocytes that are highlighted by periodic acid-Schiff stain (Figure 26.17a,b).
- End-stage cirrhosis in alpha-1 antitrypsin deficiency is indistinguishable from that associated with other causes of cirrhosis.

Autoimmune Hepatitis

Autoimmune hepatitis is a chronic necroinflammatory disorder that is characterized by circulating serum autoantibodies, hypergammaglobulinemia, and interface hepatitis on histologic examination of the liver (see Chapter 15).

Microscopic Features
- Autoimmune hepatitis is characterized by interface hepatitis seen as marked portal and periportal inflammation with lymphocytes and

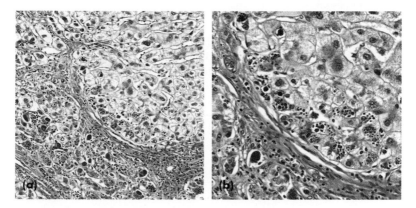

Figure 26.17 Alpha-1 antitrypsin deficiency. Photomicrographs showing eosinophilic hyaline intracytoplasmic inclusions in periportal hepatocytes. Periodic acid-Schiff, 200× (a), 400× (b).

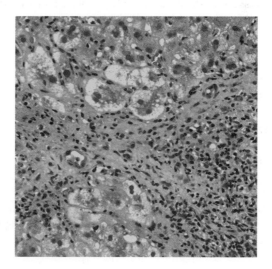

Figure 26.18 Autoimmune hepatitis. Photomicrograph showing interface hepatitis. Note the dense inflammatory infiltrate with plasma cells and lymphocytes and degeneration of hepatocytes in the periportal area. Hematoxylin and eosin, 400×. (Courtesy of Dr. Matthew Lim, Department of Pathology, Emory University, Atlanta, GA, USA.)

macrophages that spill through the limiting plates encircling periportal hepatocytes, a pattern termed "rosetting."
- Autoimmune hepatitis typically displays a marked plasma cell infiltrate (Figure 26.18), which is uncommon in other forms of hepatitis.
- Bridging necrosis and cirrhosis are similar to that seen in other chronic liver diseases.

Further Reading

Kumar, V., Abbas, A. and Fausto, N. (eds) (2010) *Robbins and Cotran Pathologic Basis of Disease*, 8th edn. Saunders Elsevier, Philadelphia.

Lee, W.M. (2004) Acetaminophen and the US Acute Liver Failure Study Group: lowering the risks of hepatic failure. *Hepatology*, 40, 6–9.

Weblinks

http://www.humpath.com/

http://library.med.utah.edu/WebPath/GIHTML/GIIDX.html

Classic Images

Abhijit Datir, William Small, and Pardeep Mittal

CHAPTER 27

Achalasia

Achalasia is an esophageal motor disorder characterized by the absence of esophageal peristalsis and failure of lower esophageal sphincter to relax with swallowing (see Chapter 2). The radiologic study of choice in the diagnosis of achalasia is a barium esophagogram (barium swallow) performed under fluoroscopic guidance. Radiographic signs of esophageal achalasia on fluoroscopic barium esophagogram (Figure 27.1) include:

- uniform dilatation of the esophagus with an air-fluid level at the level of the aortic arch;
- multiple uncoordinated tertiary contractions in early stages and absence of peristalsis in late stages;
- smooth, tapered, conical narrowing of the distal esophagus ("bird's beak" sign) at the lower esophageal sphincter;
- a narrowed segment of <3.5 cm in length and proximal dilatation (>4 cm).

A normal barium esophagogram does not exclude achalasia. The diagnosis of achalasia should be confirmed by esophageal manometry. Endoscopy is generally performed to exclude secondary causes of achalasia such as an infiltrating carcinoma at the gastroesophageal junction.

Esophageal Ulcer

Esophagitis and esophageal ulcers may be caused by gastroesophageal reflux disease, viral infections (human immunodeficiency virus, cytomegalovirus, herpes simplex virus), and medications (see Chapter 2). Fluoroscopic studies using barium are inexpensive and simple to perform

Essentials of Gastroenterology, First Edition. Edited by Shanthi V. Sitaraman, Lawrence S. Friedman.
© 2012 John Wiley & Sons, Ltd. Published 2012 by John Wiley & Sons, Ltd.

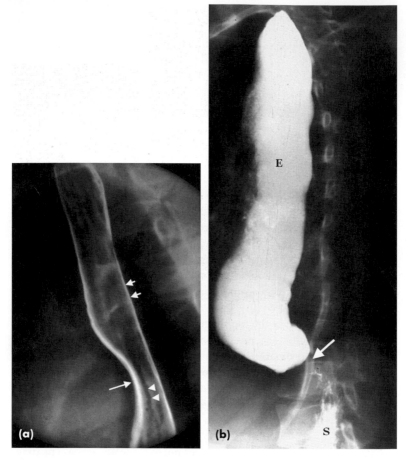

Figure 27.1 Barium esophagogram of achalasia. (a) A normal esophagogram shows smooth mucosal lining (short arrows), normal fold thickness (arrowheads) and retrocardiac impression. (b) In achalasia there is uniform dilatation of the esophagus (E) to the level of the gastroesophageal (GE) junction (arrow). Note the tapered appearance of the GE junction with the column of barium above. (S, stomach.)

and provide critical assessment of the esophagus. Barium studies are often used as an initial step in the diagnostic work-up of dysphagia and serve as a complementary test to endoscopy. The radiographic signs of esophageal ulcer or esophagitis (Figure 27.2) include:

- thickened esophageal folds (>3 mm);
- limited esophageal distensibility (asymmetric flattening);
- abnormal motility;
- mucosal plaques and nodules;

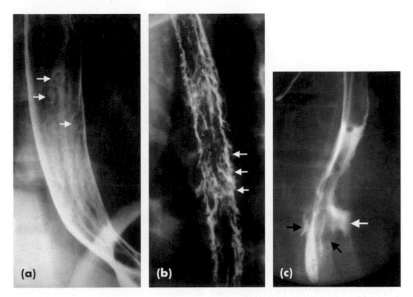

Figure 27.2 Barium esophagogram of esophageal ulcers. (a) Herpetic esophagitis is seen as multiple, small, esophageal ulcers (arrows) in the midesophagus. Note the radiolucent mound of edema surrounding the ulcers. The remainder of the mucosa is normal. (b) Esophageal candidiasis is seen as grossly irregular esophageal contour due to innumerable plaques and pseudomembranes (arrows), with trapping of barium between lesions. (c) Cytomegalovirus esophagitis is seen as a large, flat ulcer in the mid-esophagus (white arrow) with multiple satellite ulcers (black arrows).

- erosions and ulcerations;
- localized stricture(s).

Gastric Ulcer (Benign vs. Malignant)

Gastric ulcers can be benign (peptic ulcer disease) or malignant (gastric adenocarcinoma, lymphoma, metastasis). Endoscopy is the diagnostic procedure of choice in patients suspected of gastric ulcer. Nevertheless, double contrast barium study has a sensitivity of 95% for detecting malignant gastric ulcer and hence may be used as an alternative to endoscopy in selected patients for either detection or follow-up of a gastric ulcer. The radiographic signs consistent with a **benign** ulcer (Figure 27.3, Table 27.1) include:

- a smooth ulcer mound with tapering edges;
- an edematous ulcer collar with an overhanging mucosal edge;
- an ulcer projecting beyond the expected lumen;

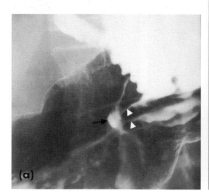
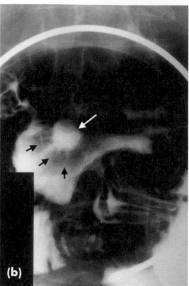

Figure 27.3 Double contrast barium radiograph of benign gastric ulcers. (a) A benign (en face) barium-filled ulcer is seen in the posterior wall of the gastric body (arrow). Thin, regular radiating folds are seen converging toward the ulcer (arrowheads). (b) A large (in profile) ulcer (white arrow) is seen on the lesser curvature; its projection from the lumen of the stomach is consistent with a benign lesion. This ulcer is surrounded by a prominent ring of edema represented by the lucent area around the crater (black arrows).

Table 27.1 Radiographic findings of benign and malignant gastric ulcers.

Radiographic findings	Benign	Malignant
Hampton line	Present	Absent
Extension beyond gastric wall	Yes	No
Folds	Smooth, even	Irregular, nodular
Ulcer shape	Round, oval, or linear	Irregular
Associated mass	Absent	Present
Carmen meniscus	Absent	Present
Healing	Complete	Usually incomplete

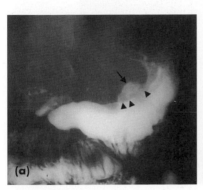
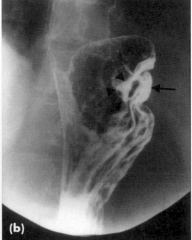

Figure 27.4 Double contrast barium radiograph of malignant gastric ulcer. (a) A malignant ulcerated mass is seen along the lesser curvature of the gastric body (arrow) with a sharply demarcating shelf (arrowheads). (b) A malignant polypoid ulcer (arrow) is seen along the greater curvature of the gastric fundus and body junction projecting into the lumen. Note the associated distorted gastric folds (arrowheads).

- radiating folds extending into the ulcer crater;
- depth of ulcer greater than width;
- sharply marginated contour;
- Hampton line (a thin, sharp, lucent line that traverses the orifice of the ulcer).

The radiographic signs of a **malignant** gastric ulcer (Figure 27.4) include:

- eccentric location of the ulcer within the tumor mound;
- width greater than depth;
- nodular, rolled, irregular, or shouldered edges;
- Carmen meniscus sign (a large flat-based, inwardly folded ulcer with heaped-up edges).

The Normal Plain Abdominal Film

A plain abdominal film (Figure 27.5) is most often used to assess for bowel obstruction or perforation in patients who present with acute abdominal pain (see Chapters 23 and 25). Relatively large amounts of gas are normally present in the stomach and colon, but only a small amount of air is seen in the small intestine. The presence of bowel gas is

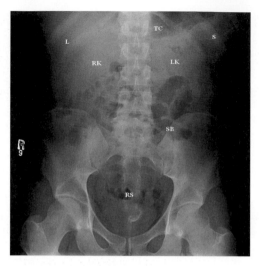

Figure 27.5 A normal plain abdominal film. (L, liver; S, spleen; RK, right kidney; LK, left kidney; TC, transverse colon; SB, small bowel; RS, rectosigmoid colon.)

helpful in assessing the position and diameter of the bowel. Air and fluid represent normal bowel contents, and the presence of three to five air–fluid levels less than 2.5 cm in length is considered normal on an upright film.

The amount of air present in a normal colon is quite variable, but sufficient gas is usually present for the colonic haustra to be identified readily. The colonic diameter is also variable, with the transverse colon measuring 5.5 cm in diameter. A colonic diameter of more than 9 cm is considered abnormal and indicates obstruction or ileus. The borders of the kidneys, psoas muscles, and bladder and the posterior borders of the liver and spleen can often be identified by the fat that surrounds them. The fat lines may be displaced due to enlargement of these organs or effaced by inflammation or fluid.

Small Intestinal Obstruction

On a plain abdominal film, the normal small intestinal lumen diameter is ≤2.5 cm for jejunum and 3.0 cm for ileum. A small bowel diameter measuring greater than 3.0 cm should raise a suspicion of obstruction (mechanical or functional) in the appropriate clinical setting (Table 27.2). The hallmark of mechanical bowel obstruction is a point of transition between dilated and nondilated bowel (Figure 27.6). Functional bowel

Table 27.2 Causes of dilated small intestine (>3 cm).

Mechanical obstruction	Functional obstruction (pseudo-obstruction)
Adhesions (75% of small bowel obstructions)	Adynamic ileus:
	After surgery
Incarcerated hernia	After trauma
Volvulus	Peritoneal inflammation
Extrinsic tumor	Ischemia
Congenital stenosis	Drugs (e.g., opiates, barbiturates)
Intraluminal lesions:	Vagotomy
Tumor	Electrolyte imbalance
Intussusception	Collagen vascular disorders:
Foreign body	Scleroderma
Gallstone ileus	Dermatomyositis
Bezoar	Malabsorption syndromes
Meconium	Chronic idiopathic pseudo-obstruction

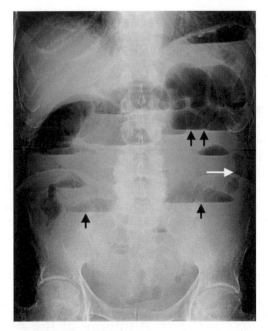

Figure 27.6 Upright abdominal film showing small intestinal obstruction. Note the dilated small bowel loops with multiple air–fluid levels (black arrows), a tell-tale sign of bowel obstruction. Note the decompressed loop of descending colon (white arrow) distal to the obstruction.

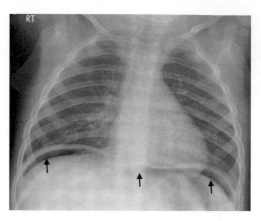

Figure 27.7 Chest radiograph showing intestinal perforation. Free intraperitoneal air along the undersurface of the left diaphragm (arrows) indicates a perforated viscus.

obstruction (called pseudo-obstruction) causes diffuse bowel dilatation with no transition point.

Intestinal perforation

The presence of free intraperitoneal air (*pneumoperitoneum*) almost always indicates perforation of a viscus, most commonly a perforated duodenal or gastric ulcer. Additional causes of pneumoperitoneum include trauma, inflammatory bowel disease, recent surgery, and infection of the peritoneal cavity with gas-producing organisms.

A plain film is valuable in the acute setting to exclude pneumoperitoneum. As little as one milliliter of free air can be detected on an erect chest X-ray or left lateral decubitus abdominal film. A small amount of free air can be detected under the right hemidiaphragm on erect films (Figure 27.7). It may be difficult, however, to differentiate free air under the left hemidiaphragm from normal air in the stomach or colon. Free air is typically seen between the liver and the abdominal wall on a lateral decubitus film. Abdominal computed tomography (CT) is usually performed to confirm perforation noted on a plain abdominal film.

Normal Cross-Sectional Anatomy of the Abdomen on Axial Computed Tomography and Coronal Magnetic Resonance Imaging

Computed tomography (CT) and magnetic resonance imaging (MRI) with and without contrast are commonly used diagnostic tests. CT and

MRI allow precise visualization of organs and structures within the abdominal and/or pelvic cavity. Figure 27.8 outlines intra-abdominal organs and structures seen on axial CT and coronal MRI.

Cholelithiasis

Gallstones can be visualized on abdominal plain films, ultrasonography, and CT. As outlined below, ultrasonography is the test of choice to detect gallstones.

Plain films

Only 10–15% of gallstones are readily visible on plain films (Figure 27.9a). Small radiopaque gallstones tend to be uniform in density while larger stones typically show a peripheral or laminated pattern of calcification.

Ultrasonography

The sensitivity and specificity of ultrasonography to detect gallstones is >95% (Figure 27.9b). Gallstones appear as echogenic foci that produce acoustic shadows and are usually mobile.

Computed Tomography

Up to 20% of gallstones are isodense with bile and not detected by CT, whereas some gallstones may be missed because of their small size.

Choledocholithiasis

Ultrasonography has varying degree of sensitivity (50–80%) but high specificity (approximately 95%) for detecting bile duct stones.

Magnetic resonance cholangiopancreatography (MRCP) (Figure 27.10a) is highly accurate in the diagnosis of choledocholithiasis with a sensitivity of 92–94% and specificity of 99%.

Signs of biliary dilatation on MRCP include the following (Figure 27.10b):

- multiple branching tubular or round structures coursing toward the porta hepatis;
- diameter of intrahepatic bile ducts larger than that of adjacent portal vein diameter;
- dilatation of bile duct >6 mm;
- gallbladder diameter >5 cm.

Acute Cholecystitis

Ultrasonography (Figure 27.11a) along with CT and scintigraphy, is used for the diagnosis of acute cholecystitis and related complications (see

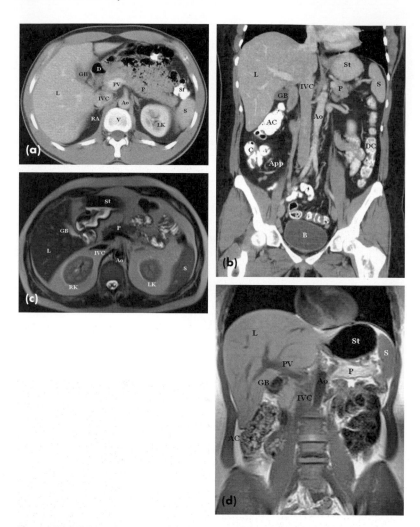

Figure 27.8 Normal cross sectional anatomy of the abdomen on axial CT and coronal MR images. (L, liver; S, spleen; GB, gallbladder; P, pancreas; RK, right kidney; LK, left kidney; RA, right adrenal; LA, left adrenal; Ao, aorta; IVC, inferior vena cava; PV, portal vein; St, stomach; D, duodenum; TI, terminal ileum; App, appendix; AC, ascending colon; Sf, splenic flexure of the colon; DC, descending colon; SC, sigmoid colon; V, vertebral body.)

Chapter 21). The radiographic features of acute cholecystitis on CT (Figure 27.11b) include:
- a distended gallbladder with wall thickening;
- presence of gallstones;
- high-density bile;

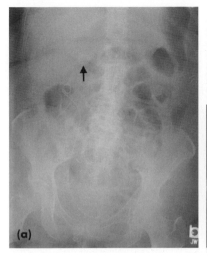
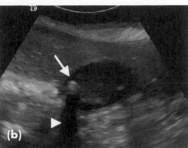

Figure 27.9 Imaging of gallstones. (a) A plain abdominal film shows a round, radiopaque calculus (arrow) in the right upper quadrant, the typical location for gallstone. (b) An ultrasonographic image demonstrates an echogenic focus in the gallbladder lumen (arrow) with posterior acoustic shadowing (arrowhead), characteristic of a gallstone.

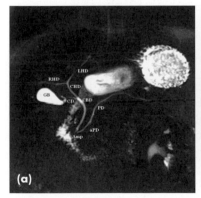
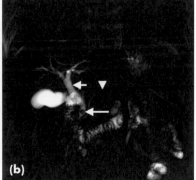

Figure 27.10 Magnetic resonance cholangiopancreatography (MRCP) of choledocholithiasis. (a) Normal MRCP demonstrates biliary system anatomy including bile duct (BD), cystic duct (CD), gallbladder (GB), common hepatic duct (CHD), right hepatic duct (RHD) and left hepatic duct (LHD), pancreatic duct (PD), accessory pancreatic duct (aPD), and duodenal ampulla (Amp). (b) Choledocholithiasis as seen on a coronal MRCP image in a patient with obstructive jaundice shows a distal bile duct stone (long arrow) with dilatation of the proximal hepatic and intrahepatic bile ducts (short arrow). Note the normal pancreatic duct (arrowhead).

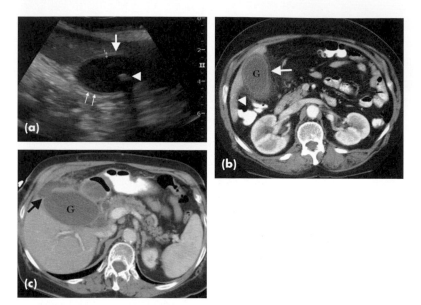

Figure 27.11 Imaging of acute cholecystitis. (a) An ultrasonographic image shows a distended gallbladder lumen with sludge, calculus (arrowhead), wall thickening (arrow), and thin rim of pericholecystic fluid (thin arrows) in a patient with acute calculous cholecystitis. (b) Axial contrast-enhanced CT image shows dilated gallbladder (G) with a thickened wall (white arrow) and pericholecystic fluid (white arrowhead). (c) CT image shows acute perforated cholecystitis with focal discontinuity in the gallbladder (G) wall (arrow) and expulsion of the bile into the pericholecystic fluid.

- inflammatory stranding in pericholecystic fat;
- blurring of interface between gallbladder and liver.
  Complications of acute cholecystitis include the following:
- **Gangrenous cholecystitis** defined as gallbladder wall necrosis with a high risk of perforation. Gangrenous cholecystitis is seen as asymmetric gallbladder wall thickening with multiple lucent layers, indicating ulceration and edema.
- **Gallbladder perforation** (Figure 27.11c) is a life-threatening complication that may lead to pericholecystic abscess and/or generalized peritonitis.
- **Emphysematous cholecystitis** is an infection of the gallbladder with gas-forming organisms. It is common in diabetic patients. On CT, emphysematous cholecystitis is seen as intramural gas with an arc-like configuration.
- **Mirizzi syndrome** refers to a condition resulting from a cystic duct stone eroding into the adjacent hepatic duct and causing obstruction.

A gallstone may be seen at the junction of the cystic and the common hepatic ducts with associated cholecystitis and biliary obstruction.

Pancreatitis

CT is used to diagnose and stage pancreatitis. A dedicated CT pancreatic protocol with both oral and intravenous contrast administration is used.

Acute Pancreatitis

The pancreas may appear normal in mild acute pancreatitis, but edema of the pancreas and surrounding fat may be seen. In acute pancreatitis (Figure 27.12a), the pancreas appears enlarged with patchy high attenuation of the surrounding fat. A small amount of fluid may be seen around the adjacent vessels with associated thickening of the fascial planes.

CT is useful in demonstrating complications associated with acute pancreatitis (see Chapter 18):

- **Liquefactive necrosis** of pancreatic parenchyma (Figure 27.12b) is seen as focal or diffuse lack of pancreatic parenchymal enhancement.
- **Pancreatic fluid collections**: acute collections may be intrapancreatic, anterior to the pararenal space, in the lesser sac, or anywhere in the abdomen.
- **Pseudocyst** (Figure 27.12c) is an encapsulated fluid collection with a distinct fibrous capsule. It requires at least 4 weeks to develop. Up to 50% of pesudocysts may need surgical, radiologic, or endoscopic drainage.
- **Infected necrosis** is seen as an area of nonenhancing necrotic tissue containing gas. Infected necrosis usually requires surgical or per-endoscopic debridement.
- **Pancreatic abscess** (Figure 27.12d) is a circumscribed collection of pus with little or no necrotic tissue. On CT, a pancreatic abscess is seen as a fluid collection with thick enhancing wall.
- **Vascular involvement** may be seen as thrombosis or erosion of a blood vessel due to a direct effect of pancreatic enzymes on peripancreatic blood vessels. Erosion of a vessel may result in acute hemorrhage or pesudoaneurysm formation.
- **Gastrointestinal involvement**: most common is duodenal necrosis or perforaton. Bile duct obstruction or stricture may also be seen.

Chronic Pancreatitis

The most common cause of chronic pancreatitis is alcohol abuse (see Chapter 19). The features of chronic pancreatitis on CT (Figure 27.13) include:

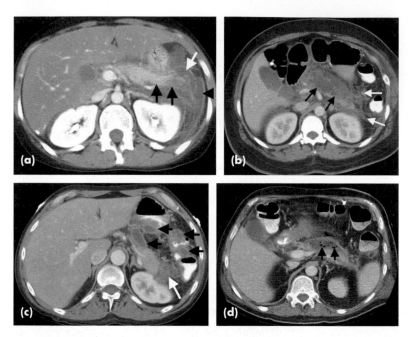

Figure 27.12 CT image of acute pancreatitis and its complications. (a) An axial contrast-enhanced CT image of acute pancreatitis shows pancreatic parenchymal thickening predominantly affecting the distal body and tail (black arrows). There is associated inflammation causing blurring of the peripancreatic fat (white arrow) and free fluid (black arrowhead). (b) An axial contrast-enhanced CT image of acute necrotizing pancreatitis shows thickened, poorly enhancing pancreatic parenchyma (black arrows) with surrounding inflammation (white arrows) consistent with pancreatic necrosis. (c) Pancreatic pseudocysts in the same patient after 4 weeks. The image shows multiple cysts around the pancreas with peripheral rim enhancement (black arrows) and residual pancreatic inflammation (white arrow). (d) An axial contrast-enhanced CT image of a pancreatic abscess shows liquefaction of the pancreatic tissue with multiple foci of air (arrows) due to abscess formation.

- parenchymal atrophy: usually generalized but may be focal;
- dilated main pancreatic duct >3 mm: the duct appears beaded with alternating areas of dilatation and narrowing;
- pancreatic calcification is usually associated with alcoholic pancreatitis; calcifications may vary from finely stippled to coarse;
- fascial thickening and chronic inflammatory changes in the surrounding tissue.

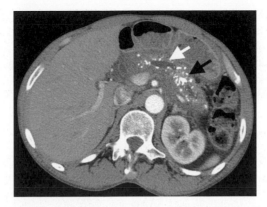

Figure 27.13 CT image of chronic pancreatitis. An axial CT image shows multiple foci of coarse pancreatic calcification (black arrow) in a patient with chronic alcoholic pancreatitis. Note the dilated pancreatic duct (white arrow).

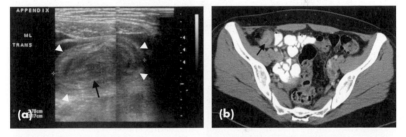

Figure 27.14 Imaging in acute appendicitis. (a) An ultrasonographic image shows a dilated appendix (arrow) with a thickened wall (arrowheads). (b) An axial CT image with oral contrast demonstrates dilated tubular appendix (arrow) with wall thickening (arrowhead), a typical CT feature of acute appendicitis.

Acute Appendicitis

Ultrasonography of the right lower quadrant is highly accurate (sensitivity and specificity approximately 90%) for diagnosing acute appendicitis (Figure 27.14a). Ultrasonography is generally used in persons with suspected acute appendicitis who have a contraindication to CT (e.g., pregnant woman). CT is the preferred imaging method for the diagnosis of acute appendicitis and its complications, with a diagnostic accuracy of 95–98% (see Chapter 25). The radiographic signs of appendicitis on CT (Figure 27.14b) include:

- appendix measuring greater than 6 mm in diameter;
- failure of appendix to fill with oral contrast or air up to its tip;
- appendicolith;
- appendicular wall enhancement with intravenous contrast;
- surrounding inflammatory changes with increased fat attenuation, fluid, cecal thickening, abscess, and extraluminal gas.

Acute Diverticulitis

Diverticulitis refers to inflammation of colonic diverticula (Figure 27.15a) and is usually associated with perforation of a diverticulum and an intramural or localized pericolic abscess. The complications of diverticulitis include bowel obstruction, bleeding, peritonitis, sinus tract development, or fistula formation.

CT findings in acute diverticulitis (Figure 27.15b) include:

- diverticular changes with associated inflammation and fat stranding;
- localized colonic wall thickening;
- pericolonic abscess;
- associated fluid that may track down to the root of the sigmoid mesentery.

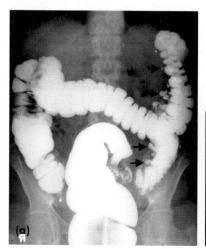
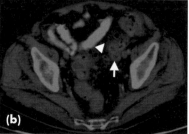

Figure 27.15 Imaging of acute diverticulitis. (a) An anteroposterior film from a barium enema series shows multiple smooth outpouchings from the descending colon (arrows) in a patient with uncomplicated diverticulosis. (b) An axial CT image with oral contrast shows a dilated, thickened colonic diverticulum (arrow) with surrounding mesenteric inflammation (arrowhead) in acute diverticulitis.

Crohn's Disease

The diagnosis of Crohn's disease is made by a combination of clinical features, imaging, endoscopy, pathology, laboratory tests, and stool studies. Contrast-enhanced imaging studies provide information on the location, extent, and severity of disease as well as complications. The hallmarks of Crohn's disease on imaging studies include aphthous ulcers, confluent deep ulcerations, predominant right colon disease, discontinuous involvement with intervening regions of normal bowel, asymmetric involvement of the bowel wall, strictures, fistulas, and sinus formation.

Small Bowel Series
Small bowel contrast studies have been largely replaced by capsule endoscopy, CT, and MRI for the diagnosis of Crohn's disease. A small bowel series can reveal aphthous ulcers, skip lesions, strictures (string sign), and entero-enteric or enterocolonic fistulas (Figure 27.16a). Enteroclysis, in which contrast material is administered slowly to the duodenum through a nasojejunal tube, is sometimes used to circumvent slow passage of contrast from the stomach into the small intestine.

Computed Tomography
CT is not only helpful in the diagnosis of Crohn's disease (Figure 27.16b) and its complications but also may be used therapeutically to guide the drainage of an abscess.

Magnetic Resonance Imaging
Small bowel MRI (MR enterography) is being used increasingly to diagnose and assess the severity of Crohn's disease and its complications (Figure 27.16c). MRI is helpful in identifying inflammatory processes in the bowel wall and submucosal inflammation and fibrosis. Assessment of submucosal disease on MRI serves as a complement to mucosal assessment using video capsule endoscopy or conventional endoscopy. In conjunction with endoscopic ultrasonography, MRI is also used to delineate the severity and extent of perianal fistulas.

Ulcerative Colitis

Clinical features, laboratory tests, stool studies, and colonoscopy with biopsies remain the mainstay of the diagnosis of ulcerative colitis. Colonoscopy is the preferred test to define extent and severity and to detect dysplasia and colon cancer. Plain abdominal films may be used to follow colonic dilatation in a patient with toxic megacolon, a

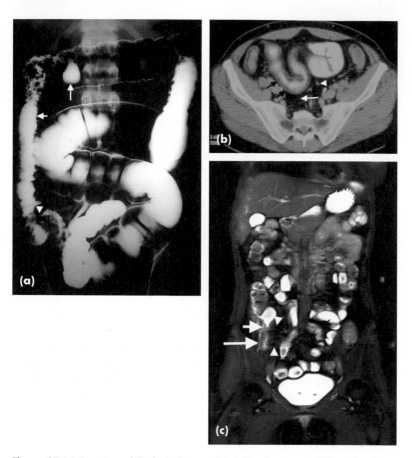

Figure 27.16 Imaging of Crohn's disease. (a) A film from a small bowel series shows marked ulceration, inflammatory changes, and narrowing of the right colon (short white arrow). Also, note the pseudodiverticulum (long arrow) and severe narrowing of the terminal ileum (arrowhead), consistent with a "string sign." (b) An axial CT image with small bowel thickening (black arrows), fibrofatty proliferation (white arrow), and mesenteric lymphadenopathy (arrowhead) in a patient with Crohn's colitis. (c) Coronal MRI in a patient with Crohn's disease affecting the terminal ileum. There is wall thickening of the terminal ileum (long white arrow) with mesenteric thickening (between arrowheads) and short-segment stricture formation (short white arrow).

complication of ulcerative colitis. Double contrast barium enema can be helpful in revealing fine mucosal details (Figure 27.17). CT and MRI are of limited use in ulcerative colitis; however, CT plays an important role in the differential diagnosis of ulcerative colitis and in the diagnosis of complications associated with ulcerative colitis. All imaging modalities

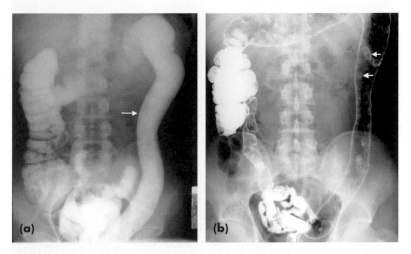

Figure 27.17 Barium enema in ulcerative colitis. Films from a barium enema shows typical features of ulcerative colitis: (a) contiguous involvement of the distal colon with loss of haustral pattern (arrow) and (b) filiform polyps (arrows).

lack specificity in this setting. For example, mucosal ulceration or bowel wall thickening depicted on barium studies is nonspecific and encountered in a variety of colitides. Barium enema should be performed cautiously in patients with severe ulcerative colitis because it may precipitate toxic megacolon.

Further Reading

Adam, A. and Dixon, A. (2007) Gastrointestinal imaging, in *Grainger and Allison's Diagnostic Radiology*, 5th edn (eds A. Adam, A.K. Dixon, R.G. Grainger, and D.J. Allison), Churchill Livingstone, Edinburgh, pp. 863–887.

Brant, W.E. (2006) Gastrointestinal tract, in *Fundamentals of Diagnostic Radiology*, 3rd edn (eds W.E. Brant and C.A. Helms), Lippincott Williams & Wilkins, Philadephia, pp. 731–764.

Weblink

http://www.radiologyeducation.com/

Classic Skin Manifestations

Melanie S. Harrison, Robert A. Swerlick, and Zakiya P. Rice

CHAPTER 28

Clinical Vignette 1

A 20-year-old man presents with a 3-month history of intermittent bright red blood per rectum. He denies constipation, abdominal pain, weight loss, or melena. His past medical history is unremarkable. Family history is notable for colonic polyps in his father, paternal uncle, and several cousins. Physical examination shows faded hyperpigmented macules concentrated around the lips and buccal mucosa. Abdominal examination reveals a soft, nontender, nondistended abdomen with no palpable masses and no hepatosplenomegaly. Bowel sounds are normal. Rectal examination reveals brown stool that is positive for occult blood. Laboratory testing shows a hemoglobin level of 8 g/dL, iron 20 μg/dL, ferritin 10 ng/mL, total iron binding capacity 394 μg/dL, and iron saturation 4.9%. Colonoscopy reveals numerous polyps ranging in size from 2 mm to 2 cm throughout the colon. Some of the polyps are ulcerated. Esophagogastroduodenoscopy (EGD) shows multiple gastric and duodenal polyps. Histologic examination of several polyps in the colon, stomach, and duodenum reveals disorganization and proliferation of the muscularis mucosa with normal overlying epithelium, suggestive of hamartomas.

Clinical Vignette 2

A 35-year-old woman presents with a 6-week history of bloody diarrhea and fatigue. She reports rectal pain with bowel movements and fecal urgency. Approximately 1 week ago, she noticed tender red lesions on both anterior shins. She denies trauma to the areas. Physical examination is remarkable for

Essentials of Gastroenterology, First Edition. Edited by Shanthi V. Sitaraman, Lawrence S. Friedman.

raised, tender, erythematous nodules on the anterior shins. Abdominal examination is significant for mild left lower quadrant tenderness without rebound tenderness or guarding. Rectal examination reveals bloody stools. Routine laboratory tests including a complete blood count and comprehensive metabolic panel are normal except for a hemoglobin level of 10 g/dL. Stool examination is positive for fecal leukocytes, but bacterial cultures, examination for ova and parasites, and a test for *Clostridium difficile* toxin are negative. Colonoscopy reveals friable mucosa with exudates involving the rectum and sigmoid colon. The remaining colonic mucosa and terminal ileum appear normal. Colonic mucosal biopsies of the affected areas reveal crypt abscesses and crypt distortion as well as inflammatory infiltrates in the lamina propria.

Erythema Nodosum

- Erythema nodosum (EN) is an inflammatory condition of the subcutaneous fat.
- Typical lesions are 1–10 cm, shiny, tender, red, nonulcerating nodules on the anterior shins (Figure 28.1). They may also be seen on the arms, face, thighs, and neck. Associated symptoms include arthralgias and fever.

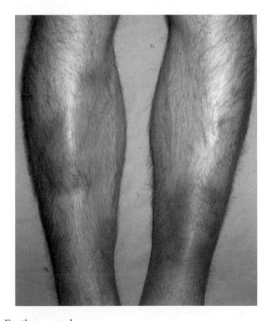

Figure 28.1 Erythema nodosum.

- The cause of EN is unknown in 30–50% of patients. In the remainder, EN may be associated with a wide variety of conditions such as autoimmune disorders (inflammatory bowel disease (IBD), Behçet's disease), pregnancy, medications (sulfonamides, oral contraceptives), and cancer.
- EN affects 5–7% of persons with IBD and has a predilection for females. EN parallels the activity of the underlying IBD and improves with treatment of the IBD.
- EN may also be associated with infectious colitis caused by *Yersinia enterocolitica*, *Shigella flexneri*, and *Campylobacter jejuni*.
- The diagnosis of EN is made by recognition of its classic appearance. Biopsy of a lesion may be performed when the diagnosis is unclear. Histologic examination reveals panniculitis with acute and chronic inflammation localized to the fibrous septae between the fat lobules of the dermis. Once a diagnosis of EN is made, a thorough work-up to elucidate the underlying cause should be performed.
- Therapy includes treatment of the underlying disease, bed rest, elevation of the legs, glucocorticoids, and topical potassium iodide.

Pyoderma Gangrenosum

- Pyoderma gangrenosum (PG) is an ulcerative cutaneous disorder.
- Lesions begin as pustules or nodules that rapidly ulcerate.
- Lesions are tender and painful, with an elevated dusky purple border (Figure 28.2).
- PG affects up to 5% of persons with ulcerative colitis and 1% of those with Crohn's disease.

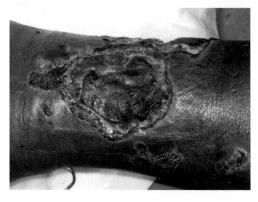

Figure 28.2 Pyoderma gangrenosum.

- Fifty percent of patients with PG will eventually be found to have ulcerative colitis or Crohn's disease, and colonoscopy should be performed in all patients with PG.
- Other systemic conditions associated with PG include hematologic malignancies and collagen vascular diseases.
- Management includes treatment of the underlying IBD, gentle local wound care and dressings, topical and/or systemic glucocorticoids, topical and/or systemic tacrolimus or pimecrolimus, and other immunosuppressive drugs. Infliximab has been shown to benefit some patients.
- Debridement or surgery should be avoided because of pathergy, a condition in which minor trauma leads to worsening of lesions, which may be resistant to healing.

Henoch–Schonlein Purpura

- Henoch–Schonlein purpura (HSP) is a systemic vasculitis characterized by palpable purpura, arthralgias, abdominal pain, and renal disease.
- Palpable purpura typically occurs on the buttocks and legs and may have vesicles or ulcerations (Figure 28.3).
- Gastrointestinal symptoms include abdominal pain, gastrointestinal hemorrhage, intussusception, and perforation.
- The diagnosis of HSP is made by immunofluorescence performed on biopsy specimens of the skin lesions within 24 hours of their appearance. Leukocytoclastic vasculitis with immunoglobulin A (IgA) deposits in the superficial capillaries is characteristic of HSP.
- Most cases of HSP are self-limiting and require no treatment apart from symptom control with analgesics for arthralgias and abdominal pain.

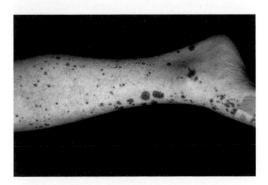

Figure 28.3 Henoch–Schonlein purpura.

Hereditary Hemorrhagic Telangiectasia (Osler–Weber–Rendu Disease)

- Hereditary hemorrhagic telangiectasia is an autosomal dominant vascular disorder characterized by telangiectasias, arteriovenous malformations, and aneurysms of the skin, lung, brain, and gastrointestinal tract (see Chapter 22).
- Epistaxis and gastrointestinal hemorrhage are common complications of the disease.
- Skin lesions are 1–3mm macular telangiectasias of the face, lips, tongue, conjunctivae, chest, fingers, and feet (Figure 28.4).
- The diagnosis is based on four criteria: spontaneous recurrent epistaxis; mucocutaneous telangiectasias; visceral involvement; and a first-degree family member with the disease. The diagnosis is confirmed by genetic testing for the endoglin or the activin receptor-like kinase type I (ALK-1) gene mutation.
- Treatment is supportive with iron supplements or blood transfusions for anemia, and ablation of telangiectasias using neodymium yttrium aluminum garnet (Nd:YAG) laser for the skin lesions and argon plasma coagulation for lesions in the gastrointestinal tract.

Peutz–Jeghers Syndrome

- Peutz–Jeghers syndrome (PJS) is an autosomal dominant hereditary intestinal polyposis syndrome characterized by the development of benign hamartomatous polyps (see Chapter 10).

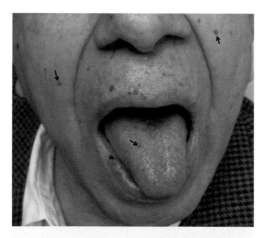

Figure 28.4 Hereditary hemorrhagic telangiectasia. Arrows point to telangiectasias. (Photo courtesy of Dr. Elise Brantley, Emory University, Atlanta, GA, USA).

- Typical cutaneous lesions in PJS include hyperpigmented papules 1–10 mm in size that occur on the lips, buccal mucosa, palms, soles, and digits, as well as around the eyes, anus, and mouth (Figure 28..5).
- Patients with PJS have a mutation in the *STK11/LKB1* gene, which encodes a serine threonine kinase.
- Hamartomatous polyps have only a small malignant potential; however, patients with PJS have an increased risk of developing carcinomas of the pancreas, liver, lungs, breast, ovaries, uterus, testicles, and other organs. Close surveillance for malignancies is advised in patients with PJS.

Acanthosis Nigricans

- Acanthosis nigricans (AN) is characterized by hyperpigmented, thickened skin typically in areas of body folds such as the neck, axilla, groin, and umbilicus (Figure 28.6). Multiple skin tags may be present.

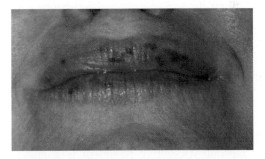

Figure 28.5 Peutz–Jeghers syndrome. Hyperpigmented papules on the lips are shown.

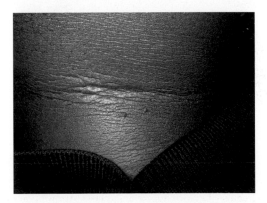

Figure 28.6 Acanthosis nigricans. Hyperpigmented, thickened skin in the neck is shown.

- AN occurs in persons >40 years of age. It may be inherited or associated with endocrine disorders, such as obesity, hypothyroidism, hyperthyroidism, acromegaly, polycystic ovary syndrome, insulin-resistant diabetes mellitus, or Cushing's sydrome.
- AN may also occur as a paraneoplastic syndrome associated with gastrointestinal (adenocarcinomas) or uterine malignancies.
- The diagnosis is made by the classic appearance of the lesion; rarely is a biopsy needed.
- Persons with AN should be screened for diabetes mellitus and, if appropriate, malignancy.
- AN usually resolves when the underlying cause is treated.

Dermatitis Herpetiformis

- Dermatitis herpetiformis (DH) is a chronic blistering skin condition. It is characterized by small, intensely pruritic, papulovesicular lesions located in a symmetrical manner on the scalp and extensor surfaces of the extremities (Figure 28.7).
- DH is associated with celiac disease and occurs in up to 25% of persons with celiac disease.
- The diagnosis of DH with celiac disease is confirmed by detection of tissue transglutaminase antibodies in serum and characteristic findings on small intestinal biopsy (see Chapter 6). The diagnosis of DH may also be made by skin biopsy and direct immunofluorescence for IgA deposits in the dermal papillae.
- Dapsone is the drug of choice to treat DH, and the lesions respond rapidly to dapsone. Definitive treatment is a gluten-free diet for celiac disease. Other medications used to treat DH include colchicine, lymecycline, nicotinamide, tetracycline, sulfamethoxypyridazine, and sulfapyridine.

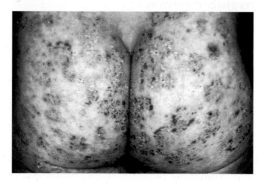

Figure 28.7 Dermatitis herpetiformis.

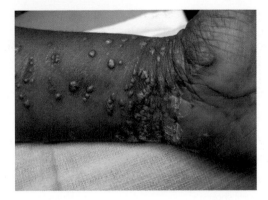

Figure 28.8 Lichen planus.

Lichen Planus

- Lichen planus (LP) is a chronic inflammatory disorder involving the oral mucosa and skin.
- Lesions are polygonal, purple, flat-topped papules with white plaques and affect the flexures of the wrist, arms, and legs (Figure 28.8).
- LP is typically found in adulthood and is more common in women than in men.
- LP is associated with chronic hepatitis C and primary biliary cirrhosis.
- The diagnosis of LP is made by skin biopsy. Direct immunofluorescence shows deposits of IgA, IgM, IgG, and complement. Deposits of fibrin and fibrinogen are present in the basement membrane.
- Treatment is with topical or systemic glucocorticoids. Azathioprine, cyclosporine, and phototherapy are alternatives.

Mixed Cryoglobulinemia

- Mixed cryoglobulinemia (MC) occurs when immune complexes deposit in blood vessels, resulting in vasculitis of small and medium-sized vessels.
- Skin manifestations of MC include palpable purpura, commonly seen on the lower extremities (Figure 28.9).
- Other findings include arthralgias, peripheral neuropathy, lymphadenopathy, hepatosplenomegaly, renal disease, and hypocomplementemia.
- MC is associated with chronic inflammatory conditions, such as hepatitis C and less commonly hepatitis B and prolonged hepatitis A, as well as connective tissue diseases.

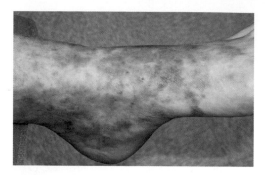

Figure 28.9 Mixed cryoglobulinemia. Palpable purpura associated with mixed cryoglobulinemia is shown.

- The diagnosis of MC is made by the detection of purpura, circulating cryoglobulins, and low complement levels.
- Skin biopsy reveals a leukoclastic vasculitis. Deposits of IgM, IgG, and complement C3 may be seen with direct immunofluorescence.
- Treatment includes initiation of antiviral therapy for chronic hepatitis C (or B) and plasma exchange.

Porphyria Cutanea Tarda

- Porphyria cutanea tarda (PCT) is a metabolic disorder caused by deficiency of urobilinogen decarboxylase, an enzyme in the heme synthesis pathway
- PCT is characterized by increased skin fragility, facial hypertrichosis, blistering, milia, and skin hyperpigmentation typically of sun-exposed areas (Figure 28.10).

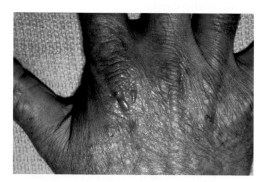

Figure 28.10 Porphyria cutanea tarda.

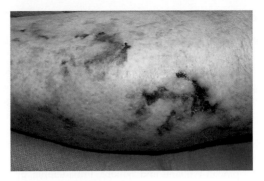

Figure 28.11 Polyarteritis nodosa.

- PCT is associated with chronic hepatitis C and hemochromatosis.
- Multiple factors can exacerbate PCT, including alcohol, iron, sunlight, and estrogens.
- The diagnosis of PCT is made by the detection of excessive uroporphyrinogen in the urine.
- Treatment includes avoidance of exacerbating factors and treatment of underlying hepatitis C or hemochromatosis. Medications such as choloroquine, deferoxamine, and thalidomide may also be used to treat PCT.

Polyarteritis Nodosa

- Polyarteritis nodosa (PN) is a vasculitis of small and medium-sized arteries.
- Cutaneous involvement in PN occurs in 25% of cases.
- Cutaneous lesions are characterized by nodules 0.5–1 cm in size along the distribution of the superficial arteries (Figure 28.11).
- PN is most commonly associated with chronic hepatitis B but may also be associated with hepatitis C virus, parvovirus B19, and human immunodeficiency virus infections.
- The diagnosis of PN is made by tissue biopsy, which reveals arteritis, or angiography, which shows aneurysms.
- Treatment is with glucocorticoids and cyclophosphamide; in >90% of patients the skin lesions resolve with treatment.

Further Reading

Habif, TP. (2009) Hypersensitivity syndromes and vasculitis, in *Clinical Dermatology*, 5th edn (ed T.P. Habif), Mosby, Philadelphia, pp. 720–726.

Mirowski, G.W. and Mark, L.A. (2010) Oral disease and oral-cutaneous manifestations of gastrointestinal and liver disease, in *Sleisenger and Fordtran's Gastrointestinal and Liver Disease: Pathophysiology/Diagnosis/Management*, 9th edn (eds M. Feldman, L.S. Friedman and L.J. Brandt), Saunders Elsevier, Philadelphia, pp. 359–368.

Yamada, T., Hasler, W.L., Inadomi, J.M., *et al.* (2005) Skin lesions associated with gastrointestinal and liver diseases, in *Handbook of Gastroenterology*, 2nd edn (ed T. Yamada), Lippincott Williams and Wilkins, Philadelphia, pp. 589–597.

Weblinks

http://dermatlas.med.jhmi.edu/derm/
http://www.dermis.net/dermisroot/en/home/index.htm

Index

Essentials of Gastroenterology, First Edition. Edited by Shanthi V. Sitaraman,
Lawrence S. Friedman.
© 2012 John Wiley & Sons, Ltd. Published 2012 by John Wiley & Sons, Ltd.